A Practical Guide to
PRESCRIPTION &
NON-PRESCRIPTION
MEDICINES
& Alternative Remedies

A Practical Guide to
PRESCRIPTION &
NON-PRESCRIPTION
MEDICINES
& Alternative Remedies

CHRISTINA BUNCE

INDEX

Published by
Arcturus Publishing Limited
for Index Books
Henson Way
Kettering
Northamptonshire
NN16 8PX

This book is intended to provide reference
information to help people understand more about the
medical treatment they have been prescribed or have purchased.
While every effort has been made to ensure this book is free from error,
the knowledge of medicines and healthcare treatment is constantly changing
for many reasons, and so it should not be considered as a substitute
for personalised advice from a qualified medical practitioner.

The publisher, the editor and their respective employees
shall not accept responsibility for injury, loss or damage occasioned
to any person acting or refraining from action as a result of material in this
book whether or not such injury, loss or damage is in any way due to
any negligent act or omission on the part of the publisher,
editor or their employees.

This edition published 2001 for Index Books Ltd

Printed and bound in Finland

Text layout and design by Moo Design

© Arcturus Publishing Limited
1–7 Shand Street, London SE1 2ES

ISBN 1 900032 78 3

CONTENTS

INTRODUCTION

Medicines have been a major force in the fight against disease for many centuries. Most of us have taken some kind of medicine to treat or ward off illness.

The range of medicines at our disposal has never been greater than it is today. We have access not only to the conventional pills and potions prescribed by doctors, but to a range of alternative, complementary and over-the-counter products which we can buy without a prior medical consultation. While this is undoubtedly a good thing, in that many people do not feel that conventional medicine meets their needs, it also means that the average consumer is faced with a bewildering array of options to choose from.

This book is designed as a guide to the most common complementary and conventional medicines. It is divided into three sections:

PRESCRIPTION MEDICINES
A list of over 450 of the most commonly prescribed medicines together with information about their actions, side effects and special precautions.

OVER-THE-COUNTER MEDICINES
An A-Z of many, but by no means all, of the most commonly used Over-the-Counter remedies for common complaints.

ALTERNATIVE REMEDIES
A guide to homeopathic and herbal medicines organised by the type of conditions they are most commonly used to treat.

IMPORTANT

If a problem persists and does not respond to over-the-counter treatment or alternative therapy, you should consult a medical professional. This book is not intended as a substitute for professional medical advice.

PRESCRIPTION MEDICINES

This section is designed to be a quick-reference guide to the medicines which are most commonly prescribed for people both at home and in hospital. It may be that you have been given information about a medicine prescribed and have forgotten it, or it may be that you want to find out more about a drug which has been prescribed for yourself or a member of the family. Whatever your motive for searching, this chapter offers basic information about each medicine in layman's language.

HOW TO USE THIS SECTION

The medicines are listed in alphabetical order, according to their most commonly used generic name, which is the official chemical name for a medicine and describes its main active ingredient. You can find the generic name on any medicine. If you cannot, your pharmacist will tell you.

Brand name: These are the names given to the product by a manufacturer. For instance, Aspirin is the generic name for the painkilling drug, while Anadin is one of the many brand names under which it is marketed.

Type of drug: This loosely classifies the drug, either by the type of action it has (eg, beta blocker) or the effect it has (eg, anticancer).

Uses: Describes what conditions the drug will be used for.

How it works: Where known, an explanation of how the drug works and what effect it has will be given.

Possible adverse effects: These are undesirable side effects that, as far as most drugs are concerned, will affect only a small number of people but which should always be reported. Some drugs, such as those which fight cancer, will nearly always have adverse effects that will be monitored closely by medical staff.

Availability: Indicates whether some strengths or form of the drug are available over-the-counter as well as on prescription. Some products which are available over-the-counter may also be prescribed by doctors and nurses in some circumstances.

Other information: Information about the drug which will be of interest to the people taking it.

CAUTIONS: These indicate whether a drug should not be prescribed, or only prescribed with extreme caution, for children or pregnant and/or breastfeeding women. It also indicates whether the drug may affect the ability to drive or operate machinery, and whether it is advisable to consume alcohol during treatment.

ACAMPROSATE CALCIUM

Brand name: Campral EC

Type of drug: Alcohol abuse deterrent

Uses: The treatment of people who have been diagnosed as having an addiction to alcohol. Usually used in conjunction with counselling, particularly for people who are at risk of starting to drink again.

How it works: It interferes with the chemicals in the brain which are thought to be involved in causing people to become dependent on alcohol.

Possible adverse effects: Diarrhoea, nausea, vomiting, stomach pain and loss of sex drive.

Availability: Available only with a prescription from a doctor.

Other information: Do not take if you have liver problems. Treatment will usually be started as soon as the patient has stopped drinking and be continued for around a year.

CAUTIONS

Children: This drug is either not recommended for children, or is recommended only for children above a certain age.

Pregnancy and breastfeeding: This drug is either not recommended for use by women who are pregnant or breastfeeding, or the precise effects are not known and it should therefore only be used with caution and under medical advice.

Alcohol: Alcohol should not be consumed, or only consumed with caution - after medical advice has been sought - while you are taking this drug.

Driving and operating machinery: There are no commonly reported problems which may impact on the ability to drive or operate machinery. However, many drugs can cause dizziness or drowsiness in a few people, so it is wise to see how the drug affects you before driving or working with dangerous machinery.

ACARBOSE
Brand name: Glucobay
Type of drug: Anti-diabetic
Uses: The treatment of diabetes in people whose condition cannot be adequately controlled by diet or other medication.
How it works: Slows down the rate at which carbohydrates are digested, with the result that high blood sugar levels, particularly following meals, are reduced.
Possible adverse effects: Wind and occasionally diarrhoea and cramps. These will be minimised if sucrose is avoided.
Availability: Available only with a prescription from a doctor.
Other information: Patients prescribed acarbose in addition to insulin or a sulphonylurea need to carry glucose rather than ordinary sucrose. Acarbose should always be taken in conjunction with the recommended diabetic diet.
CAUTIONS
Children: This drug is either not recommended for children, or is recommended only for children above a certain age.
Pregnancy and breastfeeding: This drug is either not recommended for use by women who are pregnant or breastfeeding, or the precise effects are not known and it should therefore only be used with caution and when advised by a doctor.
Alcohol: No known problems if taken with alcohol.
Driving and operating machinery: There are no commonly reported problems which may impact on the ability to drive or operate machinery. However, many drugs can cause dizziness or drowsiness in a few people, so it is wise to see how the drug affects you before driving or working with dangerous machinery.

ACEBUTOLOL

Brand name: Sectral

Type of drug: Beta-blocker

Uses: A treatment for angina, abnormal heart rhythms and high blood pressure. Can also sometimes be used as a treatment for anxiety.

How it works: Works to slow and steady the heart rate. It does not cure the underlying problem but works to control the symptoms.

Possible adverse effects: Lethargy and fatigue, cold hands and feet, nausea and vomiting, nightmares. Sometimes a slow pulse may be noticed. A rash and/or breathlessness should always be reported to a doctor.

Availability: Available only with a prescription from a doctor.

Other information: Acebutolol will not normally be prescribed for people with asthma or other lung disorders such as obstructive airways disease because it can make the conditions worse. It is likely that Acebutolol will need to be taken for long periods.

CAUTIONS

Children: This drug is either not recommended for children, or is recommended only for children above a certain age.

Pregnancy and breastfeeding: No specific problems documented, but any medication should be taken with utmost caution by women who are either pregnant or breastfeeding, and only after professional medical or pharmaceutical advice has been sought.

Alcohol: No known problems if taken with alcohol.

Driving and operating machinery: This drug may have some effect on your driving ability, so it is advisable not to drive or operate machinery while taking it.

ACEMETACIN

Brand name: Emflex

Type of drug: Anti-inflammatory

Uses: To treat the pain and inflammation of rheumatism and other musculoskeletal disorders.

How it works: Reduces pain and inflammation by blocking the production of prostaglandins, chemicals produced by the body which contribute to the inflammation associated with rheumatoid arthritis.

Possible adverse effects: Stomach and bowel upsets, headaches, blurred vision and dizziness, tinnitus.

Availability: Available only with a prescription from a doctor.

Other information: Must not be taken if allergic to aspirin. Patients on long-term treatment should have an annual eye examination.

CAUTIONS

Children: There are no commonly reported problems associated with prescribing this medication for children.

Pregnancy and breastfeeding: This drug is either not recommended for use by women who are pregnant or breastfeeding, or the precise effects are not known and it should therefore only be used with caution and under medical advice.

Alcohol: No known problems if taken with alcohol.

Driving and operating machinery: This drug may have some effect on your driving ability, so it is advisable not to drive or operate machinery while taking it.

ACETAZOLAMIDE

Brand name: Diamox, Diamox SR

Type of drug: Glaucoma treatment

Uses: Affects the chemical processes which take place in the kidneys, to produce a diuretic effect. This results in fluid being drawn out of the body.

How it works: Results in the reduction of the volume of fluid in the eye which is the main symptom of glaucoma.

Possible adverse effects: Tiredness, headache, appetite loss and tingling in the hands and feet. Stop taking the drug and call a doctor if a rash, or bruising effect, appears on the skin.

Availability: Available only with a prescription from a doctor.

Other information: People on long-term treatment may also be prescribed a potassium supplement. Blood tests will be carried out regularly.

CAUTIONS

Children: There are no commonly reported problems associated with prescribing this medication for children.

Pregnancy and breastfeeding: This drug is either not recommended for use by women who are pregnant or breastfeeding, or the precise effects are

not known and it should therefore only be used with caution and under medical advice.

Alcohol: Alcohol should not be consumed, or only consumed with caution - after medical advice has been sought - while you are taking this drug.

Driving and operating machinery: This drug may have some effect on your driving ability, so it is advisable not to drive or operate machinery while taking it.

ACICLOVIR

Brand name: Zovirax

Type of drug: Anti-viral

Uses: Antiviral drug available in cream, ointment and tablet form, used to treat herpes infections.

How it works: Attacks the herpes virus. Cream reduces the severity of cold sores and herpes. Tablets used to treat shingles. Ointment used for herpes infections affecting the eye. Can be given as an injection for severe infections.

Possible adverse effects: Cream can cause burning and stinging, or more rarely, a rash. Any rash should be discussed with a doctor.

Availability: Some preparations available over the counter.

Other information: Available as tablets, liquid, injection, cream and eye ointment. Injection not recommended for pregnant women. Always complete the full course.

CAUTIONS

Children: There are no commonly reported problems associated with prescribing this medication for children.

Pregnancy and breastfeeding: No specific problems documented, but any medication should be taken with utmost caution by women who are either pregnant or breastfeeding, and only after professional medical or pharmaceutical advice has been sought.

Alcohol: No known problems if taken with alcohol.

Driving and operating machinery: There are no commonly reported problems which may impact on the ability to drive or operate machinery. However, many drugs can cause dizziness or drowsiness in a few people, so it is wise to see how the drug affects you before driving or working with dangerous machinery.

ACITRETIN

Brand name: Neotigason

Type of drug: Oral retinoid

Uses: The treatment of extensive and severe psoriasis where other treatments have failed.

How it works: Slows down the rapid reproduction of skin cells which causes the scaling of the skin which characterises psoriasis.

Possible adverse effects: Dryness in the mouth, skin and eyes. Inflamed skin. May cause hair to thin and fall out.

Availability: Available only with a prescription from a doctor.

Other information: Usually prescribed as capsules. Avoid getting pregnant before treatment and for at least two years after taking this drug. Avoid exposure to sunlight and sunray lamps. Liver and blood tests will be conducted during treatment to monitor effects and levels of the medication.

CAUTIONS

Children: This drug is either not recommended for children, or is recommended only for children above a certain age.

Pregnancy and breastfeeding: This drug is either not recommended for use by women who are pregnant or breastfeeding, or the precise effects are not known and it should therefore only be used with caution and under medical advice.

Alcohol: No known problems if taken with alcohol.

Driving and operating machinery: There are no commonly reported problems which may impact on the ability to drive or operate machinery. However, many drugs can cause dizziness or drowsiness in a few people, so it is wise to see how the drug affects you before driving or working with dangerous machinery.

ACRIVASTINE

Brand name: Semprex

Type of drug: Antihistamine

Uses: A short acting antihistamine which is used for the treatment of hay fever and allergic skin conditions such as urticaria (hives).

How it works: It acts to control a runny nose, sneezing and other symptoms of nasal allergies, without causing the drowsiness which is a side effect of many other types of antihistamine treatment.

Possible adverse effects: Some people may experience drowsiness. On rare occasions can cause disturbances to the digestive system, headaches and dry mouth. Children and elderly people are more susceptible to the adverse effects.

Availability: Available only with a prescription from a doctor.

Other information: Has less of a sedative effect than other similar drugs, so is often prescribed for people who need to avoid becoming drowsy.

CAUTIONS

Children: This drug is either not recommended for children, or is recommended only for children above a certain age.

Pregnancy and breastfeeding: No specific problems documented, but any medication should be taken with utmost caution by women who are either pregnant or breastfeeding, and only after professional medical or pharmaceutical advice has been sought.

Alcohol: Alcohol should not be consumed, or only consumed with caution - after medical advice has been sought - while you are taking this drug.

Driving and operating machinery: There are no commonly reported problems which may impact on the ability to drive or operate machinery. However, many drugs can cause dizziness or drowsiness in a few people, so it is wise to see how the drug affects you before driving or working with dangerous machinery.

ADENOSINE

Brand name: Adenocor

Type of drug: Anti-arrhythmic

Uses: Treatment of some kinds of rapid heart beat (paroxysmal supraventricular tachycardia).

How it works: Acts on the heart muscle and arteries, causing the heart rate to slow down to normal.

Possible adverse effects: Facial flushing, difficulty in breathing and sneezing, chest pain, nausea, dizziness, headache.

Availability: Available only with a prescription from a doctor.

Other information: Usually administered as an intravenous (straight into the vein) injection in hospital. Unlikely to be given to pregnant women unless in an emergency.

CAUTIONS

Children: There are no commonly reported problems associated with prescribing this medication for children.

Pregnancy and breastfeeding: No specific problems documented, but any medication should be taken with utmost caution by women who are either pregnant or breastfeeding, and only after professional medical or pharmaceutical advice has been sought.

Alcohol: No known problems if taken with alcohol.

Driving and operating machinery: There are no commonly reported problems which may impact on the ability to drive or operate machinery. However, many drugs can cause dizziness or drowsiness in a few people, so it is wise to see how the drug affects you before driving or working with dangerous machinery.

ADRENALINE (Epinephrine)

Brand name: Ana-Guard, Epipen, Min-I-Jet adrenaline, Medihaler-Epi

Type of drug: Emergency treatment

Uses: For emergency treatment of anaphylactic shock and severe asthma attacks.

How it works: Reverses the dangerous effects of anaphylactic shock which include difficulty in breathing, a drop in blood pressure and swelling of the throat. It increases the blood supply to muscles, including those of the heart and lungs.

Possible adverse effects: Anxiety, breathlessness, restlessness, palpitations, rapid heartbeat, dizziness and cold hands and feet.

Availability: Available only with a prescription from a doctor.

Other information: Patients who have a high risk of developing anaphylaxis as a result of an allergy to food or insect stings, for instance, may be advised to carry adrenaline with them at all times and understand how to inject it in case of an emergency. Special dose syringes are available for children.

CAUTIONS

Children: There are no commonly reported problems associated with prescribing this medication for children.

Pregnancy and breastfeeding: No specific problems documented, but any medication should be taken with utmost caution by women who are

17

either pregnant or breastfeeding, and only after professional medical or pharmaceutical advice has been sought.

Alcohol: No known problems if taken with alcohol.

Driving and operating machinery: There are no commonly reported problems which may impact on the ability to drive or operate machinery. However, many drugs can cause dizziness or drowsiness in a few people, so it is wise to see how the drug affects you before driving or working with dangerous machinery.

ALBENDAZOLE

Brand name: Eskazole

Type of drug: Anti-tapeworm

Uses: In conjunction with surgery can reduce the risk of recurrence of cysts caused by Echinococcus granulosus.

How it works: Keeps the cysts which characterise the disease at bay and prevents symptoms resulting from their effect on the surrounding tissues such as the brain, liver or lungs.

Possible adverse effects: Digestive disturbances, headache, dizziness, rash and fever.

Availability: Available only with a prescription from a doctor.

Other information: Usually prescribed as tablets.

CAUTIONS

Children: There are no commonly reported problems associated with prescribing this medication for children.

Pregnancy and breastfeeding: This drug is either not recommended for use by women who are pregnant or breastfeeding, or the precise effects are not known and it should therefore only be used with caution and under medical advice.

Alcohol: No known problems if taken with alcohol.

Driving and operating machinery: There are no commonly reported problems which may impact on the ability to drive or operate machinery. However, many drugs can cause dizziness or drowsiness in a few people, so it is wise to see how the drug affects you before driving or working with dangerous machinery.

ALENDRONIC ACID

Brand name: Fosamax

Type of drug: Biphosphonate

Uses: Treatment of osteoporosis, which affects women who have passed the menopause.

How it works: Acts on the rate of bone growth which has a role in the development of osteoporosis.

Possible adverse effects: Rarely, alendronic acid can lead to severe oesophageal reactions which may cause pain on swallowing, heartburn and chest pain, which should be reported to a doctor immediately. More common adverse effects include abdominal pain and swelling, wind and headache.

Availability: Available only with a prescription from a doctor.

Other information: Usually prescribed as tablets.

The tablets should be taken at least 30 minutes before breakfast (and any other medication) with a full glass of water on an empty stomach. Patients should then stand or sit upright for 30 minutes and not lie down until after breakfast.

Because of the risk of gastric disturbance, alendronic acid is rarely given to people who have existing gastric problems such as ulcers or oesophageal disease.

CAUTIONS

Children: Not usually prescribed.

Pregnancy and breastfeeding: This drug is either not recommended for use by women who are pregnant or breastfeeding, or the precise effects are not known and it should therefore only be used with caution and under medical advice.

Alcohol: No known problems if taken with alcohol.

Driving and operating machinery: There are no commonly reported problems which may impact on the ability to drive or operate machinery. However, many drugs can cause dizziness or drowsiness in a few people, so it is wise to see how the drug affects you before driving or working with dangerous machinery.

ALFACALCIDOL

Brand name: AlphaD, One-Alpha

Type of drug: Vitamin

Uses: The prevention or treatment of some kinds of bone disease which are caused by either kidney malfunction or vitamin D-resistant rickets.

How it works: Replaces vitamin D, which is essential to healthy bone growth.

Possible adverse effects: Adverse effects usually only occur as a result of overdose and include a loss of appetite, nausea and vomiting, diarrhoea, weight loss, headache, thirst and vertigo. The drug may also cause the levels of calcium in the blood to rise, but this will be monitored by regular blood tests.

Availability: Available only with a prescription from a doctor.

Other information: Usually prescribed as tablets. Blood should be tested regularly to check calcium levels in people who are taking high doses.

CAUTIONS

Children: There are no commonly reported problems associated with prescribing this medication for children.

Pregnancy and breastfeeding: No specific problems documented, but any medication should be taken with utmost caution by women who are either pregnant or breastfeeding, and only after professional medical or pharmaceutical advice has been sought.

Alcohol: No known problems if taken with alcohol.

Driving and operating machinery: There are no commonly reported problems which may impact on the ability to drive or operate machinery. However, many drugs can cause dizziness or drowsiness in a few people, so it is wise to see how the drug affects you before driving or working with dangerous machinery.

ALLOPURINOL

Brand name: Caplenal, Cosuric, Rimapurinol, Xanthomaz, Zyloric

Type of drug: Gout treatment

Uses: Used as a preventative measure for people who suffer from gout. It is not usually prescribed to treat sudden flare-ups of the condition.

How it works: It inhibits the production of an enzyme which is crucial to the formation of crystals - made from uric acid - in the joints of the body which characterises the disease. It can also be used to reduce high uric acid levels which occur as side effects of some anti-cancer treatments.

Possible adverse effects: Adverse effects are uncommon, but there may be nausea and itching. Rarely causes drowsiness, headache, fever, a metallic taste in the mouth and fever and chills.

Availability: Available only with a prescription from a doctor.

Other information: Will often be given in conjunction with an anti-inflammatory drug, as in some cases it may increase the severity of acute attacks of the disease. Regular blood checks will be made to assess the levels of uric acid. It is advisable to drink plenty of fluids while taking this medication.

CAUTIONS

Children: This drug is either not recommended for children, or is recommended only for children above a certain age.

Pregnancy and breastfeeding: This drug is either not recommended for use by women who are pregnant or breastfeeding, or the precise effects are not known and it should therefore only be used with caution and under medical advice.

Alcohol: Alcohol should not be consumed, or only consumed with caution - after medical advice has been sought - while you are taking this drug.

Driving and operating machinery: There are no commonly reported problems which may impact on the ability to drive or operate machinery. However, many drugs can cause dizziness or drowsiness in a few people, so it is wise to see how the drug affects you before driving or working with dangerous machinery.

ALPROSTADIL

Brand name: Caverject, Viridal

Type of drug: Prostaglandin

Uses: Treatment of impotence.

How it works: When injected into the penis it results in an erection in men who are otherwise unable to obtain or maintain an erection. The erection should last no more than an hour.

Possible adverse effects: Persistent erections or scarring of the penis, pain in testicles and bottom. Female partners of men taking this drug may occasionally experience vaginal itching and burning.

Availability: Available only with a prescription from a doctor.

Other information: Given as an injection into the penis. The first dose should always be given by qualified medical personnel. Thereafter, self-administration is possible after tuition. The drug should not be used more often than once in 24 hours or more than three times a week. A qualified medical practitioner should be consulted if any erection lasts more than four hours.

Children: This drug is either not recommended for children, or is recommended only for children above a certain age.

Pregnancy and breastfeeding: This drug is either not recommended for use by women who are pregnant or breastfeeding, or the precise effects are not known and it should therefore only be used with caution and under medical advice.

Alcohol: No known problems if taken with alcohol.

Driving and operating machinery: There are no commonly reported problems which may impact on the ability to drive or operate machinery. However, many drugs can cause dizziness or drowsiness in a few people, so it is wise to see how the drug affects you before driving or working with dangerous machinery.

ALTEPLASE

Brand name: Actilyse

Type of drug: Clot-buster

Uses: Treatment of heart attacks.

How it works: If administered early enough, it works to dissolve the clots which cause heart attacks and enables oxygen to reach the affected part of the heart muscle and thus prevents it from being permanently damaged.

Possible adverse effects: Can occasionally lead to bleeding from the site of the injection, nausea, vomiting, allergic skin rash and fever.

Availability: Available only with a prescription from a doctor.

Other information: Usually administered as an intravenous infusion (also known as a drip), in hospital. It will be used with extreme caution in women who are pregnant, for people with kidney disorders or those with diabetes.

Children: There are no commonly reported problems associated with prescribing this medication for children.

Pregnancy and breastfeeding: This drug is either not recommended for use by women who are pregnant or breastfeeding, or the precise effects are not known and it should therefore only be used with caution and under medical advice.

Alcohol: No known problems if taken with alcohol.

Driving and operating machinery: There are no commonly reported problems which may impact on the ability to drive or operate machinery. However, many drugs can cause dizziness or drowsiness in a few people, so it is wise to see how the drug affects you before driving or working with dangerous machinery.

ALUMINIUM HYDROXIDE
Brand name: Alu-Cap, Aludrox
Type of drug: Antacid
Uses: Treatment of indigestion, heartburn, and sometimes diarrhoea. Also used to prevent these conditions.
How it works: Acts to neutralise the acid in the stomach which in turn reduces the irritant effect which causes the symptoms of the gastric problems.
Possible adverse effects: Side effects are rare and not usually serious, but include constipation, nausea and vomiting. Constipation is more likely in elderly people.
Availability: Available without a prescription.
Other information: Usually taken as a liquid, which should be slightly diluted with water or fruit juice.
CAUTIONS
Children: There are no commonly reported problems associated with prescribing this medication for children.
Pregnancy and breastfeeding: This drug is either not recommended for use by women who are pregnant or breastfeeding, or the precise effects are not known and it should therefore only be used with caution and under medical advice.
Alcohol: No known problems if taken with alcohol.
Driving and operating machinery: There are no commonly reported problems which may impact on the ability to drive or operate machinery. However, many drugs can cause dizziness or drowsiness in a few people, so it is wise to see how the drug affects you before driving or working with dangerous machinery.

AMANTADINE
Brand name: Symmetrel

Type of drug: Parkinsonism and anti-viral treatment

Uses: It can be used as an anti-viral drug - to treat infections of influenza type A virus, and infections of the respiratory tract. It is also used to control, although not cure, the symptoms of Parkinson's disease.

How it works: Protects against influenza A and reduces the symptoms once an infection has occurred. It affects the release of the brain chemical, dopamine, which plays a crucial part in Parkinsonism. The Parkinsonism symptoms usually diminish during the first few weeks of treatment, but the effect of the drug often wears off within six to eight weeks, after which another drug will be needed to deal with the symptoms. Occasionally the effectiveness of the drug will be restored after a break from it.

Possible adverse effects: Nervousness, agitation and confusion. Dizziness, blurred vision, loss of appetite, ankle swelling and a rash are rare side effects. The drug may cause insomnia in some people, in which case it should be taken several hours before bedtime.

Availability: Available only with a prescription from a doctor.

Other information: Usually supplied as capsules or tablets. Should be taken after meals to ensure maximum absorption. When taken as an anti-Parkinsonism treatment, it is important not to suddenly stop taking it, as this may make the symptoms of the original problem worse.

CAUTIONS

Children: There are no commonly reported problems associated with prescribing this medication for children.

Pregnancy and breastfeeding: This drug is either not recommended for use by women who are pregnant or breastfeeding, or the precise effects are not known and it should therefore only be used with caution and under medical advice.

Alcohol: Alcohol should not be consumed, or only consumed with caution - after medical advice has been sought - while you are taking this drug.

Driving and operating machinery: This drug may have some effect on your driving ability, so it is advisable not to drive or operate machinery while taking it.

AMILORIDE

Brand name: Amilospare, Berkamil, Midamor.

Type of drug: Diuretic

Uses: Helps the body to get rid of the excess fluid that is often retained as a result of heart or liver disease and which results in high blood pressure.

How it works: Encourages more fluid to be expelled from the body as urine. The effect is not noticeable until a few hours after the pill has been taken.

Possible adverse effects: Side effects are rare, but include possible digestive disturbance, confusion, muscle weakness, rash and a dry mouth.

Availability: Available only with a prescription from a doctor.

Other information: Can be taken as a pill or a liquid. It is best to take this medication in the afternoon, rather than evening, to prevent frequent trips to the toilet during the night. Foods high in potassium should be avoided. Unlikely to be used in patients who suffer from diabetes mellitus.

CAUTIONS

Children: This drug is either not recommended for children, or is recommended only for children above a certain age.

Pregnancy and breastfeeding: This drug is either not recommended for use by women who are pregnant or breastfeeding, or the precise effects are not known and it should therefore only be used with caution and under medical advice.

Alcohol: No known problems if taken with alcohol.

Driving and operating machinery: This drug may have some effect on your driving ability so it is advisable not to drive or operate machinery while taking it.

AMINOGLUTETHIMIDE

Brand name: Orimeten

Type of drug: Hormone antagonist

Uses: Treatment of advanced stages of breast cancer in women who have passed the menopause.

How it works: Interferes with the hormone actions, thereby starving certain types of cancerous tumours of the hormone they need to survive.

Possible adverse effects: Side effects usually occur within two weeks of treatment and include drowsiness and fever, which usually settle spontaneously. If a rash occurs which persists for more than five days, you should consult your doctor.

Availability: Available only with a prescription from a doctor.

Other information: Should not be used at the same time as hormonal contraception.

CAUTIONS

Children: Not usually prescribed.

Pregnancy and breastfeeding: This drug is either not recommended for use by women who are pregnant or breastfeeding, or the precise effects are not known and it should therefore only be used with caution and under medical advice.

Alcohol: Alcohol should not be consumed, or only consumed with caution - after medical advice has been sought - while you are taking this drug.

Driving and operating machinery: This drug may have some effect on your driving ability, so it is advisable not to drive or operate machinery while taking it.

AMINOPHYLLINE

Brand name: Pecram, Phyllocontin Continus

Type of drug: Bronchodilator

Uses: Treatment of reversible airways obstruction and asthma attacks.

How it works: Reverses the effects of airways obstruction and asthma to enable the sufferer to breathe more easily.

Possible adverse effects: Rapid heart beat, palpitations, nausea, gastric discomfort, headaches. Dizziness is quite common when people start taking this drug.

Availability: Available only with a prescription from a doctor.

Other information: Will usually be given as a tablet. Seek medical advice before taking any other kind of medication while taking this drug.

CAUTIONS

Children: There are no commonly reported problems associated with prescribing this medication for children.

Pregnancy and breastfeeding: This drug is either not recommended for use by women who are pregnant or breastfeeding, or the precise effects are not known and it should therefore only be used with caution.

Alcohol: Alcohol should not be consumed, or only consumed with caution - after medical advice has been sought - while you are taking this drug.

Driving and operating machinery: There are no commonly reported problems which may impact on the ability to drive or operate machinery.

However, many drugs can cause dizziness or drowsiness in a few people, so it is wise to see how the drug affects you before driving or working with dangerous machinery.

AMIODARONE
Brand name: Cordarone
Type of drug: Anti-arrhythmic
Uses: Used to prevent and treat a range of abnormal heart rhythms such as those which occur in Wolff-Parkinson-White syndrome, atrial fibrillation and ventricular fibrillation.
How it works: It slows the messages sent to the heart muscle, with the result that the heartbeat is slowed and steadied.
Possible adverse effects: Liver damage, thyroid problems and damage to the eyes and lungs. Also nausea, shortness of breath, a metallic taste in the mouth and a rash which is sensitive to light. The skin can also become more sensitive and burn easily in sunlight if not adequately protected. Eye drops may be prescribed for the few patients who may not get visual disturbances while taking this drug.
Availability: Available only with a prescription from a doctor.
Other information: This drug can cause the eyes to be dazzled by bright lights. It is worth wearing a sunscreen to prevent sensitised skin reacting to sunlight.
CAUTIONS
Children: This drug is either not recommended for children, or is recommended only for children above a certain age.
Pregnancy and breastfeeding: This drug is either not recommended for use by women who are pregnant or breastfeeding, or the precise effects are not known and it should therefore only be used with caution.
Alcohol: No known problems if taken with alcohol.
Driving and operating machinery: This drug may have some effect on your driving ability, so it is advisable not to drive or operate machinery while taking it.

AMITRIPTYLINE
Brand name: Domical, Elavil, Lentizol, Tryptizol
Type of drug: Tricyclic antidepressant

Uses: Used in the treatment of depression which has persisted for long periods. Has also been used for the treatment of anorexia or bulimia associated with depression. Occasionally used in the treatment of bedwetting.

How it works: It inhibits the re-uptake of brain chemicals, which results in a heightening of mood. It also encourages appetite and enables users to lead a more normal daily life. Its sedative effect is also useful for people who find difficulty in sleeping at nights.

Possible adverse effects: A more sedative effect than similar drugs. Drowsiness, sweating, dry mouth, dizziness and blurred vision can be experienced. The risk of nausea can be reduced if taken with food or milk. Any troublesome side effects should be reported instantly.

Availability: Available only with a prescription from a doctor.

Other information: Usually administered as a pill. The beneficial effects are reduced if taken by someone who is a heavy cigarette smoker. An overdose is dangerous and may lead to fits and abnormal heart rhythms. An overdose should be treated as an emergency situation. It is advisable to take this drug at bedtime in order to avoid daytime sedation. Alternatively, if taken early in the morning, a 'hangover' effect may be avoided. It may take four weeks before the beneficial effects of the medication are noticed.

CAUTIONS

Children: This drug is either not recommended for children, or is recommended only for children above a certain age.

Pregnancy and breastfeeding: No specific problems documented, but any medication should be taken with utmost caution by women who are either pregnant or breastfeeding, and only after professional medical or pharmaceutical advice has been sought.

Alcohol: Alcohol should not be consumed, or only consumed with caution - after medical advice has been sought - while you are taking this drug.

Driving and operating machinery: This drug may have some effect on your driving ability, so it is advisable not to drive or operate machinery while taking it.

AMLODIPINE
Brand name: Istin
Type of drug: Anti-angina and anti-hypertensive

Uses: The treatment of the chest pain associated with both chronic (ongoing) and acute (sudden worsening) angina.

How it works: Affects the electrical impulses which pass through the heart muscle and blood vessels, with the result that the heart can operate more effectively. It also dilates the blood vessels around the heart.

Possible adverse effects: May cause blood pressure to drop too low. May lead to leg and ankle swelling, which should be reported to a doctor immediately. You should also report any worsening of angina symptoms to a doctor. Can also cause dizziness and flushing.

Availability: Available only with a prescription from a doctor.

Other information: Usually given in tablet form. You should not stop taking this drug without first discussing it with your doctor.

CAUTIONS

Children: This drug is either not recommended for children, or is recommended only for children above a certain age.

Pregnancy and breastfeeding: This drug is either not recommended for use by women who are pregnant or breastfeeding, or the precise effects are not known and it should therefore only be used with caution and under medical advice.

Alcohol: Alcohol should not be consumed, or only consumed with caution - after medical advice has been sought - while you are taking this drug.

Driving and operating machinery: This drug may have some effect on your driving ability, so it is advisable not to drive or operate machinery while taking it.

AMOXYCILLIN

Brand name: Almodan, Amix, Amoram, Amoxil, Amrit, Galenamox, Rimoxallin

Type of drug: Antibiotic

Uses: Penicillin antibiotic used for a wide range of infections, including respiratory and ear infections, sinusitis, skin infections and infections of the urinary tract.

How it works: Acts fast - sometimes within one or two hours - to kill the bacteria which cause infections.

Possible adverse effects: Rash and diarrhoea are relatively common. Can also cause nausea and diarrhoea. Occasionally a severe allergic reaction can occur, which results in a high fever, swelling of the mouth and tongue, itching and breathing problems. If this happens a doctor should be consulted immediately.

Availability: Available only with a prescription from a doctor.

Other information: Usually prescribed as a pill. Can be administered intravenously (through a vein) but this will normally only happen in hospital. Maximum absorption of Amoxycillin takes place if the stomach is empty. Tablets should be chewed thoroughly or crushed and washed down with liquid to ensure the maximum beneficial effect takes place. As with any course of antibiotics the prescribed course should always be completed. You should tell your doctor any known allergy to antibiotics or anything else and whether you are on the contraceptive pill. May reduce effectiveness of contraceptive pill.

CAUTIONS

Children: There are no commonly reported problems associated with prescribing this medication for children.

Pregnancy and breastfeeding: No specific problems documented, but any medication should be taken with utmost caution by women who are either pregnant or breastfeeding, and only after professional medical or pharmaceutical advice has been sought.

Alcohol: No known problems if taken with alcohol.

Driving and operating machinery: There are no commonly reported problems which may impact on the ability to drive or operate machinery. However, many drugs can cause dizziness or drowsiness in a few people, so it is wise to see how the drug affects you before driving or working with dangerous machinery.

AMPHOTERICIN

Brand name: Abelcet, AmBisome, Amphocil, Fungilin, Fungizone

Type of drug: Anti-fungal

Uses: Drug used to fight fungal infections such as fungal meningitis, cystitis caused by candida, and fungal infections of the eye.

How it works: Treats infections caused by a fungus by damaging the outer, protective layer of the fungus.

Possible adverse effects: Rash and diarrhoea are relatively common. Occasionally a severe allergic reaction can occur, with high fever, swelling of the mouth and tongue, itching and breathing problems. Any signs of this should be reported to a doctor immediately.

Availability: Available only with a prescription from a doctor.

Other information: Administered either in tablet form or as an intravenous infusion. Treatment may last for some time. You should tell your doctor about any known allergy to antibiotics or anything else and whether you are on the pill. May reduce effectiveness of contraceptive pill.

CAUTIONS

Children: There are no commonly reported problems associated with prescribing this medication for children.

Pregnancy and breastfeeding: No specific problems documented, but any medication should be taken with utmost caution by women who are either pregnant or breastfeeding, and only after professional medical or pharmaceutical advice has been sought.

Alcohol: No known problems if taken with alcohol.

Driving and operating machinery: There are no commonly reported problems which may impact on the ability to drive or operate machinery. However, many drugs can cause dizziness or drowsiness in a few people, so it is wise to see how the drug affects you before driving or working with dangerous machinery.

ANASTROZOLE

Brand name: Arimidex

Type of drug: Anti-cancer

Uses: Treatment of breast cancer in women who have passed the menopause and for whom other treatments have not been successful.

How it works: Starves the cancer of certain hormones which are known to stimulate its growth.

Possible adverse effects: Hot flushes, sweating, vaginal irritation, thinning of the hair and gastric disturbances.

Availability: Available only with a prescription from a doctor.

Other information: Will usually only be administered in hospital by staff experienced in this kind of treatment.

CAUTIONS

Children: There are no commonly reported problems associated with prescribing this medication for children.

Pregnancy and breastfeeding: This drug is either not recommended for use by women who are pregnant or breastfeeding, or the precise effects are not known and it should therefore only be used with caution and under medical advice.

Alcohol: No known problems if taken with alcohol.

Driving and operating machinery: This drug may have some effect on your driving ability, so it is advisable not to drive or operate machinery while taking it.

ANISTREPLASE

Brand name: Eminase

Type of drug: Clot busting

Uses: The treatment of heart attacks.

How it works: Dissolves the thrombus or lump which is blocking coronary arteries and causing a heart attack to occur.

Possible adverse effects: Flushing, internal bleeding, nausea and vomiting, a sudden drop in blood pressure and heart rate.

Availability: Available only with a prescription from a doctor.

Other information: Should be used with caution by people with a history of heart rhythm problems. Use with caution if there is an increased risk of bleeding, for example following surgery or an injury. Will usually only be administered in hospital as an emergency treatment.

CAUTIONS

Children: This drug is either not recommended for children, or is recommended only for children above a certain age.

Pregnancy and breastfeeding: This drug is either not recommended for use by women who are pregnant or breastfeeding, or the precise effects are not known and it should therefore only be used with caution and under medical advice.

Alcohol: No known problems if taken with alcohol.

Driving and operating machinery: There are no commonly reported problems which may impact on the ability to drive or operate machinery. However, many drugs can cause dizziness or drowsiness in a few people, so it is wise to see how the drug affects you before driving or working with dangerous machinery.

ANTAZOLINE

Brand name: Otrivine-Antistin

Type of drug: Antihistamine

Uses: Treatment of mild allergic reactions which affect the skin or the eyes.

How it works: Counteracts the inflammatory response which occurs with allergies.

Possible adverse effects: These rarely occur, but allergy is possible, as is a headache.

Availability: Available without a prescription (over the counter).

Other information: Can be used either as a cream, or as eye drops. This drug should not be used regularly for long periods.

CAUTIONS

Children: There are no commonly reported problems associated with prescribing this medication for children.

Pregnancy and breastfeeding: No specific problems documented, but any medication should be taken with utmost caution by women who are either pregnant or breastfeeding, and only after professional medical or pharmaceutical advice has been sought.

Alcohol: No known problems if taken with alcohol.

Driving and operating machinery: There are no commonly reported problems which may impact on the ability to drive or operate machinery. However, many drugs can cause dizziness or drowsiness in a few people, so it is wise to see how the drug affects you before driving or working with dangerous machinery.

APOMORPHINE HYDROCHLORIDE

Brand name: Britaject

Type of drug: Anti-Parkinsonism

Uses: Control of some of the symptoms of Parkinsonism in patients in whom the effects of other drugs are no longer sufficient.

How it works: Helps to control some of the symptoms which have not been helped by other treatments.

Possible adverse effects: Symptoms may not improve, and can worsen. Nausea and vomiting may occur and patients may show signs of confusion.

Availability: Available only with a prescription from a doctor.

Other information: Administered as an injection. Hospital admission is necessary for at least three days prior to treatment.

CAUTIONS

Children: There are no commonly reported problems associated with prescribing this medication for children.

Pregnancy and breastfeeding: This drug is either not recommended for use by women who are pregnant or breastfeeding, or the precise effects are not known and it should therefore only be used with caution and under medical advice.

Alcohol: No known problems if taken with alcohol.

Driving and operating machinery: There are no commonly reported problems which may impact on the ability to drive or operate machinery. However, many drugs can cause dizziness or drowsiness in a few people, so it is wise to see how the drug affects you before driving or working with dangerous machinery.

APRACLONIDINE

Brand name: Iopidine

Type of drug: Eye surgery preparation

Uses: Given as preparation for surgery before an eye operation.

How it works: Controls the pressure within the eyeball to increase the safety and effectiveness of surgery.

Possible adverse effects: Dry mouth and a funny taste in the mouth, eye discomfort and headache.

Availability: Available only with a prescription from a doctor.

Other information: Administered as eye drops which will usually be administered three times a day for a month.

CAUTIONS

Children: This drug is either not recommended for children, or is recommended only for children above a certain age.

Pregnancy and breastfeeding: This drug is either not recommended for use by women who are pregnant or breastfeeding, or the precise effects are not known and it should therefore only be used with caution and under medical advice.

Alcohol: No known problems if taken with alcohol.

Driving and operating machinery: This drug may have some effect on your driving ability, so it is advisable not to drive or operate machinery while taking it.

ASPIRIN

Brand name: Angettes, Caprin, Disprin, Nu-Seals Aspirin

Type of drug: Non-opioid analgesic, anti-platelet, anti-pyretic

Uses: Treatment of a wide variety of mild to moderate pain, including menstrual pain, headache, toothache. Aspirin is an effective way of treating a fever. It is also useful to control the symptoms of colds and flu. It relieves the inflammation present in conditions such as arthritis. Aspirin is thought to be helpful in the treatment of some types of heart disease.

How it works: Acts on the hypothalamus in the brain to block the generation of pain impulses. As this part of the brain also helps to control the body temperature, it causes sweating, which helps to lower the body temperature. It interferes with the clotting mechanism in the blood, which helps with the treatment of heart and circulatory conditions.

Possible adverse effects: Can cause irritation and, with long term use, bleeding in the stomach. Can also provoke asthma attacks. Rarely it can cause Reye's syndrome in children under 12 years.

Availability: Available without a prescription (over-the-counter).

Other information: Usually taken as a tablet, but also available as suppositories. Should be taken with food or milk, to protect the stomach.

CAUTIONS

Children: This drug is either not recommended for children, or is recommended only for children above a certain age.

Pregnancy and breastfeeding: This drug is either not recommended for use by women who are pregnant or breastfeeding, or the precise effects are not known and it should therefore only be used with caution and under medical advice.

Alcohol: Alcohol should not be consumed, or only consumed with caution - after medical advice has been sought - while you are taking this drug.

Driving and operating machinery: There are no commonly reported problems which may impact on the ability to drive or operate machinery. However, many drugs can cause dizziness or drowsiness in a few people,

so it is wise to see how the drug affects you before driving or working with dangerous machinery.

ASTEMIZOLE

Brand name: Hismanal

Type of drug: Antihistamine

Uses: The treatment of hay fever and other allergic skin conditions such as chronic urticaria (hives).

How it works: Blocks the effect of histamine without having a sedative effect.

Possible adverse effects: Weight gain, and rarely, headache, nausea and rash. Occasionally palpitations can occur which should be reported to a doctor immediately.

Availability: Available without a prescription.

Other information: This medication should be discontinued if you are to have allergy testing within four weeks.

CAUTIONS

Children: This drug is either not recommended for children, or is recommended only for children above a certain age.

Pregnancy and breastfeeding: This drug is either not recommended for use by women who are pregnant or breastfeeding, or the precise effects are not known and it should therefore only be used with caution and under medical advice.

Alcohol: No known problems if taken with alcohol.

Driving and operating machinery: There are no commonly reported problems which may impact on the ability to drive or operate machinery. However, many drugs can cause dizziness or drowsiness in a few people, so it is wise to see how the drug affects you before driving or working with dangerous machinery.

ATENOLOL

Brand name: Antipressan, Atenix, Tenormin, Totamol

Type of drug: Beta-blocker

Uses: Prescribed to control hypertension (high blood pressure). Is also used to control the symptoms of angina. If administered soon after a heart attack it can be effective at minimising the damage.

How it works: Affects angina by slowing the heart rate and reducing the amount of oxygen needed by the heart. Treats angina by reducing the amount of work the heart has to do in order to effectively pump blood around the body.

Possible adverse effects: Muscle aches and tiredness are common. Headache, nausea and a rash are also possible. Any sign of palpitations should be reported immediately. Can cause breathing difficulties, so extra caution is needed for people with asthma or bronchitis.

Availability: Available only with a prescription from a doctor.

Other information: Will usually be prescribed as a tablet, although sometimes a liquid is the chosen option. Can react with a number of other medicines, so make sure your doctor is aware of all other medication.

CAUTIONS

Children: This drug is either not recommended for children, or is recommended only for children above a certain age.

Pregnancy and breastfeeding: No specific problems documented, but any medication should be taken with utmost caution by women who are either pregnant or breastfeeding, and only after professional medical or pharmaceutical advice has been sought.

Alcohol: No known problems if taken with alcohol.

Driving and operating machinery: This drug may have some effect on your driving ability, so it is advisable not to drive or operate machinery while taking it.

ATROPINE

Brand name: Lomotil, Minims Atropine

Type of drug: Anti-cholinergic and mydriatic

Uses: Atropine tablets are used to treat irritable bowel syndrome.
Atropine eye drops are used to treat uveitis, an inflammation of part of the eye.

How it works: A muscle relaxant which acts on the wall of the intestine. When used as eye drops, it enlarges the pupil in the eye.

Possible adverse effects: Blurred vision, dry mouth and thirst. Flushing and dry skin. Constipation and rash. If eye pain or palpitations occur, medical attention should be sought as a matter of urgency.

Availability: Available only with a prescription from a doctor.

Other information: An overdose should be treated as an emergency.

CAUTIONS

Children: There are no commonly reported problems associated with prescribing this medication for children.

Pregnancy and breastfeeding: This drug is either not recommended for use by women who are pregnant or breastfeeding, or the precise effects are not known and it should therefore only be used with caution and under medical advice.

Alcohol: Alcohol should not be consumed, or only consumed with caution - after medical advice has been sought - while you are taking this drug.

Driving and operating machinery: This drug may have some effect on your driving ability, so it is advisable not to drive or operate machinery while taking it.

AURANOFIN

Brand name: Ridaura

Type of drug: Gold compound

Uses: The treatment of severe rheumatoid arthritis, psoriatic arthritis and systemic lupus erythematosus.

How it works: It has an anti-inflammatory effect which suppresses, and in some cases prevents, but does not cure, adult or juvenile arthritis. The precise way it works is unknown.

Possible adverse effects: Diarrhoea, which can be treated with bran. Can cause some blood problems, so a doctor should be informed immediately if there are any signs of sore throat, fever, infection, mouth ulcers or bleeding and bruising.

Availability: Available only with a prescription from a doctor.

Other information: Pre-menopausal women should use contraception during treatment and for six months following it.

CAUTIONS

Children: This drug is either not recommended for children, or is recommended only for children above a certain age.

Pregnancy and breastfeeding: This drug is either not recommended for use by women who are pregnant or breastfeeding, or the precise effects are not known and it should therefore only be used with caution and under medical advice.

Alcohol: No known problems if taken with alcohol.

Driving and operating machinery: There are no commonly reported problems which may impact on the ability to drive or operate machinery. However, many drugs can cause dizziness or drowsiness in a few people, so it is wise to see how the drug affects you before driving or working with dangerous machinery.

AZAPROPAZONE

Brand name: Rheumox

Type of drug: Non-steroidal and anti-inflammatory

Uses: For providing pain relief.

How it works: Is absorbed rapidly to provide pain relief. Because of its anti-inflammatory qualities, azapropazone is also particularly useful in the treatment of conditions such as osteoarthritis, rheumatoid arthritis and injuries where inflammation has resulted.

Possible adverse effects: Rash, gastrointestinal disturbances. This drug can irritate the lining of the stomach, but discomfort can be avoided if it is taken with milk or at mealtimes. Can lead to worsening of asthma in some people.

Availability: Available only with a prescription from a doctor.

Other information: Do not take aspirin or other similar pain-relieving drugs whilst on this medication.

CAUTIONS

Children: There are no commonly reported problems associated with prescribing this medication for children.

Pregnancy and breastfeeding: This drug is either not recommended for use by women who are pregnant or breastfeeding, or the precise effects are not known and it should therefore only be used with caution and under medical advice.

Alcohol: Alcohol should not be consumed, or only consumed with caution - after medical advice has been sought - while you are taking this drug.

Driving and operating machinery: There are no commonly reported problems which may impact on the ability to drive or operate machinery. However, many drugs can cause dizziness or drowsiness in a few people, so it is wise to see how the drug affects you before driving or working with dangerous machinery.

AZATHIOPRINE

Brand name: Azamune, Berkaprine, Immunoprin, Imuran

Type of drug: Anti-rheumatic

Uses: Treatment of rheumatoid arthritis that has not responded to other types of medication.

How it works: Acts on the immune system and boosts the effect of other rheumatic drugs to relieve the symptoms of rheumatoid arthritis.

Possible adverse effects: Can affect the production of white blood cells, leaving patients at an increased risk of infection. Can also irritate the stomach. Any signs of side effects should be reported immediately.

Availability: Available only with a prescription from a doctor.

Other information: Can be given as tablets or as an injection. Regular blood checks will be made to assess the effect of this drug.

CAUTIONS

Children: There are no commonly reported problems associated with prescribing this medication for children.

Pregnancy and breastfeeding: This drug is either not recommended for use by women who are pregnant or breastfeeding, or the precise effects are not known and it should therefore only be used with caution and under medical advice.

Alcohol: No known problems if taken with alcohol.

Driving and operating machinery: This drug may have some effect on your driving ability, so it is advisable not to drive or operate machinery while taking it.

AZITHROMYCIN

Brand name: Zithromax

Type of drug: Antibiotic

Uses: The treatment of a wide range of infections, such as those which occur with chronic obstructive pulmonary disease, pneumonia, tonsillitis and otitis media.

How it works: Binds to part of the bacteria, preventing it from multiplying.

Possible adverse effects: Dizziness, vertigo, headache. Nausea, vomiting, diarrhoea and gastrointestinal disturbances.

Availability: Available only with a prescription from a doctor.

Other information: Should be taken on an empty stomach - one or two hours after meals.

CAUTIONS

Children: This drug is either not recommended for children, or is recommended only for children above a certain age.

Pregnancy and breastfeeding: No specific problems documented, but any medication should be taken with utmost caution by women who are either pregnant or breastfeeding, and only after professional medical or pharmaceutical advice has been sought.

Alcohol: No known problems if taken with alcohol.

Driving and operating machinery: There are no commonly reported problems which may impact on the ability to drive or operate machinery. However, many drugs can cause dizziness or drowsiness in a few people, so it is wise to see how the drug affects you before driving or working with dangerous machinery.

AZTREONAM

Brand name: Azactam

Type of drug: Antibiotic

Uses: Treatment of a wide range of severe infections including those affecting the lungs, urinary tract and skin.

How it works: Binds to the infectious organisms and kills them, thereby relieving the symptoms of the infection.

Possible adverse effects: Disturbances to the stomach, leading to diarrhoea and nausea. Any signs of a rash, reddening of the skin, or itching should be reported to a doctor as these could signify an allergic reaction.

Availability: Available only with a prescription from a doctor.

Other information: Usually given as an injection in hospital.

CAUTIONS

Children: There are no commonly reported problems associated with prescribing this medication for children.

Pregnancy and breastfeeding: This drug is either not recommended for use by women who are pregnant or breastfeeding, or the precise effects are not known and it should therefore only be used with caution and under medical advice.

Alcohol: No known problems if taken with alcohol.

Driving and operating machinery: There are no commonly reported problems which may impact on the ability to drive or operate machinery. However, many drugs can cause dizziness or drowsiness in a few people, so it is wise to see how the drug affects you before driving or working with dangerous machinery.

BACLOFEN

Brand name: Baclospas, Lioresal

Type of drug: Muscle relaxant

Uses: A drug which relaxes muscles, thereby relieving painful spasms which occur in conditions such as multiple sclerosis or which are caused by trauma such as spinal injuries. Baclofen is also a useful treatment option for seized-up or spastic muscles that can occur following brain injury, cerebral palsy or stroke.

How it works: The exact way it works is unknown, but it is thought to act on the spinal cord and inhibit the transmission of chemicals which contribute to the spasms. It relieves symptoms but does not cure the underlying condition.

Possible adverse effects: Dizziness, drowsiness, nausea, weakness. These effects are more likely to occur in patients over 40 years of age and should be reported to a doctor immediately.

Availability: Available only with a prescription from a doctor.

Other information: Administered either as tablets or as an injection - although the latter will only be given in hospital. May interfere with a diabetic's blood sugar levels. Do not take any other medication without checking with your doctor first.

CAUTIONS

Children: This drug is either not recommended for children, or is recommended only for children above a certain age.

Pregnancy and breastfeeding: This drug is either not recommended for use by women who are pregnant or breastfeeding, or the precise effects are not known and it should therefore only be used with caution and under medical advice.

Alcohol: Alcohol should not be consumed, or only consumed with caution - after medical advice has been sought - while you are taking this drug.

Driving and operating machinery: There are no commonly reported

problems which may impact on the ability to drive or operate machinery. However, many drugs can cause dizziness or drowsiness in a few people, so it is wise to see how the drug affects you before driving or working with dangerous machinery.

BECLOMETHASONE
Brand name: AeroBec, BDP Spacehaler, Beclazone, Becloforte, Becodisks, Beconase, Becotide, Filair
Type of drug: Corticosteroid
Uses: Prescribed as an inhalant to relieve the symptoms of severe asthma which has not responded to other treatments. It is also prescribed as a nasal spray to treat hay fever and as an ointment for some skin conditions.
How it works: Reduces inflammation and the production of mucus in the nose. Used as a preventative treatment for asthmatics.
Possible adverse effects: Occasionally fungal infections can occur in the mouth, but gargling with water after each inhalation will prevent this is most cases. Nasal discomfort and a sore throat are also possible.
Availability: Some preparations available over the counter.
Other information: Beclomethasone is unlikely to be prescribed for long periods for children.
CAUTIONS
Children: There are no commonly reported problems associated with prescribing this medication for children.
Pregnancy and breastfeeding: No specific problems documented, but any medication should be taken with utmost caution by women who are either pregnant or breastfeeding, and only after professional medical or pharmaceutical advice has been sought.
Alcohol: No known problems if taken with alcohol.
Driving and operating machinery: There are no commonly reported problems which may impact on the ability to drive or operate machinery. However, many drugs can cause dizziness or drowsiness in a few people, so it is wise to see how the drug affects you before driving or working with dangerous machinery.

BENDROFLUAZIDE
Brand name: Aprinox, Berkozide, Neo-NaClex

Type of drug: Diuretic

Uses: A diuretic (water pill) used to prevent the water retention, or oedema, caused by heart conditions or pre-menstrual bloating. It can also be used as a treatment for high blood pressure.

How it works: Works to encourage excess water to be eliminated from the body.

Possible adverse effects: The most serious side effect is that too much potassium can be expelled from the body. Rarely, cramps, lethargy and nausea may also occur. Any incidence should be discussed with your doctor.

Availability: Available only with a prescription from a doctor.

Other information: Administered as tablets. Blood tests will be conducted regularly to check potassium levels. Potassium pills may be prescribed if the levels are too low.

CAUTIONS

Children: This drug is either not recommended for children, or is recommended only for children above a certain age.

Pregnancy and breastfeeding: This drug is either not recommended for use by women who are pregnant or breastfeeding, or the precise effects are not known and it should therefore only be used with caution and under medical advice.

Alcohol: No known problems if taken with alcohol.

Driving and operating machinery: There are no commonly reported problems which may impact on the ability to drive or operate machinery. However, many drugs can cause dizziness or drowsiness in a few people, so it is wise to see how the drug affects you before driving or working with dangerous machinery.

BENZHEXOL

Brand name: Artane, Broflex

Type of drug: Anti-Parkinsonism

Uses: Anti-Parkinsonism drug, used to control the symptoms of Parkinson's disease and other conditions that cause tremor. Also used to treat the tremor which can be experienced as a side effect of some medicines used for psychiatric disorders.

How it works: Goes some way towards correcting the imbalance between two chemicals in the brain - dopamine and acetylcholine - which lead to Parkinsonian symptoms. It boosts the response to treatment of people already using another similar medicine, Levodopa.

Possible adverse effects: Dry mouth, nausea, dizziness and blurred vision. Occasionally it can affect the bladder, making it difficult to pass water, in which case medical advice should be sought immediately.

Availability: Available only with a prescription from a doctor.

Other information: Regular checks will be made on blood pressure, eyes and heart whilst taking this drug.

CAUTIONS

Children: This drug is either not recommended for children, or is recommended only for children above a certain age.

Pregnancy and breastfeeding: This drug is either not recommended for use by women who are pregnant or breastfeeding, or the precise effects are not known and it should therefore only be used with caution and under medical advice.

Alcohol: Alcohol should not be consumed, or only consumed with caution - after medical advice has been sought - while you are taking this drug.

Driving and operating machinery: This drug may have some effect on your driving ability, so it is advisable not to drive or operate machinery while taking it.

BENZOIC ACID

Brand name: Benzoic Acid Ointment, Compound, BP

Type of drug: Anti-fungal

Uses: The treatment of ringworm - athlete's foot.

How it works: When applied to the affected area it destroys the fungus which causes the problem.

Possible adverse effects: Rarely occur.

Availability: Available with or without a prescription.

Other information: Available as a cream.

CAUTIONS

Children: There are no commonly reported problems associated with prescribing this medication for children.

Pregnancy and breastfeeding: No specific problems documented, but any medication should be taken with utmost caution by women who are

either pregnant or breastfeeding, and only after professional medical or pharmaceutical advice has been sought.

Alcohol: No known problems if taken with alcohol.

Driving and operating machinery: There are no commonly reported problems which may impact on the ability to drive or operate machinery. However, many drugs can cause dizziness or drowsiness in a few people, so it is wise to see how the drug affects you before driving or working with dangerous machinery.

BENZOYL PEROXIDE

Brand name: Acetoxyl, Acnecide, Acnegel, Benoxyl, Nericur, Panoxyl, Quinoped

Type of drug: Acne and fungal skin infection treatment

Uses: Used mainly to treat moderate acne.

How it works: Lifts off the top layer of skin which helps to unblock the sebaceous glands.

Possible adverse effects: A drying effect, leading to stinging or redness on the skin which may feel uncomfortable. If the skin starts to peel, the cream should be applied less frequently.

Availability: Available with or without a prescription.

Other information: Available as a cream, lotion or gel. May bleach any clothing it comes into contact with. Avoid contact with the eyes and mouth. Should not be used for more than six weeks at a time unless under medical supervision.

CAUTIONS

Children: This drug is either not recommended for children, or is recommended only for children above a certain age.

Pregnancy and breastfeeding: No specific problems documented, but any medication should be taken with utmost caution by women who are either pregnant or breastfeeding, and only after professional medical or pharmaceutical advice has been sought.

Alcohol: No known problems if taken with alcohol.

Driving and operating machinery: There are no commonly reported problems which may impact on the ability to drive or operate machinery. However, many drugs can cause dizziness or drowsiness in a few people, so it is wise to see how the drug affects you before driving or working with dangerous machinery.

BETAHISTINE
Brand name: Serc
Type of drug: Meniere's disease treatment
Uses: Most frequently used to control the nausea and vertigo attacks which are symptomatic of Meniere's disease. It can also be used to control the sound of ringing in the ears experienced by people with tinnitus.
How it works: Thought to improve the blood flow through the small blood vessels in the ear, with the result that the pressure in the inner ear is reduced.
Possible adverse effects: Nausea and indigestion. Rarely, a rash can occur, which should be reported to a doctor.
Availability: Available only with a prescription from a doctor.
Other information: Not successful in all cases. An overdose should be treated as an emergency.

CAUTIONS
Children: This drug is either not recommended for children, or is recommended only for children above a certain age.
Pregnancy and breastfeeding: This drug is either not recommended for use by women who are pregnant or breastfeeding, or the precise effects are not known and it should therefore only be used with caution and under medical advice.
Alcohol: No known problems if taken with alcohol.
Driving and operating machinery: There are no commonly reported problems which may impact on the ability to drive or operate machinery. However, many drugs can cause dizziness or drowsiness in a few people, so it is wise to see how the drug affects you before driving or working with dangerous machinery.

BETAMETHASONE
Brand name: Betnelan, Betnesol, Betnovate, Diprosone, Vista-Methasone
Type of drug: Corticosteroid
Uses: Main use is as an anti-inflammatory when it is given as an injection straight into the affected joints in order to alleviate the symptoms of arthritis. Is also given by mouth as part of the treatment of conditions affecting the pituitary and adrenal glands and some blood disorders. Can be applied to the skin to treat eczema and psoriasis.

How it works: Stimulates the production of enzymes in the body, which reduces the inflammation associated with arthritis and other inflammatory conditions.

Possible adverse effects: Most reactions to this drug are related to the dose and can be alleviated with adjustment. Indigestion is common and should always be reported to a doctor. Long term, large doses can lead to symptoms such as peptic ulcers, muscle weakness, delicate skin.

Availability: Available only with a prescription from a doctor.

Other information: There is a significant difference in strength between the topical preparations (creams and ointments) and those which are given in tablet or injection form. It is not recommended that oral courses of medication are stopped suddenly.

CAUTIONS

Children: This drug is either not recommended for children, or is recommended only for children above a certain age.

Pregnancy and breastfeeding: This drug is either not recommended for use by women who are pregnant or breastfeeding, or the precise effects are not known and it should therefore only be used with caution and under medical advice.

Alcohol: Alcohol should not be consumed, or only consumed with caution - after medical advice has been sought - while you are taking this drug.

Driving and operating machinery: There are no commonly reported problems which may impact on the ability to drive or operate machinery. However, many drugs can cause dizziness or drowsiness in a few people, so it is wise to see how the drug affects you before driving or working with dangerous machinery.

BETHANECHOL CHLORIDE

Brand name: Myotonine

Type of drug: Cholinergic

Uses: The treatment of people who are unable to pass urine and for whom catheterisation (the passing of a tube into the bladder) is not an option.

How it works: Stimulates the nerves in the urinary tract, forcing the bladder to contract and enabling urination to take place.

Possible adverse effects: Sweating, slow pulse and intestinal discomfort.

Availability: Available only with a prescription from a doctor.

Other information: Can be given in either injection or tablet form. Will usually be given when the patient has an empty stomach.

CAUTIONS

Children: There are no commonly reported problems associated with prescribing this medication for children.

Pregnancy and breastfeeding: This drug is either not recommended for use by women who are pregnant or breastfeeding, or the precise effects are not known and it should therefore only be used with caution and under medical advice.

Alcohol: No known problems if taken with alcohol.

Driving and operating machinery: There are no commonly reported problems which may impact on the ability to drive or operate machinery. However, many drugs can cause dizziness or drowsiness in a few people, so it is wise to see how the drug affects you before driving or working with dangerous machinery.

BEZAFIBRATE

Brand name: Bezalip, Bezalip-Mono

Type of drug: Lipid lowering

Uses: To lower the level of fats (lipids) in the blood which are thought to contribute to coronary heart disease, which can lead to angina, heart attacks and stroke.

How it works: Bezafibrate is prescribed with the aim of reducing the level of cholesterol in the blood as a way of preventing the onset of coronary heart disease in people who are known to have high cholesterol levels in the blood.

Possible adverse effects: Nausea, appetite loss, gastric pain. Usually short-term. Any episodes of gastric pain should be reported to a doctor.

Availability: Available only with a prescription from a doctor.

Other information: Should to be taken in conjunction with a low fat diet. Blood tests will be performed regularly to assess the effect on the level of fat in the blood.

CAUTIONS

Children: This drug is either not recommended for children, or is recommended only for children above a certain age.

Pregnancy and breastfeeding: This drug is either not recommended for use by women who are pregnant or breastfeeding, or the precise effects are not known and it should therefore only be used with caution and under medical advice.

Alcohol: No known problems if taken with alcohol.

Driving and operating machinery: There are no commonly reported problems which may impact on the ability to drive or operate machinery. However, many drugs can cause dizziness or drowsiness in a few people, so it is wise to see how the drug affects you before driving or working with dangerous machinery.

BICALUTAMIDE

Brand name: Casodex

Type of drug: Anti-cancer

Uses: The treatment of cancer of the prostate in patients who have advanced stages of the disease.

How it works: Changes the chemical composition of the tissue where the cancer is growing.

Possible adverse effects: Hot flushes, constipation, nausea, diarrhoea are relatively common, as is a pain in the back or pelvic area.

Availability: Available only with a prescription from a doctor.

Other information: This drug should be taken at approximately the same time each day.

CAUTIONS

Children: This drug is either not recommended for children, or is recommended only for children above a certain age.

Pregnancy and breastfeeding: This drug is either not recommended for use by women who are pregnant or breastfeeding, or the precise effects are not known and it should therefore only be used with caution and under medical advice.

Alcohol: No known problems if taken with alcohol.

Driving and operating machinery: There are no commonly reported problems which may impact on the ability to drive or operate machinery. However, many drugs can cause dizziness or drowsiness in a few people, so it is wise to see how the drug affects you before driving or working with dangerous machinery.

BROMOCRIPTINE

Brand name: Parlodel

Type of drug: Fertility

Uses: The treatment of both male and female infertility and a variety of period problems. It is also effective for some people who are in the later stages of Parkinsonism, particularly those for whom other courses of treatment have not worked.

How it works: Prevents the pituitary gland from producing a hormone which causes some types of female infertility, breast problems and menstrual disorders. It is also used to prevent women who do not wish to breast-feed from producing milk. Stimulates the production of chemicals in the central nervous system which counteract the symptoms of Parkinsonism.

Possible adverse effects: Nausea and vomiting are the most common but these can be minimised by taking the medication at mealtimes.

Availability: Available only with a prescription from a doctor.

Other information: Regular blood and gynaecological tests will be conducted to assess the effectiveness of the drug.

CAUTIONS

Children: This drug is either not recommended for children, or is recommended only for children above a certain age.

Pregnancy and breastfeeding: This drug is either not recommended for use by women who are pregnant or breastfeeding, or the precise effects are not known and it should therefore only be used with caution.

Alcohol: Alcohol should not be consumed, or only consumed with caution - after medical advice has been sought - while you are taking this drug.

Driving and operating machinery: This drug may have some effect on your driving ability, so it is advisable not to drive or operate machinery while taking it.

BUDESONIDE

Brand name: Pulmicort

Type of drug: Anti-inflammatory

Uses: Prescribed to control the symptoms of hay fever and asthma.

How it works: Precise action is not known but it controls some of the chemicals which are involved in the development of the conditions.

Possible adverse effects: Nasal irritation, cough, nose bleeds and headache.

Availability: Available only with a prescription from a doctor.

Other information: Will be prescribed as an inhaler. The prescribed dose should not be exceeded. It is important that patients use the correct technique when taking this medication - if in doubt check with a medical professional. This drug will not achieve its maximum level of effectiveness until it has been used for a few weeks.

CAUTIONS

Children: This drug is either not recommended for children, or is recommended only for children above a certain age.

Pregnancy and breastfeeding: This drug is either not recommended for use by women who are pregnant or breastfeeding, or the precise effects are not known and it should therefore only be used with caution and under medical advice.

Alcohol: No known problems if taken with alcohol.

Driving and operating machinery: There are no commonly reported problems which may impact on the ability to drive or operate machinery. However, many drugs can cause dizziness or drowsiness in a few people, so it is wise to see how the drug affects you before driving or working with dangerous machinery.

BUMETANIDE

Brand name: Burinex

Type of drug: Diuretic

Uses: Used to reduce fluid retention in people who have problems such as heart failure and cirrhosis of the liver. It can also be used for people with kidney problems, unlike most diuretics.

How it works: Encourages elimination of excess fluid.

Possible adverse effects: Most side effects are due to the loss of potassium and the rapid loss of fluid and include dizziness, lethargy and muscle cramps. For this reason, bumetanide is usually given in conjunction with potassium supplements. Any sign of a rash should be reported immediately.

Availability: Available only with a prescription from a doctor.

Other information: A diet high in fresh fruit and vegetables should be taken. Regular blood tests will be taken to monitor effectiveness.

CAUTIONS

Children: There are no commonly reported problems associated with prescribing this medication for children.

Pregnancy and breastfeeding: No specific problems documented, but any medication should be taken with utmost caution by women who are either pregnant or breastfeeding, and only after professional medical or pharmaceutical advice has been sought.

Alcohol: Alcohol should not be consumed, or only consumed with caution - after medical advice has been sought - while you are taking this drug.

Driving and operating machinery: This drug may have some effect on your driving ability, so it is advisable not to drive or operate machinery while taking it.

BUPRENORPHINE

Brand name: Temgesic

Type of drug: Painkiller

Uses: The alleviation of moderate to severe pain.

How it works: The precise way it works is unknown, but it is thought to neutralise the effect of the chemicals which transmit the pain messages.

Possible adverse effects: Dizziness, drowsiness, headache, vertigo, nausea.

Availability: Available only with a prescription from a doctor.

Other information: Will usually be prescribed as a pill which needs to be taken sublingually - allowed to dissolve under the tongue.

CAUTIONS

Children: There are no commonly reported problems associated with prescribing this medication for children.

Pregnancy and breastfeeding: This drug is either not recommended for use by women who are pregnant or breastfeeding, or the precise effects are not known and it should therefore only be used with caution and under medical advice.

Alcohol: Alcohol should not be consumed, or only consumed with caution - after medical advice has been sought - while you are taking this drug.

Driving and operating machinery: This drug may have some effect on your driving ability, so it is advisable not to drive or operate machinery while taking it.

BUSERELIN

Brand name: Suprefact

Type of drug: Hormone

Uses: The treatment of types of prostate cancer which depend on hormones to grow. Also used to treat endometriosis.

How it works: Deprives prostate cancer of the hormones it needs for growth. For endometriosis, it blocks the production of hormones by the ovaries and stops periods.

Possible adverse effects: In men - hot flushes, nasal irritation due to nasal spray, loss of sex drive, depression, vomiting, diarrhoea. In women - hot flushes, dry vagina, emotional swings, sore breasts and changes in breast size.

Availability: Available only with a prescription from a doctor.

Other information: Barrier methods of contraception should be used during treatment to prevent unwanted pregnancy.

CAUTIONS

Children: Not usually prescribed.

Pregnancy and breastfeeding: This drug is either not recommended for use by women who are pregnant or breastfeeding, or the precise effects are not known and it should therefore only be used with caution and under medical advice.

Alcohol: No known problems if taken with alcohol.

Driving and operating machinery: There are no commonly reported problems which may impact on the ability to drive or operate machinery. However, many drugs can cause dizziness or drowsiness in a few people, so it is wise to see how the drug affects you before driving or working with dangerous machinery.

CABERGOLINE

Brand name: Dostinex

Type of drug: Dopamine receptor stimulant

Uses: To halt or prevent the production of a mother's milk soon after childbirth - this is usually necessary in people who have pituitary gland disorders, a symptom of which may be a vast over-production of milk.

How it works: Inhibits the release of prolactin by the pituitary gland, which alleviates the symptoms.

Possible adverse effects: Headache, vertigo, dizziness, breast pain, weakness.

Availability: Available only with a prescription from a doctor.

Other information: Prescribed as tablets. Use a barrier method of contraception whilst being treated with this drug.

CAUTIONS

Children: This drug is either not recommended for children, or is recommended only for children above a certain age.

Pregnancy and breastfeeding: This drug is either not recommended for use by women who are pregnant or breastfeeding, or the precise effects are not known and it should therefore only be used with caution and under medical advice.

Alcohol: No known problems if taken with alcohol.

Driving and operating machinery: This drug may have some effect on your driving ability, so it is advisable not to drive or operate machinery while taking it.

CALCIPOTRIOL

Brand name: Dovonex

Type of drug: Synthetic vitamin

Uses: A cream, ointment or lotion for external use only, to treat moderate and severe psoriasis.

How it works: Reduces the production of skin cells that cause the symptoms of skin thickening and scaling associated with psoriasis.

Possible adverse effects: The skin may be irritated initially but this usually wears off. Long term, heavy use may affect calcium levels in the blood.

Availability: Available only with a prescription from a doctor.

Other information: The drug is not normally used for longer than six weeks. Regular blood tests may be required to check calcium levels for people on long term treatment.

CAUTIONS

Children: This drug is either not recommended for children, or is recommended only for children above a certain age.

Pregnancy and breastfeeding: No specific problems documented, but any medication should be taken with utmost caution by women who are either pregnant or breastfeeding, and only after professional medical or pharmaceutical advice has been sought.

Alcohol: No known problems if taken with alcohol.

Driving and operating machinery: There are no commonly reported problems which may impact on the ability to drive or operate machinery. However, many drugs can cause dizziness or drowsiness in a few people, so it is wise to see how the drug affects you before driving or working with dangerous machinery.

CALCITONIN

Brand name: Calcitare

Type of drug: Thyroid hormone

Uses: An injection to relieve pain of Paget's disease and other bony disorders. Is useful for the treatment of osteoporosis. Relieves bony problems in the ear which are causing deafness. It can also be administered in the form of a nasal spray.

How it works: It regulates the blood calcium level in bones.

Possible adverse effects: Nausea, vomiting, tingling of hands, flushing, unpleasant taste and allergies.

Availability: Available only with a prescription from a doctor.

Other information: A skin test should be carried out before use to test for allergic reactions.

CAUTIONS

Children: This drug is either not recommended for children, or is recommended only for children above a certain age.

Pregnancy and breastfeeding: This drug is either not recommended for use by women who are pregnant or breastfeeding, or the precise effects are not known and it should therefore only be used with caution and under medical advice.

Alcohol: No known problems if taken with alcohol.

Driving and operating machinery: There are no commonly reported problems which may impact on the ability to drive or operate machinery. However, many drugs can cause dizziness or drowsiness in a few people, so it is wise to see how the drug affects you before driving or working with dangerous machinery.

CALCIUM POLYSTYRENE SULPONATE

Brand name: Calcium Resonium

Type of drug: Potassium removing

Uses: To treat people who have excess potassium in the blood due to a urinary disorder or as a result of kidney dialysis.

How it works: Once in the intestine, it exchanges calcium ions for potassium ions, thus reducing the amount of potassium in the body.

Possible adverse effects: Too much calcium in the blood or too little potassium. Because the drug is given as a resin it can cause a blockage in the intestine.

Availability: Available only with a prescription from a doctor.

Other information: Regular blood tests will be taken to monitor the effect of the drug.

CAUTIONS

Children: This drug is either not recommended for children, or is recommended only for children above a certain age.

Pregnancy and breastfeeding: This drug is either not recommended for use by women who are pregnant or breastfeeding, or the precise effects are not known and it should therefore only be used with caution and under medical advice.

Alcohol: No known problems if taken with alcohol.

Driving and operating machinery: There are no commonly reported problems which may impact on the ability to drive or operate machinery. However, many drugs can cause dizziness or drowsiness in a few people, so it is wise to see how the drug affects you before driving or working with dangerous machinery.

CAPREOMYCIN

Brand name: Capastat

Type of drug: Antibiotic

Uses: An injection to treat tuberculosis when other forms of drug treatment have failed.

How it works: It reduces the development of resistant bacteria.

Possible adverse effects: Vertigo, tinnitus and rashes are possible side effects.

Availability: Available only with a prescription from a doctor.

Other information: This drug will be used with caution in people who have impaired hearing or impaired kidney function.

CAUTIONS

Children: There are no commonly reported problems associated with prescribing this medication for children.

Pregnancy and breastfeeding: This drug is either not recommended for use by women who are pregnant or breastfeeding, or the precise effects are not known and it should therefore only be used with caution and under medical advice.

Alcohol: No known problems if taken with alcohol.

Driving and operating machinery: There are no commonly reported problems which may impact on the ability to drive or operate machinery. However, many drugs can cause dizziness or drowsiness in a few people, so it is wise to see how the drug affects you before driving or working with dangerous machinery.

CAPTOPRIL

Brand name: Acepril, Capoten

Type of drug: ACE inhibitor

Uses: To treat and lower, high blood pressure and heart failure.

How it works: It relaxes the muscles around the blood vessels, which allows the blood vessels to dilate, thereby easing blood flow, and reducing blood pressure.

Possible adverse effects: A fall in blood pressure, dizziness, palpitations, stomach upsets, dry cough, unpleasant taste and rashes, though they usually disappear fairly quickly.

Availability: Available only with a prescription from a doctor.

Other information: The first dose should be taken while lying down as there is a risk of falling due to the sudden drop in blood pressure.

CAUTIONS

Children: This drug is either not recommended for children, or is recommended only for children above a certain age.

Pregnancy and breastfeeding: This drug is either not recommended for use by women who are pregnant or breastfeeding, or the precise effects are not known and it should therefore only be used with caution and under medical advice.

Alcohol: Alcohol should not be consumed, or only consumed with caution - after medical advice has been sought - while you are taking this drug.

Driving and operating machinery: This drug may have some effect on your driving ability, so it is advisable not to drive or operate machinery while taking it.

CARBACHOL

Brand name: Isopto carbachol

Type of drug: Cholinergic

Uses: To reduce the pressure inside the eye in patients with glaucoma. It is also given after abdominal surgery to people having difficulty in emptying their bladders.

How it works: Causes contraction of the sphincter muscle in the iris and in the bladder.

Possible adverse effects: Headaches, brow pain and eye pain. Blurred vision initially.

Availability: Available only with a prescription from a doctor.

Other information: Do not wear soft contact lenses during treatment.

CAUTIONS

Children: There are no commonly reported problems associated with prescribing this medication for children.

Pregnancy and breastfeeding: This drug is either not recommended for use by women who are pregnant or breastfeeding, or the precise effects are not known and it should therefore only be used with caution and under medical advice.

Alcohol: No known problems if taken with alcohol.

Driving and operating machinery: This drug may have some effect on your driving ability, so it is advisable not to drive or operate machinery while taking it.

CARBAMAZEPINE

Brand name: Tegretol

Type of drug: Anti-convulsant and anti-psychotic

Uses: For the treatment of epilepsy. It is also used for severe nerve pain and for certain behaviour or psychological disorders.

How it works: Reduces the possible occurrences of fits caused by abnormal signals to the brain.

Possible adverse effects: Headache, dizziness, blurred vision, nausea, tiredness.

Availability: Available only with a prescription from a doctor.

Other information: Considered a particularly suitable drug for treating children, because the side effects occur less frequently than with similar drugs.

CAUTIONS

Children: There are no commonly reported problems associated with prescribing this medication for children.

Pregnancy and breastfeeding: This drug is either not recommended for use by women who are pregnant or breastfeeding, or the precise effects are not known and it should therefore only be used with caution and under medical advice.

Alcohol: Alcohol should not be consumed, or only consumed with caution - after medical advice has been sought - while you are taking this drug.

Driving and operating machinery: This drug may have some effect on your driving ability, so it is advisable not to drive or operate machinery while taking it.

CARBARYL

Brand name: Carylderm, Clinicide, Derbac C, Suleo-C

Type of drug: Insecticide treatment

Uses: A solution in the form of a lotion or shampoo that is used to treat head lice.

How it works: As an insecticide it functions by interfering with the nervous system of the lice, causing their death through paralysis.

Possible adverse effects: Skin irritations are the mostly likely side effect from using this product, so it should not be used more than once a week, for three weeks only.

Availability: Available only with a prescription from a doctor.

Other information: Should not be used for long periods. Several different preparations should be used to treat head lice, as the lice become easily resistant to insecticides.

CAUTIONS

Children: There are no commonly reported problems associated with prescribing this medication for children.

Pregnancy and breastfeeding: No specific problems documented, but any medication should be taken with utmost caution by women who are either pregnant or breastfeeding, and only after professional medical or pharmaceutical advice has been sought.

Alcohol: No known problems if taken with alcohol.

Driving and operating machinery: There are no commonly reported problems which may impact on the ability to drive or operate machinery. However, many drugs can cause dizziness or drowsiness in a few people, so it is wise to see how the drug affects you before driving or working with dangerous machinery.

CARBENOXOLONE

Brand name: Bioplex, Bioral

Type of drug: Anti-ulcer

Uses: Originally used for the treatment of gastric and duodenal ulcers, now mainly used for treating mouth ulcers.

How it works: It stimulates the production of mucus and also protects the mucosal barrier from gastric juices and so aids the healing of ulcers.

Possible adverse effects: May cause salt and water retention which can lead to swelling and blood pressure problems.

Availability: Prescription needed for mouthwash but not for gel.

Other information: For patients with heart disease, kidney disease or low blood potassium, use with caution.

CAUTIONS

Children: This drug is either not recommended for children, or is recommended only for children above a certain age.

Pregnancy and breastfeeding: This drug is either not recommended for use by women who are pregnant or breastfeeding, or the precise effects are not known and it should therefore only be used with caution and under medical advice.

Alcohol: Alcohol should not be consumed, or only consumed with caution - after medical advice has been sought - while you are taking this drug.

Driving and operating machinery: There are no commonly reported

problems which may impact on the ability to drive or operate machinery. However, many drugs can cause dizziness or drowsiness in a few people, so it is wise to see how the drug affects you before driving or working with dangerous machinery.

CARBIMAZOLE

Brand name: Neo-Mercazole

Type of drug: Anti-thyroid

Uses: Used for people with an overactive thyroid or after thyroid surgery.

How it works: It reduces the production of thyroid hormones.

Possible adverse effects: Nausea, headaches, joint pain, and skin rashes.

Availability: Available only with a prescription from a doctor.

Other information: Sore throat, mouth ulcers or fevers should be reported to a doctor immediately.

CAUTIONS

Children: There are no commonly reported problems associated with prescribing this medication for children.

Pregnancy and breastfeeding: This drug is either not recommended for use by women who are pregnant or breastfeeding, or the precise effects are not known and it should therefore only be used with caution and under medical advice.

Alcohol: No known problems if taken with alcohol.

Driving and operating machinery: This drug may have some effect on your driving ability, so it is advisable not to drive or operate machinery while taking it.

CARBOCISTEINE

Brand name: Mucodyne

Type of drug: Mucolytic

Uses: To facilitate expectoration in patients with excess sticky sputum. Also used to treat glue ear in children.

How it works: It facilitates expectoration by reducing sputum viscosity.

Possible adverse effects: Nausea, stomach upsets and rashes.

Availability: Available only with a prescription from a doctor.

Other information: Do not use if the patient is suffering from an active peptic ulcer.

CAUTIONS

Children: There are no commonly reported problems associated with prescribing this medication for children.

Pregnancy and breastfeeding: This drug is either not recommended for use by women who are pregnant or breastfeeding, or the precise effects are not known and it should therefore only be used with caution and under medical advice.

Alcohol: No known problems if taken with alcohol.

Driving and operating machinery: There are no commonly reported problems which may impact on the ability to drive or operate machinery. However, many drugs can cause dizziness or drowsiness in a few people, so it is wise to see how the drug affects you before driving or working with dangerous machinery.

CARBOPROST

Brand name: Hemabate

Type of drug: Prostaglandin

Uses: To treat haemorrhage after childbirth due to the failure of the womb to contract.

How it works: Stimulates the uterus to contract, as it does during labour.

Possible adverse effects: Nausea, vomiting, and diarrhoea. Pain and redness at the site of the injection.

Availability: Available only with a prescription from a doctor.

Other information: Will only be administered in hospital, as an injection.

CAUTIONS

Children: Unlikely to be prescribed.

Pregnancy and breastfeeding: This drug is either not recommended for use by women who are pregnant or breastfeeding, or the precise effects are not known and it should therefore only be used with caution and under medical advice.

Alcohol: No known problems if taken with alcohol.

Driving and operating machinery: There are no commonly reported problems which may impact on the ability to drive or operate machinery. However, many drugs can cause dizziness or drowsiness in a few people, so it is wise to see how the drug affects you before driving or working with dangerous machinery.

CARISOPRODOL

Brand name: Carisoma

Type of drug: Muscle relaxant

Uses: To relieve chronic muscular spasms.

How it works: Prescribed as pills which have a sedative effect on muscles, thus causing them to relax.

Possible adverse effects: Drowsiness is the most commonly experienced side effect. It can also cause nausea, headache, flushes and rashes, insomnia and depressive reactions.

Availability: Available only with a prescription from a doctor.

Other information: Not suitable for long term use. Also use with caution in conjunction with sleeping drugs, sedatives, anti-depressants and oral contraceptives. Should be stored away from direct heat and light. Do not take more than the prescribed dose.

CAUTIONS

Children: This drug is either not recommended for children, or is recommended only for children above a certain age.

Pregnancy and breastfeeding: This drug is either not recommended for use by women who are pregnant or breastfeeding, or the precise effects are not known and it should therefore only be used with caution and under medical advice.

Alcohol: Alcohol should not be consumed, or only consumed with caution — after medical advice has been sought - while you are taking this drug.

Driving and operating machinery: This drug may have some effect on your driving ability, so it is advisable not to drive or operate machinery while taking it.

CARNITINE

Brand name: Carnitor

Type of drug: Thyroid hormone

Uses: To treat a deficiency of carnitine, a chemical which is vital in the process of changing fat to energy, due to genetic defects or dialysis.

How it works: It helps to transport long-chain fatty acids into cells to be burned to produce energy.

Possible adverse effects: Nausea, vomiting, stomach pain and diarrhoea.

Availability: Available only with a prescription from a doctor.

Other information: Use with caution if there is impaired kidney function.

CAUTIONS

Children: There are no commonly reported problems associated with prescribing this medication for children.

Pregnancy and breastfeeding: This drug is either not recommended for use by women who are pregnant or breastfeeding, or the precise effects are not known and it should therefore only be used with caution and under medical advice.

Alcohol: No known problems if taken with alcohol.

Driving and operating machinery: There are no commonly reported problems which may impact on the ability to drive or operate machinery. However, many drugs can cause dizziness or drowsiness in a few people, so it is wise to see how the drug affects you before driving or working with dangerous machinery.

CARVEDILOL

Brand name: Eucardic

Type of drug: Alpha- and beta-blocker

Uses: A drug to treat high blood pressure and heart failure.

How it works: It acts to dilate the blood vessels throughout the body, with the result that blood pressure is lowered.

Possible adverse effects: Dizziness - particularly on standing up - possibility of disturbed vision, headache, fatigue and stomach upsets.

Availability: Available only with a prescription from a doctor.

Other information: Prescribed as tablets. Dosage must not be stopped or interrupted without medical approval. Contact lens wearers may experience problems from dry eyes.

CAUTIONS

Children: This drug is either not recommended for children, or is recommended only for children above a certain age.

Pregnancy and breastfeeding: This drug is either not recommended for use by women who are pregnant or breastfeeding, or the precise effects are not known and it should therefore only be used with caution and under medical advice.

Alcohol: No known problems if taken with alcohol.

Driving and operating machinery: This drug may have some effect on your driving ability, so it is advisable not to drive or operate machinery while taking it.

CEFACLOR

Brand name: Distaclor

Type of drug: Antibiotic

Uses: Antibiotic used to treat a variety of bacterial infections of the respiratory tract, sinuses, skin, soft tissue, ear and urinary tract.

How it works: Attacks a wide range of infective organisms.

Possible adverse effects: Diarrhoea is the most common side effect, but should not be severe. Other serious side effects may indicate an allergic reaction and should be reported.

Availability: Available only with a prescription from a doctor.

Other information: Take the full course of the drug even if the infection appears to have cleared up.

CAUTIONS

Children: There are no commonly reported problems associated with prescribing this medication for children.

Pregnancy and breastfeeding: This drug is either not recommended for use by women who are pregnant or breastfeeding, or the precise effects are not known and it should therefore only be used with caution and under medical advice.

Alcohol: No known problems if taken with alcohol.

Driving and operating machinery: There are no commonly reported problems which may impact on the ability to drive or operate machinery. However, many drugs can cause dizziness or drowsiness in a few people, so it is wise to see how the drug affects you before driving or working with dangerous machinery.

CEPHALEXIN

Brand name: Ceporex, Keflex

Type of drug: Antibiotic

Uses: Antibiotic most commonly used for treatment of bronchitis, cystitis and some skin infections.

How it works: Targeted at specific, rather than a wide range of infections.

Possible adverse effects: Diarrhoea. May trigger an allergic reaction in people who are sensitive to penicillin.

Availability: Available only with a prescription from a doctor.

Other information: May reduce the effect of oral contraceptives.

CAUTIONS

Children: There are no commonly reported problems associated with prescribing this medication for children.

Pregnancy and breastfeeding: This drug is either not recommended for use by women who are pregnant or breastfeeding, or the precise effects are not known and it should therefore only be used with caution and under medical advice.

Alcohol: No known problems if taken with alcohol.

Driving and operating machinery: There are no commonly reported problems which may impact on the ability to drive or operate machinery. However, many drugs can cause dizziness or drowsiness in a few people, so it is wise to see how the drug affects you before driving or working with dangerous machinery.

CETIRIZINE

Brand name: Zirtek

Type of drug: Antihistamine

Uses: The treatment of hayfever and other similar allergies.

How it works: Inhibits the production of histamine which leads to the symptoms of an allergic reaction.

Possible adverse effects: Drowsiness, dizziness, headaches and stomach upsets.

Availability: Prescription needed for liquid but not for tablets.

Other information: Can be prescribed as tablets or as a syrup.

CAUTIONS

Children: This drug is either not recommended for children, or is recommended only for children above a certain age.

Pregnancy and breastfeeding: This drug is either not recommended for use by women who are pregnant or breastfeeding, or the precise effects are not known and it should therefore only be used with caution and under medical advice.

Alcohol: Alcohol should not be consumed, or only consumed with caution - after medical advice has been sought - while you are taking this drug.

Driving and operating machinery: This drug may have some effect on

your driving ability, so it is advisable not to drive or operate machinery while taking it.

CHENODEOXYCHOLIC ACID

Brand name: Chendol, Chenofalk

Type of drug: Gallstones treatment

Uses: An orally prescribed drug to treat gallstones.

How it works: Reduces the levels of cholesterol in the blood, which encourages the gallstones to dissolve, usually within 18 months.

Possible adverse effects: Diarrhoea which can often be controlled by a reduction in dosage.

Availability: Available only with a prescription from a doctor.

Other information: The benefits of this drug are increased by weight loss and a low-fat, high-fibre diet.

CAUTIONS

Children: This drug is either not recommended for children, or is recommended only for children above a certain age.

Pregnancy and breastfeeding: This drug is either not recommended for use by women who are pregnant or breastfeeding, or the precise effects are not known and it should therefore only be used with caution and under medical advice.

Alcohol: No known problems if taken with alcohol.

Driving and operating machinery: There are no commonly reported problems which may impact on the ability to drive or operate machinery. However, many drugs can cause dizziness or drowsiness in a few people, so it is wise to see how the drug affects you before driving or working with dangerous machinery.

CHLORAL HYDRATE

Brand name: Noctec, Welldorm Elixir; [chloral betaine] Welldorm tablets

Type of drug: Sleep inducing

Uses: For short term treatment of sleeplessness.

How it works: Acts on the central nervous system to induce drowsiness.

Possible adverse effects: Headache, nausea, dizziness, drowsiness, nightmares. Can irritate and upset the stomach.

Availability: Available only with a prescription from a doctor.

Other information: If taking the drug for longer than four weeks, do not suddenly stop taking it. Withdrawal symptoms may well occur, so a gradual reduction in dosage is recommended.

CAUTIONS

Children: There are no commonly reported problems associated with prescribing this medication for children.

Pregnancy and breastfeeding: This drug is either not recommended for use by women who are pregnant or breastfeeding, or the precise effects are not known and it should therefore only be used with caution and under medical advice.

Alcohol: Alcohol should not be consumed, or only consumed with caution - after medical advice has been sought - while you are taking this drug.

Driving and operating machinery: This drug may have some effect on your driving ability, so it is advisable not to drive or operate machinery while taking it.

CHLORAMBUCIL

Brand name: Leukeran

Type of drug: Anti-cancer

Uses: For treating various cancers, in particular leukaemia, ovarian cancer and Hodgkin's disease.

How it works: Acts on the DNA within the cell to prevent the cancerous cells from multiplying.

Possible adverse effects: Nausea, vomiting, diarrhoea and rashes.

Availability: Available only with a prescription from a doctor.

Other information: Blood will be taken regularly to monitor the effect of this medication. Also best to avoid aspirin derivatives. A barrier contraceptive is also advised.

CAUTIONS

Children: There are no commonly reported problems associated with prescribing this medication for children.

Pregnancy and breastfeeding: This drug is either not recommended for use by women who are pregnant or breastfeeding, or the precise effects are not known and it should therefore only be used with caution and under medical advice.

Alcohol: No known problems if taken with alcohol.

Driving and operating machinery: There are no commonly reported problems which may impact on the ability to drive or operate machinery. However, many drugs can cause dizziness or drowsiness in a few people, so it is wise to see how the drug affects you before driving or working with dangerous machinery.

CHLORAMPHENICOL

Brand name: Chloromycetin, Kemicetine, Minims Chloramphenicol, Sno-Phenicol

Type of drug: Antibiotic

Uses: Used topically to treat acne, ear and eye infections. Occasionally administered by mouth or injection to treat more serious conditions such as meningitis, typhoid or pneumonia.

How it works: Treats infection by bacterial organisms.

Possible adverse effects: Can very occasionally cause blood disorders and is usually only used after other treatments have failed.

Availability: Available only with a prescription from a doctor.

Other information: Take the full course of the drug even if the infection has cleared up.

CAUTIONS

Children: There are no commonly reported problems associated with prescribing this medication for children.

Pregnancy and breastfeeding: This drug is either not recommended for use by women who are pregnant or breastfeeding, or the precise effects are not known and it should therefore only be used with caution and under medical advice.

Alcohol: No known problems if taken with alcohol.

Driving and operating machinery: There are no commonly reported problems which may impact on the ability to drive or operate machinery. However, many drugs can cause dizziness or drowsiness in a few people, so it is wise to see how the drug affects you before driving or working with dangerous machinery.

CHLORDIAZEPOXIDE

Brand name: Librium, Tropium

Type of drug: Anti-anxiety

Uses: To treat anxiety and tension and to encourage sleep. It can also be used to treat the symptoms of alcohol withdrawal. Also helps to ease muscular spasms.

How it works: Depresses activity in the part of the brain which is thought to control anxiety and tension by changing the chemical activity there.

Possible adverse effects: Drowsiness, confusion, nausea, constipation, menstrual irregularities and decreased libido.

Availability: Available only with a prescription from a doctor.

Other information: Not suitable for a long-term solution as the drug can be habit-forming, but it also loses its effectiveness after a time. Treatment is usually limited to two weeks.

CAUTIONS

Children: This drug is either not recommended for children, or is recommended only for children above a certain age.

Pregnancy and breastfeeding: This drug is either not recommended for use by women who are pregnant or breastfeeding, or the precise effects are not known and it should therefore only be used with caution and under medical advice.

Alcohol: Alcohol should not be consumed, or only consumed with caution - after medical advice has been sought - while you are taking this drug.

Driving and operating machinery: This drug may have some effect on your driving ability, so it is advisable not to drive or operate machinery while taking it.

CHLORMETHIAZOLE

Brand name: Heminevrin

Type of drug: Hypnotic

Uses: As a treatment for epilepsy, insomnia and the symptoms of alcohol withdrawal.

How it works: Has a hypnotic, sedative-like, effect.

Possible adverse effects: Nasal congestion accompanied by sneezing, headache, nausea, vomiting, stomach upsets.

Availability: Available only with a prescription from a doctor.

Other information: Not suitable for patients with chest problems or for alcoholics who continue to drink.

CAUTIONS

Children: There are no commonly reported problems associated with prescribing this medication for children.

Pregnancy and breastfeeding: This drug is either not recommended for use by women who are pregnant or breastfeeding, or the precise effects are not known and it should therefore only be used with caution and under medical advice.

Alcohol: Alcohol should not be consumed, or only consumed with caution - after medical advice has been sought - while you are taking this drug.

Driving and operating machinery: This drug may have some effect on your driving ability, so it is advisable not to drive or operate machinery while taking it.

CHLOROQUINE

Brand name: Avloclor, Nivaquine

Type of drug: Anti-malarial and anti-rheumatic

Uses: For prevention and treatment of malaria. It is also used to treat rheumatoid arthritis.

How it works: An oral dose usually clears up the infection within a few days. Injections may be needed for a severe attack.

Possible adverse effects: Nausea, headache, diarrhoea and abdominal pain.

Availability: No prescription needed for malarial prevention.

Other information: Prolonged use of the drug could lead to serious damage of the retina which could progress to blindness. Regular eye checks should be carried out.

CAUTIONS

Children: There are no commonly reported problems associated with prescribing this medication for children.

Pregnancy and breastfeeding: No specific problems documented, but any medication should be taken with utmost caution by women who are either pregnant or breastfeeding, and only after professional medical or pharmaceutical advice has been sought.

Alcohol: No known problems if taken with alcohol.

Driving and operating machinery: This drug may have some effect on your driving ability, so it is advisable not to drive or operate machinery while taking it.

CHLORPHENIRAMINE

Brand name: Calimal, Piriton, Rimarin

Type of drug: Antihistamine

Uses: To help treat the symptoms of hayfever, allergic conjunctivitis, hives and other allergic swellings.

How it works: It relieves the symptoms of itching and swelling through anti-cholinergic action which suppresses mucus secretion.

Possible adverse effects: Drowsiness, excitability in children and possibly rashes.

Availability: Available over the counter without a prescription.

Other information: Tablets should be swallowed whole, not crushed or chewed.

CAUTIONS

Children: There are no commonly reported problems associated with prescribing this medication for children.

Pregnancy and breastfeeding: This drug is either not recommended for use by women who are pregnant or breastfeeding, or the precise effects are not known and it should therefore only be used with caution and under medical advice.

Alcohol: Alcohol should not be consumed, or only consumed with caution - after medical advice has been sought - while you are taking this drug.

Driving and operating machinery: This drug may have some effect on your driving ability, so it is advisable not to drive or operate machinery while taking it.

CHLORPROMAZINE

Brand name: Chloractil, Largactil

Type of drug: Anti-psychotic

Uses: Used to treat schizophrenia, mania and other conditions which result in confused or abnormal behaviour.

How it works: Has an anti-psychotic effect which reduces aggression and promotes more tranquil behaviour.

Possible adverse effects: Drowsiness, increase in weight, blurred vision, dizziness and tremors.

Availability: Available only with a prescription from a doctor.

Other information: Avoid exposure to sunlight. Take drug exactly as prescribed.

CAUTIONS

Children: This drug is either not recommended for children, or is recommended only for children above a certain age.

Pregnancy and breastfeeding: This drug is either not recommended for use by women who are pregnant or breastfeeding, or the precise effects are not known and it should therefore only be used with caution and under medical advice.

Alcohol: Alcohol should not be consumed, or only consumed with caution - after medical advice has been sought - while you are taking this drug.

Driving and operating machinery: This drug may have some effect on your driving ability, so it is advisable not to drive or operate machinery while taking it.

CHLORPROPAMIDE

Brand name: Diabinese, Glymese

Type of drug: Anti-diabetic

Uses: Taken by mouth to treat maturity onset diabetes.

How it works: Lowers blood sugar levels by increasing the production of insulin and encouraging the uptake of sugar into the body.

Possible adverse effects: Rare, but include feeling faint, weakness, sweating and confusion.

Availability: Available only with a prescription from a doctor.

Other information: Regular monitoring of urine and blood sugar is required.

CAUTIONS

Children: This drug is either not recommended for children, or is recommended only for children above a certain age.

Pregnancy and breastfeeding: This drug is either not recommended for use by women who are pregnant or breastfeeding, or the precise effects are not known and it should therefore only be used with caution and under medical advice.

Alcohol: Alcohol should not be consumed, or only consumed with caution - after medical advice has been sought - while you are taking this drug.

Driving and operating machinery: There are no commonly reported problems which may impact on the ability to drive or operate machinery.

However, many drugs can cause dizziness or drowsiness in a few people, so it is wise to see how the drug affects you before driving or working with dangerous machinery.

CHLORTETRACYCLINE
Brand name: Aureomycin
Type of drug: Antibiotic
Uses: Used to treat bacterial and chlamydial infections of the eye.
How it works: Available as an ointment to treat eye infections which do not respond to other antibiotics. Occasionally it may be necessary to take tablets to combat infections which have spread.
Possible adverse effects: Unlikely to occur.
Availability: Available only with a prescription from a doctor.
Other information: Always complete the course of treatment prescribed.
CAUTIONS
Children: There are no commonly reported problems associated with prescribing this medication for children.
Pregnancy and breastfeeding: This drug is either not recommended for use by women who are pregnant or breastfeeding, or the precise effects are not known and it should therefore only be used with caution and under medical advice.
Alcohol: No known problems if taken with alcohol.
Driving and operating machinery: There are no commonly reported problems which may impact on the ability to drive or operate machinery. However, many drugs can cause dizziness or drowsiness in a few people, so it is wise to see how the drug affects you before driving or working with dangerous machinery.

CHOLESTYRAMINE
Brand name: Questran, Questran Light
Type of drug: Lipid lowering
Uses: To treat people who have high levels of cholesterol or fat in their blood, and who are at risk from heart disease.
How it works: It is a resin that binds acids in the intestine to prevent their reabsorption. This action results in a reduction of cholesterol levels in the blood.

Possible adverse effects: Can cause nausea, constipation and general abdominal discomfort.

Availability: Available only with a prescription from a doctor.

Other information: Vitamin absorption is reduced while taking this drug, so vitamin supplements of A, D and K are advised. Regular blood checks will help monitor the cholesterol level.

CAUTIONS

Children: This drug is either not recommended for children, or is recommended only for children above a certain age.

Pregnancy and breastfeeding: No specific problems documented, but any medication should be taken with utmost caution by women who are either pregnant or breastfeeding, and only after professional medical or pharmaceutical advice has been sought.

Alcohol: Alcohol should not be consumed, or only consumed with caution - after medical advice has been sought - while you are taking a course of this drug.

Driving and operating machinery: There are no commonly reported problems which may impact on the ability to drive or operate machinery. However, many drugs can cause dizziness or drowsiness in a few people, so it is wise to see how the drug affects you before driving or working with dangerous machinery.

CHORIONIC GONADOTROPHIN

Brand name: Pregnyl, Profasi, Choragon

Type of drug: Infertility treatment

Uses: The treatment of female infertility where the problem is due to an inability to ovulate.

How it works: It encourages the ovaries to produce hormones which are essential to conception and stimulates ovulation, which usually occurs within 18 hours of administration by injection.

Possible adverse effects: Abdominal pain or swelling may occur but this should pass off soon after treatment.

Availability: Available only with a prescription from a doctor.

Other information: Patients offered this treatment should be aware of the increased likelihood of multiple births as several eggs may be released at once.

CAUTIONS

Children: Unlikely to be prescribed.

Pregnancy and breastfeeding: This drug is either not recommended for use by women who are pregnant or breastfeeding, or the precise effects are not known and it should therefore only be used with caution and under medical advice.

Alcohol: Alcohol should not be consumed, or only consumed with caution - after medical advice has been sought - while you are taking this drug.

Driving and operating machinery: This drug may have some effect on your driving ability, so it is advisable not to drive or operate machinery while taking it.

CILAZAPRIL

Brand name: Vascace

Type of drug: ACE inhibitor

Uses: Used, in conjunction with other drugs, to treat high blood pressure and chronic heart failure.

How it works: It is rapidly metabolised in the stomach and enables the blood vessels to dilate, with the result that blood pressure is lowered.

Possible adverse effects: Headache, dizziness, fatigue, rash, dry cough.

Availability: Available only with a prescription from a doctor.

Other information: Use with caution if patients have impaired kidney or liver function.

CAUTIONS

Children: There are no commonly reported problems associated with prescribing this medication for children.

Pregnancy and breastfeeding: This drug is either not recommended for use by women who are pregnant or breastfeeding, or the precise effects are not known and it should therefore only be used with caution and under medical advice.

Alcohol: No known problems if taken with alcohol.

Driving and operating machinery: There are no commonly reported problems which may impact on the ability to drive or operate machinery. However, many drugs can cause dizziness or drowsiness in a few people, so it is wise to see how the drug affects you before driving or working with dangerous machinery.

CIMETIDINE

Brand name: Acitak, Dyspamet, Galenamet, Peptimax, Phimetin, Tagamet, Ultec, Zita

Type of drug: Anti-ulcer

Uses: To treat ulcers of the stomach and duodenum.

How it works: This drug reduces the secretion of gastric acid, and pepsin - an enzyme which helps in the digestion of protein. It thereby promotes healing of the stomach lining where the ulcers occur.

Possible adverse effects: Headaches, dizziness, confusion, hallucinations and sometimes diarrhoea.

Availability: Available with a prescription or without (over the counter).

Other information: Patients receiving anti-coagulants and anti-convulsant drugs need to take extra caution with this drug.

CAUTIONS

Children: There are no commonly reported problems associated with prescribing this medication for children.

Pregnancy and breastfeeding: This drug is either not recommended for use by women who are pregnant or breastfeeding, or the precise effects are not known and it should therefore only be used with caution and under medical advice.

Alcohol: No known problems if taken with alcohol.

Driving and operating machinery: There are no commonly reported problems which may impact on the ability to drive or operate machinery. However, many drugs can cause dizziness or drowsiness in a few people, so it is wise to see how the drug affects you before driving or working with dangerous machinery.

CINNARIZINE

Brand name: Cinaziere, Stugeron, Stugeron Forte

Type of drug: Anti-emetic

Uses: A drug to treat travel sickness; also to help control the symptoms of labyrinthitis and Meniere's disease. It is also used to improve circulation.

How it works: An antihistamine which is effective at preventing nausea caused by the motion of travel.

Possible adverse effects: Drowsiness is the main side effect; however, sometimes the reverse can occur and people become over-stimulated by the drug and unable to sleep.

Availability: Available with or without a prescription.

Other information: Discuss with your doctor before taking this drug at the same time as anti-depressants or sedatives.

CAUTIONS

Children: There are no commonly reported problems associated with prescribing this medication for children.

Pregnancy and breastfeeding: No specific problems documented, but any medication should be taken with utmost caution by women who are either pregnant or breastfeeding, and only after professional medical or pharmaceutical advice has been sought.

Alcohol: Alcohol should not be consumed, or only consumed with caution - after medical advice has been sought - while you are taking this drug.

Driving and operating machinery: This drug may have some effect on your driving ability, so it is advisable not to drive or operate machinery while taking it.

CIPROFIBRATE

Brand name: Modalim

Type of drug: Lipid lowering

Uses: Used to lower blood cholesterol and fat levels.

How it works: Lowers the levels of fat in the blood, with the result that the risk of developing coronary artery disease is low.

Possible adverse effects: Stomach upsets, dizziness, headache and fatigue. Possible hair loss and impotence. Any unexplained muscle weakness or pain should be reported immediately.

Availability: Available only with a prescription from a doctor.

Other information: A barrier method of contraception should be used whilst on this medication. Use with great caution in patients with any impairment of liver or kidney function.

CAUTIONS

Children: There are no commonly reported problems associated with prescribing this medication for children.

Pregnancy and breastfeeding: This drug is either not recommended for use by women who are pregnant or breastfeeding, or the precise effects are

not known and it should therefore only be used with caution and under medical advice.

Alcohol: No known problems if taken with alcohol.

Driving and operating machinery: There are no commonly reported problems which may impact on the ability to drive or operate machinery. However, many drugs can cause dizziness or drowsiness in a few people, so it is wise to see how the drug affects you before driving or working with dangerous machinery.

CIPROFLOXACIN

Brand name: Ciproxin, Ciloxan

Type of drug: Anti-bacterial

Uses: To treat infections of the chest, intestine and urinary tract. Also a single dose treatment for gonorrhoea.

How it works: Acts on the DNA of the bacteria to stop them replicating.

Possible adverse effects: Nausea, vomiting, diarrhoea and abdominal pain occasionally.

Availability: Available only with a prescription from a doctor.

Other information: Patients are advised to drink plenty of fluids while taking this drug.

CAUTIONS

Children: This drug is either not recommended for children, or is recommended only for children above a certain age.

Pregnancy and breastfeeding: This drug is either not recommended for use by women who are pregnant or breastfeeding, or the precise effects are not known and it should therefore only be used with caution and under medical advice.

Alcohol: Alcohol should not be consumed, or only consumed with caution - after medical advice has been sought - while you are taking this drug.

Driving and operating machinery: This drug may have some effect on your driving ability, so it is advisable not to drive or operate machinery while taking it.

CISAPRIDE

Brand name: Alimix, Prepulsid

Type of drug: Motility stimulant

Uses: To treat stomach problems such as indigestion, heartburn, and gastro-oesophageal reflux.

How it works: Stimulates movement of the gut, so that the acid which is causing the problem passes through the gastrointestinal system more quickly.

Possible adverse effects: Abdominal cramps and diarrhoea.

Availability: Available only with a prescription from a doctor.

Other information: Patients with heart conditions need to exercise caution if taking this drug.

CAUTIONS

Children: There are no commonly reported problems associated with prescribing this medication for children.

Pregnancy and breastfeeding: This drug is either not recommended for use by women who are pregnant or breastfeeding, or the precise effects are not known and it should therefore only be used with caution and under medical advice.

Alcohol: Alcohol should not be consumed, or only consumed with caution - after medical advice has been sought - while you are taking this drug.

Driving and operating machinery: This drug may have some effect on your driving ability, so it is advisable not to drive or operate machinery while taking it.

CISPLATIN

Brand name: Cisplatin

Type of drug: Anti-cancer

Uses: An effective treatment for cancer of the ovaries and testicular cancer in particular. Also for cancers of the bladder, head, neck and lung, and for bone cancer in children.

How it works: Acts on the DNA of the cancer cells to prevent them replicating.

Possible adverse effects: Severe nausea and vomiting, impairment of kidney function. Also tinnitus and damage to hearing.

Availability: Available only with a prescription from a doctor.

Other information: This drug is usually administered as an injection. Anti-emetics are often given at the same time if nausea and vomiting are very severe.

CAUTIONS

Children: There are no commonly reported problems associated with prescribing this medication for children.

Pregnancy and breastfeeding: This drug is either not recommended for use by women who are pregnant or breastfeeding, or the precise effects are not known and it should therefore only be used with caution and under medical advice.

Alcohol: No known problems if taken with alcohol.

Driving and operating machinery: There are no commonly reported problems which may impact on the ability to drive or operate machinery. However, many drugs can cause dizziness or drowsiness in a few people, so it is wise to see how the drug affects you before driving or working with dangerous machinery.

CITALOPRAM

Brand name: Cipramil

Type of drug: Antidepressant

Uses: To treat depression and anxiety.

How it works: Lifts the mood, enabling people to take part in normal activities of daily living.

Possible adverse effects: Nausea, vomiting, stomach upsets and diarrhoea. Appetite and weight changes, insomnia, dizziness and drowsiness.

Availability: Available only with a prescription from a doctor.

Other information: Use with caution if patient has kidney, heart or epileptic problems. Also do not take if in a manic phase of manic depression.

CAUTIONS

Children: This drug is either not recommended for children, or is recommended only for children above a certain age.

Pregnancy and breastfeeding: This drug is either not recommended for use by women who are pregnant or breastfeeding, or the precise effects are not known and it should therefore only be used with caution and under medical advice.

Alcohol: No known problems if taken with alcohol.

Driving and operating machinery: There are no commonly reported

problems which may impact on the ability to drive or operate machinery. However, many drugs can cause dizziness or drowsiness in a few people, so it is wise to see how the drug affects you before driving or working with dangerous machinery.

CLARITHROMYCIN

Brand name: Klaricid

Type of drug: Antibiotic

Uses: To treat respiratory tract infections such as tonsillitis and bronchitis.

How it works: Attaches itself to the bacteria, preventing them from replicating.

Possible adverse effects: Headaches, nausea, diarrhoea, abdominal discomfort.

Availability: Available only with a prescription from a doctor.

Other information: Do not stop before the end of the prescribed course. Use with caution in patients with impaired kidney function.

CAUTIONS

Children: This drug is either not recommended for children, or is recommended only for children above a certain age.

Pregnancy and breastfeeding: This drug is either not recommended for use by women who are pregnant or breastfeeding, or the precise effects are not known and it should therefore only be used with caution and under medical advice.

Alcohol: No known problems if taken with alcohol.

Driving and operating machinery: There are no commonly reported problems which may impact on the ability to drive or operate machinery. However, many drugs can cause dizziness or drowsiness in a few people, so it is wise to see how the drug affects you before driving or working with dangerous machinery.

CLINDAMYCIN

Brand name: Dalacin C

Type of drug: Antibiotic

Uses: Used to treat joint and bone infections such as osteomyelitis and other severe infections like peritonitis.

How it works: Inhibits the replication of the bacteria and kills them.

Possible adverse effects: Abdominal discomfort, nausea, and vomiting. Rashes and occasionally a thrush infection may develop. If severe diarrhoea or colitis results, stop use immediately.

Availability: Available only with a prescription from a doctor.

Other information: Capsules should be taken with a full glass of water.

CAUTIONS

Children: There are no commonly reported problems associated with prescribing this medication for children.

Pregnancy and breastfeeding: This drug is either not recommended for use by women who are pregnant or breastfeeding, or the precise effects are not known and it should therefore only be used with caution and under medical advice.

Alcohol: No known problems if taken with alcohol.

Driving and operating machinery: There are no commonly reported problems which may impact on the ability to drive or operate machinery. However, many drugs can cause dizziness or drowsiness in a few people so it is wise to see how the drug affects you before driving or working with dangerous machinery.

CLOBETASONE

Brand name: Eumovate, Trimovate

Type of drug: Corticosteroid

Uses: Used to treat eczema, psoriasis and dermatitis.

How it works: Has an anti-inflammatory, anti-pus forming and vasoconstrictive action which removes the discomfort of the condition.

Possible adverse effects: Worsening of skin condition, thinning of the skin if used for excessively long periods.

Availability: Available only with a prescription from a doctor.

Other information: A water-based cream is usually prescribed for moist or weeping eczema; an ointment is more likely for dry and scaly patches.

CAUTIONS

Children: There are no commonly reported problems associated with prescribing this medication for children.

Pregnancy and breastfeeding: No specific problems documented, but any medication should be taken with utmost caution by women who are

either pregnant or breastfeeding, and only after professional medical or pharmaceutical advice has been sought.

Alcohol: No known problems if taken with alcohol.

Driving and operating machinery: There are no commonly reported problems which may impact on the ability to drive or operate machinery. However, many drugs can cause dizziness or drowsiness in a few people, so it is wise to see how the drug affects you before driving or working with dangerous machinery.

CLOFIBRATE

Brand name: Atromid-S

Type of drug: Lipid lowering

Uses: To reduce cholesterol and fats in the blood and prevent associated heart and circulation problems from developing.

How it works: Affects the production of the fats which circulate in the blood to the point where cholesterol levels are lowered.

Possible adverse effects: Nausea, appetite loss, fatigue and headaches.

Availability: Available only with a prescription from a doctor.

Other information: Use with caution if patient suffers from impairment of the kidney function.

CAUTIONS

Children: There are no commonly reported problems associated with prescribing this medication for children.

Pregnancy and breastfeeding: This drug is either not recommended for use by women who are pregnant or breastfeeding, or the precise effects are not known and it should therefore only be used with caution and under medical advice.

Alcohol: No known problems if taken with alcohol.

Driving and operating machinery: There are no commonly reported problems which may impact on the ability to drive or operate machinery. However, many drugs can cause dizziness or drowsiness in a few people, so it is wise to see how the drug affects you before driving or working with dangerous machinery.

CLOMIPHENE

Brand name: Clomid, Serophene

Type of drug: Infertility treatment

Uses: Treatment of infertility in women where ovulation is not taking place because of inadequate levels of the necessary hormones.

How it works: Following a five-day course of tablets, the release of eggs (ovulation) is stimulated by the increased levels of the necessary hormones.

Possible adverse effects: Hot flushes and abdominal discomfort, headaches, insomnia and depression. Visual impairment is possible but rare.

Availability: Available only with a prescription from a doctor.

Other information: Multiple pregnancies are a possible result of this treatment. Must not be used for longer than six monthly cycles, otherwise the risk of ovarian cancer may be increased.

CAUTIONS

Children: This drug is either not recommended for children, or is recommended only for children above a certain age.

Pregnancy and breastfeeding: This drug is either not recommended for use by women who are pregnant or breastfeeding, or the precise effects are not known and it should therefore only be used with caution and under medical advice.

Alcohol: No known problems if taken with alcohol.

Driving and operating machinery: There are no commonly reported problems which may impact on the ability to drive or operate machinery. However, many drugs can cause dizziness or drowsiness in a few people, so it is wise to see how the drug affects you before driving or working with dangerous machinery.

CLOMIPRAMINE

Brand name: Anafranil, Anafranil SR

Type of drug: Tricyclic antidepressant

Uses: Long term treatment of depression, irrational fears and obsessive behaviour.

How it works: Changes the chemical balance in the brain to lift the mood, increases the appetite and stimulates an improved interest in day-to-day living.

Possible adverse effects: Dry mouth, constipation, drowsiness, hot flushes and dizziness.

Availability: Available only with a prescription from a doctor.

Other information: Avoid using over-the-counter medications that contain antihistamines and decongestants.

CAUTIONS

Children: This drug is either not recommended for children, or is recommended only for children above a certain age.

Pregnancy and breastfeeding: This drug is either not recommended for use by women who are pregnant or breastfeeding, or the precise effects are not known and it should therefore only be used with caution and under medical advice.

Alcohol: Alcohol should not be consumed, or only consumed with caution - after medical advice has been sought - while you are taking this drug.

Driving and operating machinery: This drug may have some effect on your driving ability, so it is advisable not to drive or operate machinery while taking it.

CLONAZEPAM

Brand name: Rivotril

Type of drug: Anti-epilepsy

Uses: Prevention and treatment of epileptic fits, particularly in children.

How it works: Has an anti-convulsant action that helps to prevent muscle spasms and seizures.

Possible adverse effects: Drowsiness and dizziness.

Availability: Available only with a prescription from a doctor.

Other information: The anticonvulsant effect tends to lessen after several months of use.

CAUTIONS

Children: There are no commonly reported problems associated with prescribing this medication for children.

Pregnancy and breastfeeding: This drug is either not recommended for use by women who are pregnant or breastfeeding, or the precise effects are not known and it should therefore only be used with caution and under medical advice.

Alcohol: Alcohol should not be consumed, or only consumed with caution - after medical advice has been sought - while you are taking this drug.

Driving and operating machinery: This drug may have some effect on

your driving ability, so it is advisable not to drive or operate machinery while taking it.

CLONIDINE

Brand name: Catapres, Catapres Perlongets, Dixarit

Type of drug: Anti-hypertensive, anti-migraine

Uses: To help prevent migraine attacks; also used for controlling menopausal flushing and helping with drug withdrawal symptoms.

How it works: Reduces the impulses from the brain that are thought to raise the blood pressure and increases activity in the area which is thought to decrease blood pressure.

Possible adverse effects: Drowsiness, dizziness, fatigue, nausea and dry mouth. Most side effects decrease during long term therapy.

Availability: Available only with a prescription from a doctor.

Other information: Patient should be informed to report any excessive weight gain. Do not stop taking this drug suddenly except on medical advice.

CAUTIONS

Children: This drug is either not recommended for children, or is recommended only for children above a certain age.

Pregnancy and breastfeeding: This drug is either not recommended for use by women who are pregnant or breastfeeding, or the precise effects are not known and it should therefore only be used with caution and under medical advice.

Alcohol: Alcohol should not be consumed, or only consumed with caution - after medical advice has been sought - while you are taking this drug.

Driving and operating machinery: This drug may have some effect on your driving ability, so it is advisable not to drive or operate machinery while taking it.

CLOTRIMAZOLE

Brand name: Canesten, Masnoderm, Mycil Gold

Type of drug: Anti-fungal

Uses: Used to treat tinea, ringworm, candida, thrush, infections of the mouth, vagina or penis. Also useful to control skin and outer ear infections.

How it works: When applied as a cream, powder or solution to the infected area it kills and inhibits the growth of the fungi which are causing the infection.

Possible adverse effects: Nausea, abdominal cramps, skin irritation.

Availability: Available with or without a prescription.

Other information: If irritation occurs discontinue use.

CAUTIONS

Children: There are no commonly reported problems associated with prescribing this medication for children.

Pregnancy and breastfeeding: No specific problems documented, but any medication should be taken with utmost caution by women who are either pregnant or breastfeeding, and only after professional medical or pharmaceutical advice has been sought.

Alcohol: No known problems if taken with alcohol.

Driving and operating machinery: There are no commonly reported problems which may impact on the ability to drive or operate machinery. However, many drugs can cause dizziness or drowsiness in a few people, so it is wise to see how the drug affects you before driving or working with dangerous machinery.

CLOZAPINE

Brand name: Clozaril

Type of drug: Anti-psychotic

Uses: To treat people with schizophrenia who have not responded to other treatments.

How it works: Helps to control the symptoms of the disorder, with the result that the sufferer can hopefully live a more conventionally normal life.

Possible adverse effects: Drowsiness, confusion, fatigue, dry mouth, constipation, blurred vision and nausea.

Availability: Available only with a prescription from a doctor.

Other information: It can take up to three weeks for the benefits of this drug to be felt. Regular blood tests are required as this drug can produce a life-threatening fall in the white blood count.

CAUTIONS

Children: This drug is either not recommended for children, or is recommended only for children above a certain age.

Pregnancy and breastfeeding: This drug is either not recommended for use by women who are pregnant or breastfeeding, or the precise effects are not known and it should therefore only be used with caution and under medical advice.

Alcohol: Alcohol should not be consumed, or only consumed with caution - after medical advice has been sought - while you are taking this drug.

Driving and operating machinery: This drug may have some effect on your driving ability, so it is advisable not to drive or operate machinery while taking it.

CO-AMILOFRUSE

Brand name: Fru-Co, Frumil, Lasoride, Burinex A

Type of drug: Diuretic

Uses: Used to treat oedema associated with heart failure; also high blood pressure and liver and kidney disease. It is also used when it is particularly important to avoid a fall in blood potassium levels.

How it works: Inhibits salt reabsorption in the kidneys, with the result that fluid is expelled from the body more effectively.

Possible adverse effects: Stomach and bowel upsets. Rashes.

Availability: Available only with a prescription from a doctor.

Other information: Should be used with caution by patients with kidney and liver impairments and those with diabetes.

CAUTIONS

Children: There are no commonly reported problems associated with prescribing this medication for children.

Pregnancy and breastfeeding: This drug is either not recommended for use by women who are pregnant or breastfeeding, or the precise effects are not known and it should therefore only be used with caution and under medical advice.

Alcohol: No known problems if taken with alcohol.

Driving and operating machinery: There are no commonly reported problems which may impact on the ability to drive or operate machinery. However, many drugs can cause dizziness or drowsiness in a few people, so it is wise to see how the drug affects you before driving or working with dangerous machinery.

CO-AMILOZIDE

Brand name: Amil-Co, Moduret 25, Moduretic, Navispare

Type of drug: Diuretic

Uses: Used to treat high blood pressure, congestive heart failure and liver complaints.

How it works: Encourages the expulsion of excess fluid from the body, thereby reducing the blood pressure.

Possible adverse effects: Rashes and over-sensitivity to sunlight, blood disorders and gout.

Availability: Available only with a prescription from a doctor.

Other information: Caution must be used if treating patients with liver and kidney impairments and diabetics.

CAUTIONS

Children: There are no commonly reported problems associated with prescribing this medication for children.

Pregnancy and breastfeeding: This drug is either not recommended for use by women who are pregnant or breastfeeding, or the precise effects are not known and it should therefore only be used with caution and under medical advice.

Alcohol: No known problems if taken with alcohol.

Driving and operating machinery: There are no commonly reported problems which may impact on the ability to drive or operate machinery. However, many drugs can cause dizziness or drowsiness in a few people, so it is wise to see how the drug affects you before driving or working with dangerous machinery.

CO-AMOXICLAV

Brand name: Augmentin

Type of drug: Antibiotic

Uses: Used to treat infections of the respiratory tract, genito-urinary, abdominal infections and severe dental infection.

How it works: Kills the bacteria which are causing the infection.

Possible adverse effects: Liver damage, skin disorders and dizziness and headaches are all possible side effects. Patients must be warned about becoming jaundiced, which can occur up to six weeks after stopping the drug.

Availability: Available only with a prescription from a doctor.

Other information: Should not be used for more than two weeks at a time.

CAUTIONS

Children: There are no commonly reported problems associated with prescribing this medication for children.

Pregnancy and breastfeeding: No specific problems documented, but any medication should be taken with utmost caution by women who are either pregnant or breastfeeding, and only after professional medical or pharmaceutical advice has been sought.

Alcohol: No known problems if taken with alcohol.

Driving and operating machinery: There are no commonly reported problems which may impact on the ability to drive or operate machinery. However, many drugs can cause dizziness or drowsiness in a few people, so it is wise to see how the drug affects you before driving or working with dangerous machinery.

CO-PROXAMOL

Brand name: Cosalgesic, Distalgesic

Type of drug: Painkiller

Uses: Painkiller used to relieve mild to moderate pain.

How it works: Controls pain that has not responded to paracetamol or other mild painkillers.

Possible adverse effects: Side effects are rare, but can include dizziness and nausea. Can be habit forming if taken for long periods.

Availability: Available only with a prescription from a doctor.

Other information: Overdose is dangerous because breathing can be affected.

CAUTIONS

Children: This drug is either not recommended for children, or is recommended only for children above a certain age.

Pregnancy and breastfeeding: This drug is either not recommended for use by women who are pregnant or breastfeeding, or the precise effects are not known and it should therefore only be used with caution and under medical advice.

Alcohol: Alcohol should not be consumed, or only consumed with caution

- after medical advice has been sought - while you are taking this drug.

Driving and operating machinery: This drug may have some effect on your driving ability, so it is advisable not to drive or operate machinery while taking it.

CO-TRIMOXAZOLE

Brand name: Bactrim, Chemotrim, Comixco, Fectrim, Laratrim, Septrin
Type of drug: Anti-bacterial
Uses: The treatment of stubborn infections, particularly of the lung and bladder. Can also be used as treatment for some types of pneumonia.
How it works: Uses the combined force of two antibacterial drugs to combat the infection.
Possible adverse effects: Nausea, vomiting and rash.
Availability: Available only with a prescription from a doctor.
Other information: Long term use of this drug could lead to folic acid deficiency, so supplements should be taken. It is also important to drink plenty of fluids. Blood tests will be taken to monitor blood composition.
CAUTIONS
Children: There are no commonly reported problems associated with prescribing this medication for children.
Pregnancy and breastfeeding: This drug is either not recommended for use by women who are pregnant or breastfeeding, or the precise effects are not known and it should therefore only be used with caution and under medical advice.
Alcohol: No known problems if taken with alcohol.
Driving and operating machinery: There are no commonly reported problems which may impact on the ability to drive or operate machinery. However, many drugs can cause dizziness or drowsiness in a few people, so it is wise to see how the drug affects you before driving or working with dangerous machinery.

CODEINE

Brand name: Codeine
Type of drug: Opioid analgesic, anti-diarrhoeal, cough suppressant
Uses: Painkiller for treatment of mild to moderate pain and occasionally to prevent coughing.

How it works: Acts as a mild opium-type painkiller, similar to morphine, to treat mild to moderate pain.

Possible adverse effects: Constipation is common. Other side effects such as nausea and drowsiness are rare and will usually stop if the dose is reduced.

Availability: Available only with a prescription from a doctor.

Other information: Can be habit forming if taken for long periods; usually only prescribed for short term relief . Can be supplied in either tablet, liquid or injection form.

CAUTIONS

Children: There are no commonly reported problems associated with prescribing this medication for children.

Pregnancy and breastfeeding: This drug is either not recommended for use by women who are pregnant or breastfeeding, or the precise effects are not known and it should therefore only be used with caution and under medical advice.

Alcohol: Alcohol should not be consumed, or only consumed with caution - after medical advice has been sought - while you are taking this drug.

Driving and operating machinery: This drug may have some effect on your driving ability, so it is advisable not to drive or operate machinery while taking it.

COLCHICINE

Brand name: Colchicine

Type of drug: Gout treatment

Uses: Used to relieve joint pain and inflammation in attacks of gout.

How it works: Decreases the deposits of uric acid in the joints which lead to the symptoms of the condition.

Possible adverse effects: Nausea, vomiting and abdominal pain. Possible diarrhoea. Any side effects should be reported.

Availability: Available only with a prescription from a doctor.

Other information: This drug is most effective when taken at the first sign of an attack.

CAUTIONS

Children: This drug is either not recommended for children, or is recommended only for children above a certain age.

Pregnancy and breastfeeding: This drug is either not recommended for use by women who are pregnant or breastfeeding, or the precise effects are not known and it should therefore only be used with caution and under medical advice.

Alcohol: Alcohol should not be consumed, or only consumed with caution - after medical advice has been sought - while you are taking this drug.

Driving and operating machinery: There are no commonly reported problems which may impact on the ability to drive or operate machinery. However, many drugs can cause dizziness or drowsiness in a few people, so it is wise to see how the drug affects you before driving or working with dangerous machinery.

CONJUGATED OESTROGENS

Brand name: Premarin

Type of drug: Hormone

Uses: These naturally occurring female sex hormones are used to relieve the symptoms of the menopause and to treat and prevent osteoporosis and breast cancer.

How it works: When given by mouth, they relieve the hot flushes and sweating.

Possible adverse effects: Nausea, sore breasts and weight changes.

Availability: Available only with a prescription from a doctor.

Other information: The drug is taken in a cyclic dosing schedule.

CAUTIONS

Children: This drug is either not recommended for children, or is recommended only for children above a certain age.

Pregnancy and breastfeeding: This drug is either not recommended for use by women who are pregnant or breastfeeding, or the precise effects are not known and it should therefore only be used with caution and under medical advice.

Alcohol: No known problems if taken with alcohol.

Driving and operating machinery: There are no commonly reported problems which may impact on the ability to drive or operate machinery. However, many drugs can cause dizziness or drowsiness in a few people, so it is wise to see how the drug affects you before driving or working with dangerous machinery.

CYCLOPENTHIAZIDE

Brand name: Navidrex

Type of drug: Diuretic

Uses: The treatment of water retention which occurs with some liver and kidney disorders, pre-menstrual problems and long-term heart failure.

How it works: Has a diuretic effect which results in excess water being removed from the body and prevents it from being absorbed into the tissues, causing oedema.

Possible adverse effects: The drug causes the body to lose potassium, in which case supplements will be prescribed. It can also cause loss of appetite and nausea.

Availability: Available only with a prescription from a doctor.

Other information: A diet rich in potassium or potassium supplements is recommended while taking this drug. Blood tests will be taken regularly to monitor potassium levels.

CAUTIONS

Children: There are no commonly reported problems associated with prescribing this medication for children.

Pregnancy and breastfeeding: No specific problems documented, but any medication should be taken with utmost caution by women who are either pregnant or breastfeeding, and only after professional medical or pharmaceutical advice has been sought.

Alcohol: Alcohol should not be consumed, or only consumed with caution - after medical advice has been sought - while you are taking this drug.

Driving and operating machinery: There are no commonly reported problems which may impact on the ability to drive or operate machinery. However, many drugs can cause dizziness or drowsiness in a few people, so it is wise to see how the drug affects you before driving or working with dangerous machinery.

CYCLOPENTOLATE

Brand name: Minims cyclopentolate, Mydrilate

Type of drug: Anticholinergic

Uses: Used for dilating the pupil of the eye for examination purposes.

How it works: The drug prevents the sphincter muscle of the eye from responding.

Possible adverse effects: Stinging and irritation of the eye and possible conjunctivitis. Headaches and confusion.

Availability: Available only with a prescription from a doctor.

Other information: A darker pigmented eye is more resistant; care should be taken not to overdose.

CAUTIONS

Children: There are no commonly reported problems associated with prescribing this medication for children.

Pregnancy and breastfeeding: No specific problems documented, but any medication should be taken with utmost caution by women who are either pregnant or breastfeeding, and only after professional medical or pharmaceutical advice has been sought.

Alcohol: No known problems if taken with alcohol.

Driving and operating machinery: This drug may have some effect on your driving ability, so it is advisable not to drive or operate machinery while taking it.

CYCLOPHOSPHAMIDE

Brand name: Endoxana

Type of drug: Anti-cancer

Uses: Used for treating cancers, in particular leukaemia, lymphomas and tumours. Can also be used to treat rheumatoid arthritis.

How it works: Prevents the cancer cells from dividing and therefore reproducing. Also kills the cells.

Possible adverse effects: Nausea, vomiting and diarrhoea. Abdominal pain and possible anorexia. Reversible hair loss. Because this drug reduces the production of blood cells, abnormal bleeding may occur and resistance to infection is reduced.

Availability: Available only with a prescription from a doctor.

Other information: Patients to inform the doctor if any fever or infection occurs. A barrier contraceptive is recommended during treatment.

CAUTIONS

Children: There are no commonly reported problems associated with prescribing this medication for children.

Pregnancy and breastfeeding: This drug is either not recommended for use by women who are pregnant or breastfeeding, or the precise effects are

not known and it should therefore only be used with caution and under medical advice.

Alcohol: No known problems if taken with alcohol.

Driving and operating machinery: There are no commonly reported problems which may impact on the ability to drive or operate machinery. However, many drugs can cause dizziness or drowsiness in a few people, so it is wise to see how the drug affects you before driving or working with dangerous machinery.

CYCLOSERINE

Brand name: Cycloserine, Seromycin

Type of drug: Antibiotic

Uses: Used to treat pulmonary tuberculosis; it is usually given in combination with other drugs.

How it works: Has one of two actions on the bacteria, depending on the susceptibility of the organism; it can either retard the multiplication of the bacteria or kill them.

Possible adverse effects: Headache, dizziness, drowsiness, confusion and depression. A rash or any other unusual effects should be reported to a doctor.

Availability: Available only with a prescription from a doctor.

Other information: Treatment is likely to be continued for up to two years. This medication should be taken after meals to minimise irritation of the stomach.

CAUTIONS

Children: There are no commonly reported problems associated with prescribing this medication for children.

Pregnancy and breastfeeding: This drug is either not recommended for use by women who are pregnant or breastfeeding, or the precise effects are not known and it should therefore only be used with caution and under medical advice.

Alcohol: Alcohol should not be consumed, or only consumed with caution - after medical advice has been sought - while you are taking this drug.

Driving and operating machinery: This drug may have some effect on your driving ability, so it is advisable not to drive or operate machinery while taking it.

CYCLOSPORIN

Brand name: Neoral, Sandimmun

Type of drug: Immunosuppressant

Uses: Given to prevent organ rejection following transplants. It is also prescribed in severe cases of eczema and psoriasis and rheumatoid arthritis where other drugs have failed to help.

How it works: Suppresses the body's ability to defend itself against infection and what it perceives as foreign matter. It is therefore used after transplant surgery of organs such as the heart, kidney, and liver to reduce the occurrence of organ rejection.

Possible adverse effects: Nausea, headaches, confusion, overgrowth of gums, fatigue, anaemia and diarrhoea. Increased susceptibility to infection.

Availability: Available only with a prescription from a doctor.

Other information: It is important that kidney, liver and blood levels are regularly monitored. Patients should report any unusual symptoms immediately.

CAUTIONS

Children: This drug is either not recommended for children, or is recommended only for children above a certain age.

Pregnancy and breastfeeding: This drug is either not recommended for use by women who are pregnant or breastfeeding, or the precise effects are not known and it should therefore only be used with caution and under medical advice.

Alcohol: No known problems if taken with alcohol.

Driving and operating machinery: There are no commonly reported problems which may impact on the ability to drive or operate machinery. However, many drugs can cause dizziness or drowsiness in a few people, so it is wise to see how the drug affects you before driving or working with dangerous machinery.

CYPROTERONE ACETATE

Brand name: Androcur, Cyprostat

Type of drug: Hormone

Uses: Used for treating prostate cancer and severe acne in women. Used in individuals who have misdirected male libido. Also used with oestrogen as a contraceptive, though not normally prescribed.

How it works: Cyproterone Acetate is a synthetic sex hormone that has effects similar to those of the female hormone progesterone. It is used to correct an imbalance of hormones which are thought to contribute to the above conditions.

Possible adverse effects: Reduces sex drive and stops sperm production. May cause testicles to shrink and be painful, and produce swelling of the breasts. Weight changes will probably occur. These effects usually diminish during treatment.

Availability: Available only with a prescription from a doctor.

Other information: Should not be used by patients who have a history of thrombosis, diabetes or anaemia.

CAUTIONS

Children: This drug is either not recommended for children, or is recommended only for children above a certain age.

Pregnancy and breastfeeding: This drug is either not recommended for use by women who are pregnant or breastfeeding, or the precise effects are not known and it should therefore only be used with caution and under medical advice.

Alcohol: Alcohol should not be consumed, or only consumed with caution - after medical advice has been sought - while you are taking this drug.

Driving and operating machinery: This drug may have some effect on your driving ability, so it is advisable not to drive or operate machinery while taking it.

CYTARABINE

Brand name: Cytosar

Type of drug: Anti-cancer

Uses: Used to treat several types of acute leukaemia.

How it works: Prevents the cancer cells from replicating.

Possible adverse effects: Nausea, vomiting, diarrhoea, mouth ulcers and skin rashes can occur. Increased susceptibility to infection.

Availability: Available only with a prescription from a doctor.

Other information: Blood tests should be regularly carried out to monitor the impact of treatment. Large amounts of fluid should be drunk during treatment.

CAUTIONS

Children: There are no commonly reported problems associated with prescribing this medication for children.

Pregnancy and breastfeeding: This drug is either not recommended for use by women who are pregnant or breastfeeding, or the precise effects are not known and it should therefore only be used with caution and under medical advice.

Alcohol: No known problems if taken with alcohol.

Driving and operating machinery: There are no commonly reported problems which may impact on the ability to drive or operate machinery. However, many drugs can cause dizziness or drowsiness in a few people, so it is wise to see how the drug affects you before driving or working with dangerous machinery.

DACARBAZINE

Brand name: DTIC-Dome

Type of drug: Anti-cancer

Uses: Used to treat malignant melanomas and Hodgkin's disease.

How it works: Administered as an injection to prevent the cancer cells from replicating.

Possible adverse effects: Severe nausea and vomiting, together with a loss of appetite, are relatively common. A flu-like illness may occur a week after treatment. Reduced ability to fight off infection. Loss of hair, which will grow back after treatment. Any sign of bleeding should be reported immediately.

Availability: Available only with a prescription from a doctor.

Other information: Patient should avoid people with infections and all products containing aspirin.

CAUTIONS

Children: There are no commonly reported problems associated with prescribing this medication for children.

Pregnancy and breastfeeding: This drug is either not recommended for use by women who are pregnant or breastfeeding, or the precise effects are not known and it should therefore only be used with caution and under medical advice.

Alcohol: No known problems if taken with alcohol.

Driving and operating machinery: There are no commonly reported problems which may impact on the ability to drive or operate machinery. However, many drugs can cause dizziness or drowsiness in a few people, so it is wise to see how the drug affects you before driving or working with dangerous machinery.

DALTEPARIN SODIUM

Brand name: Fragmin

Type of drug: Anticoagulant

Uses: Used to prevent the formation of blood clots in the veins of patients undergoing surgery and who have been identified as being at high risk.

How it works: Alters the clotting mechanism of the blood to make the formation of clots less likely.

Possible adverse effects: Rashes. Unusual bruising may occur which can indicate bleeding and should be reported immediately.

Availability: Available only with a prescription from a doctor.

Other information: Avoid any products containing aspirin.

CAUTIONS

Children: This drug is either not recommended for children, or is recommended only for children above a certain age.

Pregnancy and breastfeeding: This drug is either not recommended for use by women who are pregnant or breastfeeding, or the precise effects are not known and it should therefore only be used with caution and under medical advice.

Alcohol: No known problems if taken with alcohol.

Driving and operating machinery: There are no commonly reported problems which may impact on the ability to drive or operate machinery. However, many drugs can cause dizziness or drowsiness in a few people, so it is wise to see how the drug affects you before driving or working with dangerous machinery.

DANAZOL

Brand name: Danol

Type of drug: Synthetic hormone

Uses: Treatment of endometriosis, breast pain, male breast swelling and lumpy breasts in women.

How it works: It reduces the growth rate of abnormal breast tissue which causes discomfort in both men and women. It causes the abnormal endometrial tissue which occurs in endometriosis to be destroyed.

Possible adverse effects: Mainly occur when high doses are prescribed; they include swelling of the feet and ankles, weight gain, acne, and in women, unusual hair growth and voice changes. Nausea, rash, dizziness and flushing may also occur. Menstrual periods will usually be disrupted or halted.

Availability: Available only with a prescription from a doctor.

Other information: A barrier contraceptive should be used during treatment.

CAUTIONS

Children: This drug is either not recommended for children, or is recommended only for children above a certain age.

Pregnancy and breastfeeding: This drug is either not recommended for use by women who are pregnant or breastfeeding, or the precise effects are not known and it should therefore only be used with caution and under medical advice.

Alcohol: No known problems if taken with alcohol.

Driving and operating machinery: There are no commonly reported problems which may impact on the ability to drive or operate machinery. However, many drugs can cause dizziness or drowsiness in a few people, so it is wise to see how the drug affects you before driving or working with dangerous machinery.

DANTHRON

Brand name: Ailax, Capsuvac, Codalax, Normax

Type of drug: Laxative

Uses: To treat constipation particularly in the elderly, the terminally ill and patients with serious heart conditions, where straining would be dangerous.

How it works: Increases intestinal motility, which enables the stool to be passed more easily.

Possible adverse effects: Abdominal cramps, nausea and vomiting. Avoid prolonged contact with skin, as irritation can occur. Urine may be coloured red.

Availability: Available only with a prescription from a doctor.

Other information: Must not be used if bowel is obstructed.

CAUTIONS

Children: This drug is either not recommended for children, or is recommended only for children above a certain age.

Pregnancy and breastfeeding: This drug is either not recommended for use by women who are pregnant or breastfeeding, or the precise effects are not known and it should therefore only be used with caution and under medical advice.

Alcohol: No known problems if taken with alcohol.

Driving and operating machinery: There are no commonly reported problems which may impact on the ability to drive or operate machinery. However, many drugs can cause dizziness or drowsiness in a few people, so it is wise to see how the drug affects you before driving or working with dangerous machinery.

DANTROLENE

Brand name: Dantrium

Type of drug: Muscle relaxant

Uses: It is used to help relieve muscular spasms produced by conditions such as stroke, multiple sclerosis and injuries of the spinal cord.

How it works: Acts on the skeletal muscles to produce a relaxant effect.

Possible adverse effects: Drowsiness, dizziness, weakness and fatigue. Headaches and insomnia.

Availability: Available only with a prescription from a doctor.

Other information: It is advised to avoid excessive exposure to sunlight.

CAUTIONS

Children: This drug is either not recommended for children, or is recommended only for children above a certain age.

Pregnancy and breastfeeding: This drug is either not recommended for use by women who are pregnant or breastfeeding, or the precise effects are not known and it should therefore only be used with caution and under medical advice.

Alcohol: Alcohol should not be consumed, or only consumed with caution - after medical advice has been sought - while you are taking this drug.

Driving and operating machinery: This drug may have some effect on your driving ability, so it is advisable not to drive or operate machinery while taking it.

DESFERRIOXAMINE

Brand name: Desferal

Type of drug: Antidote for iron poisoning

Uses: Used in treating iron poisoning, usually due to multiple blood transfusions. Also when there is too much aluminium in the body due to kidney dialysis.

How it works: The drug joins with the iron and the combination is then excreted in the urine.

Possible adverse effects: Abdominal pain, diarrhoea, shock and a drop in blood pressure, dizziness, allergic skin reactions.

Availability: Available only with a prescription from a doctor.

Other information: Treatment should be stopped if the patient develops an infection.

CAUTIONS

Children: There are no commonly reported problems associated with prescribing this medication for children.

Pregnancy and breastfeeding: This drug is either not recommended for use by women who are pregnant or breastfeeding, or the precise effects are not known and it should therefore only be used with caution.

Alcohol: No known problems if taken with alcohol.

Driving and operating machinery: There are no commonly reported problems which may impact on the ability to drive or operate machinery. However, many drugs can cause dizziness or drowsiness in a few people so it is wise to see how the drug affects you before driving or working with dangerous machinery.

DESIPRAMINE

Brand name: Pertofran

Type of drug: Antidepressant

Uses: The treatment of depression

How it works: Changes the balance of the chemicals in the brain which have an impact on mood, leaving the sufferer more able to lead a normal day-to-day life.

Possible adverse effects: Drowsiness, dizziness, anxiety, confusion and dry mouth.

Availability: Available only with a prescription from a doctor.

Other information: May increase photosensitivity, so it is advisable to avoid excessive sunlight during treatment. Patient should also lie down for 30 minutes after each dose to avoid excessive dizziness.

CAUTIONS

Children: This drug is either not recommended for children, or is recommended only for children above a certain age.

Pregnancy and breastfeeding: No specific problems documented, but any medication should be taken with utmost caution by women who are either pregnant or breastfeeding, and only after professional medical or pharmaceutical advice has been sought.

Alcohol: Alcohol should not be consumed, or only consumed with caution - after medical advice has been sought - while you are taking this drug.

Driving and operating machinery: There are no commonly reported problems which may impact on the ability to drive or operate machinery. However, many drugs can cause dizziness or drowsiness in a few people, so it is wise to see how the drug affects you before driving or working with dangerous machinery.

DESMOPRESSIN

Brand name: DDAVP, Desmospray, Desmotabs

Type of drug: Antidiuretic hormone

Uses: Treatment of diabetes insipidus and nocturnal bedwetting (enuresis) in children.

How it works: A synthetic hormone that replaces a hormone which is lacking in people with diabetes insipidus. It also controls the production of urine by correcting the patient's hormonal deficiency.

Possible adverse effects: Fluid retention, headache, nausea, vomiting.

Availability: Available only with a prescription from a doctor.

Other information: Fluid intake must be strictly observed.

CAUTIONS

Children: There are no commonly reported problems associated with prescribing this medication for children.

Pregnancy and breastfeeding: This drug is either not recommended for use by women who are pregnant or breastfeeding, or the precise effects are not known and it should therefore only be used with caution and under medical advice.

Alcohol: Alcohol should not be consumed, or only consumed with caution - after medical advice has been sought - while you are taking this drug.

Driving and operating machinery: There are no commonly reported problems which may impact on the ability to drive or operate machinery. However, many drugs can cause dizziness or drowsiness in a few people, so it is wise to see how the drug affects you before driving or working with dangerous machinery.

DEXAMETHASONE

Brand name: Decadron

Type of drug: Corticosteroid

Uses: To treat rheumatic, allergic and inflammatory disorders such as rheumatoid arthritis, asthma and emphysema. Drops are used to treat eye inflammation.

How it works: Reduces the inflammation which occurs with the above condition.

Possible adverse effects: In the short term not too many side effects, but long-term use of corticosteroids can have many side effects.

Availability: Available only with a prescription from a doctor.

Other information: People taking this drug are advised not to wear soft contact lenses.

CAUTIONS

Children: There are no commonly reported problems associated with prescribing this medication for children.

Pregnancy and breastfeeding: This drug is either not recommended for use by women who are pregnant or breastfeeding, or the precise effects are not known and it should therefore only be used with caution and under medical advice.

Alcohol: Alcohol should not be consumed, or only consumed with caution - after medical advice has been sought - while you are taking this drug.

Driving and operating machinery: There are no commonly reported

problems which may impact on the ability to drive or operate machinery. However, many drugs can cause dizziness or drowsiness in a few people, so it is wise to see how the drug affects you before driving or working with dangerous machinery.

DEXAMPHETAMINE

Brand name: Dexadrine

Type of drug: Amphetamine

Uses: Used to treat narcolepsy, an uncontrollable tendency to fall asleep.

How it works: Acts on the nervous system to have a stimulant effect in adults, increasing alertness. However, this drug can have a sedative effect on children, so it is sometimes used to calm hyperactive children.

Possible adverse effects: Insomnia, dizziness, headache.

Availability: Available only with a prescription from a doctor.

Other information: Not to be given if there is a history of drug or alcohol abuse. Not for people with glaucoma.

CAUTIONS

Children: There are no commonly reported problems associated with prescribing this medication for children.

Pregnancy and breastfeeding: This drug is either not recommended for use by women who are pregnant or breastfeeding, or the precise effects are not known and it should therefore only be used with caution and under medical advice.

Alcohol: Alcohol should not be consumed, or only consumed with caution - after medical advice has been sought - while you are taking this drug.

Driving and operating machinery: This drug may have some effect on your driving ability, so it is advisable not to drive or operate machinery while taking it.

DEXFENFLURAMINE

Brand name: Adifax

Type of drug: Appetite suppressant

Uses: The treatment of severe obesity.

How it works: Suppresses the appetite.

Possible adverse effects: Nausea, constipation or diarrhoea, drowsiness, dizziness, headache. Heart problems.

Availability: Available only with a prescription from a doctor.

Other information: This drug is no longer available on the NHS.

CAUTIONS

Children: This drug is either not recommended for children, or is recommended only for children above a certain age.

Pregnancy and breastfeeding: This drug is either not recommended for use by women who are pregnant or breastfeeding, or the precise effects are not known and it should therefore only be used with caution and under medical advice.

Alcohol: Alcohol should not be consumed, or only consumed with caution - after medical advice has been sought - while you are taking this drug.

Driving and operating machinery: There are no commonly reported problems which may impact on the ability to drive or operate machinery. However, many drugs can cause dizziness or drowsiness in a few people, so it is wise to see how the drug affects you before driving or working with dangerous machinery.

DEXTROMETHORPHAN

Brand name: Boots Nirolex Lozenges, Contac Coughcaps, Robitussin Dry Cough

Type of drug: Cough suppressant

Uses: A medicine for treating persistent dry coughs that interrupt sleep.

How it works: It suppresses the cough reflux and sedates.

Possible adverse effects: Drowsiness.

Availability: Available with or without a prescription (over the counter).

Other information: Should not be taken for longer than two days.

CAUTIONS

Children: There are no commonly reported problems associated with prescribing this medication for children.

Pregnancy and breastfeeding: This drug is either not recommended for use by women who are pregnant or breastfeeding, or the precise effects are not known and it should therefore only be used with caution and under medical advice.

Alcohol: Alcohol should not be consumed, or only consumed with caution - after medical advice has been sought - while you are taking this drug.

Driving and operating machinery: This drug may have some effect on

your driving ability, so it is advisable not to drive or operate machinery while taking it.

DEXTROMORAMIDE

Brand name: Palfium

Type of drug: Opioid analgesic

Uses: For relieving severe pain.

How it works: Acts quickly to relieve pain for approximately two to three hours.

Possible adverse effects: Nausea, vomiting, sweating, dizziness, faintness due to a fall in blood pressure and insomnia.

Availability: Available only with a prescription from a doctor.

Other information: The patient will need to lie down after being administered the first few doses.

CAUTIONS

Children: There are no commonly reported problems associated with prescribing this medication for children.

Pregnancy and breastfeeding: This drug is either not recommended for use by women who are pregnant or breastfeeding, or the precise effects are not known and it should therefore only be used with caution and under medical advice.

Alcohol: Alcohol should not be consumed, or only consumed with caution - after medical advice has been sought - while you are taking this drug.

Driving and operating machinery: This drug may have some effect on your driving ability, so it is advisable not to drive or operate machinery while taking it.

DIAZEPAM

Brand name: Atensine, Dialar, Diazemuls, Rimapam, Stesolid, Tensium, Valclair, Valium

Type of drug: Benzodiazepine anti-anxiety drug, anticonvulsant

Uses: To treat tension, nervousness and insomnia. It can also be used to treat epileptic fits.

How it works: Stimulates a chemical in the brain that helps control emotion and has a muscle-relaxant effect.

Possible adverse effects: Drowsiness and unsteadiness. Confusion.

Availability: Available only with a prescription from a doctor.

Other information: It can be habit forming and if taken over a longer time its effect diminishes.

CAUTIONS

Children: There are no commonly reported problems associated with prescribing this medication for children.

Pregnancy and breastfeeding: This drug is either not recommended for use by women who are pregnant or breastfeeding, or the precise effects are not known and it should therefore only be used with caution and under medical advice.

Alcohol: Alcohol should not be consumed, or only consumed with caution - after medical advice has been sought - while you are taking this drug.

Driving and operating machinery: This drug may have some effect on your driving ability, so it is advisable not to drive or operate machinery while taking it.

DIAZOXIDE

Brand name: Eudemine

Type of drug: Anti-hypertensive

Uses: To treat a severe rise in blood pressure associated with kidney disease. It is also used to treat low blood sugar.

How it works: Relaxes the smooth muscles, enabling the blood vessels to expand, thereby lowering the blood pressure. Inhibits the production of insulin, which keeps blood sugar levels low.

Possible adverse effects: Rapid beating of the heart (palpitations), raised blood sugar, fall in blood pressure, fluid and salt retention.

Availability: Available only with a prescription from a doctor.

Other information: Blood sugar levels should be checked regularly.

CAUTIONS

Children: There are no commonly reported problems associated with prescribing this medication for children.

Pregnancy and breastfeeding: This drug is either not recommended for use by women who are pregnant or breastfeeding, or the precise effects are not known and it should therefore only be used with caution and under medical advice.

Alcohol: No known problems if taken with alcohol.

Driving and operating machinery: There are no commonly reported problems which may impact on the ability to drive or operate machinery. However, many drugs can cause dizziness or drowsiness in a few people, so it is wise to see how the drug affects you before driving or working with dangerous machinery.

DICLOFENAC
Brand name: Diclomax SR, Motifene, Rhumalgan, Volraman, Voltarol
Type of drug: Anti-inflammatory
Uses: Used to treat the mild to moderate pain of rheumatoid arthritis and osteoarthritis, gout, menstrual pain and post-operative pain.
How it works: Has an anti-inflammatory effect and similar pain killing actions to paracetamol.
Possible adverse effects: Irritation of the stomach, dizziness, drowsiness, irritability and insomnia.
Availability: Available only with a prescription from a doctor.
Other information: Salt intake should be restricted during treatment with this drug.
CAUTIONS
Children: This drug is either not recommended for children, or is recommended only for children above a certain age.
Pregnancy and breastfeeding: This drug is either not recommended for use by women who are pregnant or breastfeeding, or the precise effects are not known and it should therefore only be used with caution and under medical advice.
Alcohol: Alcohol should not be consumed, or only consumed with caution - after medical advice has been sought - while you are taking this drug.
Driving and operating machinery: There are no commonly reported problems which may impact on the ability to drive or operate machinery. However, many drugs can cause dizziness or drowsiness in a few people, so it is wise to see how the drug affects you before driving or working with dangerous machinery.

DICYCLOMINE
Brand name: Merbentyl

Type of drug: Anti-emetic and anti-psychotic

Uses: To relieve the symptoms of irritable bowel syndrome.

How it works: Relaxes the muscles in order to relieve the painful abdominal cramps associated with the above conditions. It does not cure the underlying condition.

Possible adverse effects: Headaches, drowsiness and insomnia.

Availability: Available only with a prescription from a doctor.

Other information: This medication is usually taken in conjunction with other drugs and treatments such as dietary changes.

CAUTIONS

Children: There are no commonly reported problems associated with prescribing this medication for children.

Pregnancy and breastfeeding: This drug is either not recommended for use by women who are pregnant or breastfeeding, or the precise effects are not known and it should therefore only be used with caution and under medical advice.

Alcohol: Alcohol should not be consumed, or only consumed with caution - after medical advice has been sought - while you are taking this drug.

Driving and operating machinery: This drug may have some effect on your driving ability, so it is advisable not to drive or operate machinery while taking it.

DIDANOSINE (ddI)

Brand name: Videx

Type of drug: Anti-viral drug for AIDS

Uses: To lessen the impact of AIDS-related infections.

How it works: Delays the onset of AIDS by boosting the body's ability to fight infection. The severity of infections associated with the disease is lessened. It is not a cure for the underlying disease.

Possible adverse effects: Headaches, nausea, vomiting, abdominal pain, tingling or numbness in the hands or feet. Fatigue is also common.

Availability: Available only with a prescription from a doctor.

Other information: Long-term effects are not known, so regular blood and other tests will be conducted during treatment. The drug should be taken on an empty stomach.

Children: This drug is either not recommended for children, or is recommended only for children above a certain age.

Pregnancy and breastfeeding: This drug is either not recommended for use by women who are pregnant or breastfeeding, or the precise effects are not known and it should therefore only be used with caution and under medical advice.

Alcohol: Alcohol should not be consumed, or only consumed with caution - after medical advice has been sought - while you are taking this drug.

Driving and operating machinery: There are no commonly reported problems which may impact on the ability to drive or operate machinery. However, many drugs can cause dizziness or drowsiness in a few people, so it is wise to see how the drug affects you before driving or working with dangerous machinery.

DIFLUNISAL

Brand name: Dolobid

Type of drug: Nonsteroidal anti-inflammatory

Uses: To alleviate the symptoms of rheumatic diseases and menstrual pain.

How it works: Works in a similar way to aspirin to relieve pain and reduce inflammation.

Possible adverse effects: Stomach pains, nausea, vomiting, diarrhoea, indigestion, dizziness, insomnia, headache and fatigue.

Availability: Available only with a prescription from a doctor.

Other information: Do not use if allergic to aspirin, or have active peptic ulcers. Take medication whole.

CAUTIONS

Children: This drug is either not recommended for children, or is recommended only for children above a certain age.

Pregnancy and breastfeeding: This drug is either not recommended for use by women who are pregnant or breastfeeding, or the precise effects are not known and it should therefore only be used with caution and under medical advice.

Alcohol: No known problems if taken with alcohol.

Driving and operating machinery: There are no commonly reported problems which may impact on the ability to drive or operate machinery.

However, many drugs can cause dizziness or drowsiness in a few people, so it is wise to see how the drug affects you before driving or working with dangerous machinery.

DIGOXIN
Brand name: Lanoxin
Type of drug: Heart disorder treatment.
Uses: To treat congestive heart failure and heart rhythm problems.
How it works: Slows down the heart, with the effect that it pumps blood more effectively.
Possible adverse effects: Side effects are usually caused by excessive dosage and include nausea, vomiting, diarrhoea, abdominal pain, headache, visual disturbances, fatigue and drowsiness. Any sign of palpitations should be reported immediately.
Availability: Available only with a prescription from a doctor.
Other information: Patient needs to be aware that it is not advisable to take other over-the-counter products that are high in sodium. In case of an overdose, seek medical advice immediately.
CAUTIONS
Children: There are no commonly reported problems associated with prescribing this medication for children.
Pregnancy and breastfeeding: No specific problems documented, but any medication should be taken with utmost caution by women who are either pregnant or breastfeeding, and only after professional medical or pharmaceutical advice has been sought.
Alcohol: No known problems if taken with alcohol.
Driving and operating machinery: There are no commonly reported problems which may impact on the ability to drive or operate machinery. However, many drugs can cause dizziness or drowsiness in a few people, so it is wise to see how the drug affects you before driving or working with dangerous machinery.

DIHYDROCODEINE
Brand name: Codydramol, DF 118, DHC Continus, Paramol, Remedeine
Type of drug: Opioid analgesic
Uses: To relieve mild to moderate pain; also used as a cough suppressant.

How it works: Acts to block the part of the brain that perceives pain.

Possible adverse effects: Nausea, vomiting, headache, dizziness and constipation.

Availability: Available only with a prescription from a doctor.

Other information: Can occasionally produce dependence similar to that of morphine.

CAUTIONS

Children: This drug is either not recommended for children, or is recommended only for children above a certain age.

Pregnancy and breastfeeding: This drug is either not recommended for use by women who are pregnant or breastfeeding, or the precise effects are not known and it should therefore only be used with caution and under medical advice.

Alcohol: Alcohol should not be consumed, or only consumed with caution - after medical advice has been sought - while you are taking this drug.

Driving and operating machinery: There are no commonly reported problems which may impact on the ability to drive or operate machinery. However, many drugs can cause dizziness or drowsiness in a few people, so it is wise to see how the drug affects you before driving or working with dangerous machinery.

DILTIAZEM

Brand name: Adizem, Angiozem, Britiazim, Calcicard, Dilzem, Slozem, Tildiem

Type of drug: Calcium channel blocker, anti-hypertensive

Uses: Treatment of angina and high blood pressure.

How it works: Interferes with the electrical signals of the heart and dilates the blood vessels, thus reducing the pressure within them.

Possible adverse effects: Dizziness, headache, nausea and slowed heartbeat, usually controlled by dosage change.

Availability: Available only with a prescription from a doctor.

Other information: Continue with drug even if feeling well. Report symptoms of dizziness.

CAUTIONS

Children: This drug is either not recommended for children, or is recommended only for children above a certain age.

Pregnancy and breastfeeding: This drug is either not recommended for use by women who are pregnant or breastfeeding, or the precise effects are not known and it should therefore only be used with caution and under medical advice.

Alcohol: Alcohol should not be consumed, or only consumed with caution - after medical advice has been sought - while you are taking this drug.

Driving and operating machinery: This drug may have some effect on your driving ability, so it is advisable not to drive or operate machinery while taking it.

DIMENHYDRINATE

Brand name: Dramamine

Type of drug: Antihistamine

Uses: To prevent and relieve motion sickness. Also can help relieve nausea, vomiting and vertigo and disorders of the inner ear.

How it works: Depresses the sensitivity of the part of the inner ear which controls balance and is closely linked to the vomiting centre in the brain.

Possible adverse effects: Most common side effect is drowsiness, sometimes blurred vision.

Availability: Available with or without a prescription (over the counter).

Other information: For motion sickness take 30 minutes before travelling.

CAUTIONS

Children: There are no commonly reported problems associated with prescribing this medication for children.

Pregnancy and breastfeeding: This drug is either not recommended for use by women who are pregnant or breastfeeding, or the precise effects are not known and it should therefore only be used with caution and under medical advice.

Alcohol: Alcohol should not be consumed, or only consumed with caution - after medical advice has been sought - while you are taking this drug.

Driving and operating machinery: This drug may have some effect on your driving ability, so it is advisable not to drive or operate machinery while taking it.

DIPHENOXYLATE

Brand name: None

Type of drug: Opioid antidiarrhoeal

Uses: Treatment for violent bouts of diarrhoea.

How it works: Reduces contractions of the bowel and therefore the frequency of bowel movements. It is not suitable for diarrhoea caused by infection or poisons.

Possible adverse effects: Bloated abdomen and nausea, rashes, drowsiness and dizziness. There is risk of addiction because it is chemically related to the opiate painkillers.

Availability: Available only with a prescription from a doctor.

Other information: Available in tablet or liquid form. An adequate level of liquid must be taken during bouts of diarrhoea.

CAUTIONS

Children: This drug is either not recommended for children, or is recommended only for children above a certain age.

Pregnancy and breastfeeding: This drug is either not recommended for use by women who are pregnant or breastfeeding, or the precise effects are not known and it should therefore only be used with caution and under medical advice.

Alcohol: Alcohol should not be consumed, or only consumed with caution - after medical advice has been sought - while you are taking this drug.

Driving and operating machinery: This drug may have some effect on your driving ability, so it is advisable not to drive or operate machinery while taking it.

DIPIPANONE

Brand name: Diconal

Type of drug: Opioid analgesic

Uses: For moderate pain relief.

How it works: Alleviates the pain at the same time as producing a less sedative effect than many similar drugs.

Possible adverse effects: Nausea, vomiting, dizziness, constipation. Can occasionally cause dependence.

Availability: Available only with a prescription from a doctor.

Other information: Should not be used by patients with severe respiratory disorders.

CAUTIONS

Children: This drug is either not recommended for children, or is recommended only for children above a certain age.

Pregnancy and breastfeeding: No specific problems documented, but any medication should be taken with utmost caution by women who are either pregnant or breastfeeding, and only after professional medical or pharmaceutical advice has been sought.

Alcohol: No known problems if taken with alcohol.

Driving and operating machinery: There are no commonly reported problems which may impact on the ability to drive or operate machinery. However, many drugs can cause dizziness or drowsiness in a few people, so it is wise to see how the drug affects you before driving or working with dangerous machinery.

DIPIVEFRINE

Brand name: Propine
Type of drug: Sympathomimetic
Uses: To treat open-angle glaucoma.
How it works: Reduces the pressure inside the eye.
Possible adverse effects: Stinging of the eyes.
Availability: Available only with a prescription from a doctor.
Other information: Do not wear soft contact lenses.

CAUTIONS

Children: There are no commonly reported problems associated with prescribing this medication for children.

Pregnancy and breastfeeding: No specific problems documented, but any medication should be taken with utmost caution by women who are either pregnant or breastfeeding, and only after professional medical or pharmaceutical advice has been sought.

Alcohol: No known problems if taken with alcohol.

Driving and operating machinery: This drug may have some effect on your driving ability, so it is advisable not to drive or operate machinery while taking it.

DIPYRIDAMOLE

Brand name: Cerebrovase, Modaplate, Persantin

Type of drug: Anti-platelet

Uses: To prevent thrombosis (the formation of blood clots).

How it works: It 'thins' the blood in patients who have had heart valve replacement surgery, and reduces the possibility of blood clots.

Possible adverse effects: Nausea, headache, dizziness, faintness.

Availability: Available only with a prescription from a doctor.

Other information: Patient may have to take drug for several months. Antacids should only be taken at the same time as this drug on the advice of a doctor.

CAUTIONS

Children: There are no commonly reported problems associated with prescribing this medication for children.

Pregnancy and breastfeeding: This drug is either not recommended for use by women who are pregnant or breastfeeding, or the precise effects are not known and it should therefore only be used with caution and under medical advice.

Alcohol: No known problems if taken with alcohol.

Driving and operating machinery: This drug may have some effect on your driving ability, so it is advisable not to drive or operate machinery while taking it.

DISODIUM PAMIDRONATE

Brand name: Aredia

Type of drug: Bisphosphonate

Uses: The treatment of Paget's disease and osteoporosis and bone pain associated with breast cancer.

How it works: Reduces blood calcium levels which are associated with the above conditions.

Possible adverse effects: Nausea, diarrhoea, muscle and joint pains, flu-like symptoms.

Availability: Available only with a prescription from a doctor.

Other information: Calcium and vitamin D supplements are recommended.

CAUTIONS

Children: There are no commonly reported problems associated with prescribing this medication for children.

Pregnancy and breastfeeding: This drug is either not recommended for use by women who are pregnant or breastfeeding, or the precise effects are not known and it should therefore only be used with caution and under medical advice.

Alcohol: No known problems if taken with alcohol.

Driving and operating machinery: This drug may have some effect on your driving ability, so it is advisable not to drive or operate machinery while taking it.

DISOPYRAMIDE

Brand name: Dirythmin SA, Rythmodan

Type of drug: Anti-arrhythmia

Uses: To treat disorders of heart rhythm such as tachycardia (rapid pulse) and atrial fibrillation.

How it works: Reduces the activity of the heart muscle and acts on the electrical impulses in the heart to encourage a normal heart rhythm.

Possible adverse effects: Stomach and bowel upsets, dry mouth, blurred vision.

Availability: Available only with a prescription from a doctor.

Other information: Blood pressure level, blood sugar and potassium levels must be watched out for and monitored.

CAUTIONS

Children: There are no commonly reported problems associated with prescribing this medication for children.

Pregnancy and breastfeeding: This drug is either not recommended for use by women who are pregnant or breastfeeding, or the precise effects are not known and it should therefore only be used with caution.

Alcohol: No known problems if taken with alcohol.

Driving and operating machinery: There are no commonly reported problems which may impact on the ability to drive or operate machinery. However, many drugs can cause dizziness or drowsiness in a few people, so it is wise to see how the drug affects you before driving or working with dangerous machinery.

DISULFIRAM

Brand name: Antabuse

Type of drug: Alcohol abuse deterrent

Uses: To treat people who are chronically addicted to alcohol.

How it works: Works as a deterrent. If alcohol is taken at the same time as disulfiram, the two react to produce unpleasant effects such as palpitations, nausea and fainting. Unconsciousness may also occur.

Possible adverse effects: Drowsiness, fatigue, nausea and vomiting.

Availability: Available only with a prescription from a doctor.

Other information: Alcohol in any form must not be consumed under any circumstances. The patient is advised to carry a card warning of the effects of this drug.

CAUTIONS

Children: This drug is either not recommended for children, or is recommended only for children above a certain age.

Pregnancy and breastfeeding: This drug is either not recommended for use by women who are pregnant or breastfeeding, or the precise effects are not known and it should therefore only be used with caution and under medical advice.

Alcohol: Alcohol should not be consumed, or only consumed with caution - after medical advice has been sought - while you are taking this drug.

Driving and operating machinery: This drug may have some effect on your driving ability, so it is advisable not to drive or operate machinery while taking it.

DITHRANOL

Brand name: Dithrocream, Micanol, Psorin

Type of drug: Psoriasis treatment

Uses: To treat moderate to severe psoriasis.

How it works: Restores excessive skin growth to normal; sometimes accompanied by ultraviolet treatments to boost its effect.

Possible adverse effects: Skin irritation.

Availability: Available with or without a prescription (over-the-counter).

Other information: The cream/ointment can be applied for short periods each day and then washed off. May stain clothes and linen. Keep away from the eyes and nose. Beneficial effect may not be felt for a few weeks.

CAUTIONS

Children: This drug is either not recommended for children, or is recommended only for children above a certain age.

Pregnancy and breastfeeding: No specific problems documented, but any medication should be taken with utmost caution by women who are either pregnant or breastfeeding, and only after professional medical or pharmaceutical advice has been sought.

Alcohol: No known problems if taken with alcohol.

Driving and operating machinery: There are no commonly reported problems which may impact on the ability to drive or operate machinery. However, many drugs can cause dizziness or drowsiness in a few people, so it is wise to see how the drug affects you before driving or working with dangerous machinery.

DOBUTAMINE

Brand name: Dobutrex, Posiject

Type of drug: Sympathomimetic

Uses: The treatment of heart failure following a heart attack, heart surgery and shock.

How it works: Stimulates heart muscle without increasing the heart rate.

Possible adverse effects: Rapid beating of heart. An unexpected rise in blood pressure may indicate an overdose.

Availability: Available only with a prescription from a doctor.

Other information: Usually only administered in intensive care units in hospital. Use with caution for patients with very low blood pressure.

CAUTIONS

Children: There are no commonly reported problems associated with prescribing this medication for children.

Pregnancy and breastfeeding: No specific problems documented, but any medication should be taken with utmost caution by women who are either pregnant or breastfeeding, and only after professional medical or pharmaceutical advice has been sought.

Alcohol: No known problems if taken with alcohol.

Driving and operating machinery: There are no commonly reported problems which may impact on the ability to drive or operate machinery. However, many drugs can cause dizziness or drowsiness in a few people, so it is wise to see how the drug affects you before driving or working with dangerous machinery.

DOMPERIDONE

Brand name: Motilium

Type of drug: Anti-emetic

Uses: Treatment of nausea and vomiting caused by gastrointestinal problems or as side effects from other medication.

How it works: Stops nausea without causing sedation.

Possible adverse effects: This drug is used because side effects from it are rare.

Availability: Available only with a prescription from a doctor.

Other information: Not prescribed for long-term treatment.

CAUTIONS

Children: There are no commonly reported problems associated with prescribing this medication for children.

Pregnancy and breastfeeding: This drug is either not recommended for use by women who are pregnant or breastfeeding, or the precise effects are not known and it should therefore only be used with caution and under medical advice.

Alcohol: No known problems if taken with alcohol.

Driving and operating machinery: There are no commonly reported problems which may impact on the ability to drive or operate machinery. However, many drugs can cause dizziness or drowsiness in a few people, so it is wise to see how the drug affects you before driving or working with dangerous machinery.

DOPEXAMINE

Brand name: Dopacard

Type of drug: Sympathomimetic

Uses: Used to treat heart failure, particularly that associated with heart surgery.

How it works: Acts on the cardiac muscle and dilates the cardiac blood vessels to improve the flow of blood to the heart.

Possible adverse effects: Rapid beating of the heart; high doses may cause nausea, vomiting, headache, anginal pain.

Availability: Available only with a prescription from a doctor.

Other information: Usually administered in an intensive care unit in hospital.

CAUTIONS

Children: There are no commonly reported problems associated with prescribing this medication for children.

Pregnancy and breastfeeding: This drug is either not recommended for use by women who are pregnant or breastfeeding, or the precise effects are not known and it should therefore only be used with caution and under medical advice.

Alcohol: Alcohol should not be consumed, or only consumed with caution - after medical advice has been sought - while you are taking this drug.

Driving and operating machinery: There are no commonly reported problems which may impact on the ability to drive or operate machinery. However, many drugs can cause dizziness or drowsiness in a few people, so it is wise to see how the drug affects you before driving or working with dangerous machinery.

DORNASE ALFA

Brand name: Pulmozyme

Type of drug: Mucolytic enzyme

Uses: To treat cystic fibrosis.

How it works: Improves pulmonary function and helps to reduce the frequency of moderate to severe respiratory infections in patients with cystic fibrosis. The enzyme helps to breakdown and remove the sticky secretions of the lungs.

Possible adverse effects: Sore throat, hoarseness, voice changes, skin rash.

Availability: Available only with a prescription from a doctor.

Other information: The drug is administered through inhalation using a jet-nebuliser.

CAUTIONS

Children: There are no commonly reported problems associated with prescribing this medication for children.

Pregnancy and breastfeeding: This drug is either not recommended for use by women who are pregnant or breastfeeding, or the precise effects are not known and it should therefore only be used with caution and under medical advice.

Alcohol: No known problems if taken with alcohol.

Driving and operating machinery: There are no commonly reported problems which may impact on the ability to drive or operate machinery. However, many drugs can cause dizziness or drowsiness in a few people, so it is wise to see how the drug affects you before driving or working with dangerous machinery.

DORZOLAMIDE

Brand name: Trusopt

Type of drug: Anti-glaucoma

Uses: To treat raised pressure in the eyes in open-angled glaucoma.

How it works: Inhibits the production of aqueous humour (the jelly-like fluid within the eye), thus reducing the pressure within the eye.

Possible adverse effects: Stinging and sore eyes, blurred vision, headache.

Availability: Available only with a prescription from a doctor.

Other information: Do not wear soft contact lenses.

CAUTIONS

Children: There are no commonly reported problems associated with prescribing this medication for children.

Pregnancy and breastfeeding: This drug is either not recommended for use by women who are pregnant or breastfeeding, or the precise effects are not known and it should therefore only be used with caution and under medical advice.

Alcohol: No known problems if taken with alcohol.

Driving and operating machinery: There are no commonly reported problems which may impact on the ability to drive or operate machinery. However, many drugs can cause dizziness or drowsiness in a few people, so it is wise to see how the drug affects you before driving or working with dangerous machinery.

DOTHIEPIN

Brand name: Dothapax, Prepadine, Prothiaden

Type of drug: Tricyclic antidepressant

Uses: A long-term treatment for depression.

How it works: Improves mood and interest in day-to-day living and encourages sleep if taken at night.

Possible adverse effects: Drowsiness, sweating and dry mouth sometimes occur during early days of treatment.

Availability: Available only with a prescription from a doctor.

Other information: Can take several weeks for full beneficial effects to be realised.

CAUTIONS

Children: This drug is either not recommended for children, or is recommended only for children above a certain age.

Pregnancy and breastfeeding: This drug is either not recommended for use by women who are pregnant or breastfeeding, or the precise effects are not known and it should therefore only be used with caution and under medical advice.

Alcohol: Alcohol should not be consumed, or only consumed with caution - after medical advice has been sought - while you are taking this drug.

Driving and operating machinery: This drug may have some effect on your driving ability, so it is advisable not to drive or operate machinery while taking it.

DOXAZOSIN

Brand name: Cardura

Type of drug: Vasodilator and anti-hypertensive

Uses: To treat high blood pressure (hypertension) and sometimes used for the treatment of enlarged prostate gland.

How it works: Dilates blood vessels, allowing more blood to pass.

Possible adverse effects: Dizziness on standing up. Headache, nausea and general fatigue.

Availability: Available only with a prescription from a doctor.

Other information: The first treatment will cause a marked drop in blood pressure which will cause the patient to feel faint and dizzy.

CAUTIONS

Children: This drug is either not recommended for children, or is recommended only for children above a certain age.

Pregnancy and breastfeeding: This drug is either not recommended for use by women who are pregnant or breastfeeding, or the precise effects are not known and it should therefore only be used with caution and under medical advice.

Alcohol: Alcohol should not be consumed, or only consumed with caution - after medical advice has been sought - while you are taking this drug.

Driving and operating machinery: This drug may have some effect on your driving ability, so it is advisable not to drive or operate machinery while taking it.

DOXORUBICIN

Brand name: Doxorubicin

Type of drug: Anti-cancer

Uses: Used to treat many types of leukaemia, Hodgkin's disease, and many other cancers.

How it works: Acts on the DNA within the cancer cells to prevent them from replicating.

Possible adverse effects: Nausea and vomiting are the most common side effects of this drug after initial injection. Urine may be stained red. Lowered resistance to infection.

Availability: Available only with a prescription from a doctor.

Other information: Blood will be carefully monitored to assess the impact of the drug. Patients should stay away from people with infections during a course of this treatment.

CAUTIONS

Children: There are no commonly reported problems associated with prescribing this medication for children.

Pregnancy and breastfeeding: This drug is either not recommended for use by women who are pregnant or breastfeeding, or the precise effects are not known and it should therefore only be used with caution and under medical advice.

Alcohol: No known problems if taken with alcohol.

Driving and operating machinery: There are no commonly reported problems which may impact on the ability to drive or operate machinery. However, many drugs can cause dizziness or drowsiness in a few people, so it is wise to see how the drug affects you.

DOXYCYCLINE

Brand name: Cyclodox, Demix, Doxylar, Nordox, Ramysis, Vibramycin

Type of drug: Antibiotic

Uses: Treatment of urinary, respiratory, eye, prostate and gut infections. Occasionally used for malaria and acne.

How it works: Antibiotic.

Possible adverse effects: Rarely causes nausea, vomiting and increased sensitivity to sun which may result in a rash.

Availability: Available only with a prescription from a doctor.

Other information: Avoid excessive exposure to sunlight.

CAUTIONS

Children: There are no commonly reported problems associated with prescribing this medication for children.

Pregnancy and breastfeeding: This drug is either not recommended for use by women who are pregnant or breastfeeding, or the precise effects are not known and it should therefore only be used with caution and under medical advice.

Alcohol: No known problems if taken with alcohol.

Driving and operating machinery: There are no commonly reported problems which may impact on the ability to drive or operate machinery. However, many drugs can cause dizziness or drowsiness in a few people, so it is wise to see how the drug affects you before driving or working with dangerous machinery.

DROPERIDOL

Brand name: Droleptan

Type of drug: Anti-emetic and anti-psychotic

Uses: The treatment of severe cases of anxiety and as an anti-emetic following surgery or chemotherapy.

How it works: Alters the balance of chemicals in the brain to block feelings of nausea and produce a calming effect.

Possible adverse effects: Drowsiness

Availability: Available only with a prescription from a doctor.

Other information: Usually given as an injection.

CAUTIONS

Children: There are no commonly reported problems associated with prescribing this medication for children.

Pregnancy and breastfeeding: This drug is either not recommended for use by women who are pregnant or breastfeeding, or the precise effects are

not known and it should therefore only be used with caution and under medical advice.

Alcohol: Alcohol should not be consumed, or only consumed with caution - after medical advice has been sought - while you are taking this drug.

Driving and operating machinery: This drug may have some effect on your driving ability, so it is advisable not to drive or operate machinery while taking it.

DYDROGESTERONE

Brand name: Duphaston, Duphaston HRT

Type of drug: Female sex hormone

Uses: Treatment of menstrual disorders and as part of hormone replacement therapy (HRT).

How it works: Synthetic hormone similar to progesterone.

Possible adverse effects: Irregular periods and bleeding between periods.

Availability: Available only with a prescription from a doctor.

Other information: Dosage is taken on selective days during the menstrual cycle.

CAUTIONS

Children: This drug is either not recommended for children, or is recommended only for children above a certain age.

Pregnancy and breastfeeding: No specific problems documented, but any medication should be taken with utmost caution by women who are either pregnant or breastfeeding, and only after professional medical or pharmaceutical advice has been sought.

Alcohol: No known problems if taken with alcohol.

Driving and operating machinery: This drug may have some effect on your driving ability, so it is advisable not to drive or operate machinery while taking it.

ECONAZOLE

Brand name: Econacort, Ecostatin, Gyno-Pevaryl, Pevaryl

Type of drug: Antifungal

Uses: Used to treat fungal infections of the skin, thrush of the vagina and infected nappy rash.

How it works: Alters the membranes of the fungal cells with the result that they can no longer multiply and the infection is halted.

Possible adverse effects: Skin irritation.

Availability: Available with or without a prescription.

Other information: Wash hands well after application of drug.

CAUTIONS

Children: There are no commonly reported problems associated with prescribing this medication for children.

Pregnancy and breastfeeding: This drug is either not recommended for use by women who are pregnant or breastfeeding, or the precise effects are not known and it should therefore only be used with caution and under medical advice.

Alcohol: No known problems if taken with alcohol.

Driving and operating machinery: There are no commonly reported problems which may impact on the ability to drive or operate machinery. However, many drugs can cause dizziness or drowsiness in a few people, so it is wise to see how the drug affects you before driving or working with dangerous machinery.

EFORMOTEROL

Brand name: Foradil, Oxis

Type of drug: Bronchodilator

Uses: The treatment of moderate to severe asthma.

How it works: It has a bronchodilating action - by relaxing the muscles surrounding the airways in the lungs it can relieve the symptoms of asthma.

Possible adverse effects: A fine tremor, palpitations and headaches.

Availability: Available only with a prescription from a doctor.

Other information: Levels of potassium in the blood will be regularly monitored.

CAUTIONS

Children: There are no commonly reported problems associated with prescribing this medication for children.

Pregnancy and breastfeeding: This drug is either not recommended for use by women who are pregnant or breastfeeding, or the precise effects are not known and it should therefore only be used with caution and under medical advice.

Alcohol: No known problems if taken with alcohol.

Driving and operating machinery: There are no commonly reported problems which may impact on the ability to drive or operate machinery. However, many drugs can cause dizziness or drowsiness in a few people, so it is wise to see how the drug affects you before driving or working with dangerous machinery.

ENALAPRIL

Brand name: Innovace
Type of drug: Vasodilator and anti-hypertensive
Uses: Treatment of hypertension and heart failure.
How it works: Dilates the blood vessels, with the result that the pressure within them is lowered.
Possible adverse effects: Dizziness and headache which usually subside after initial treatment. Possible rashes.
Availability: Available only with a prescription from a doctor.
Other information: After first treatment patient will have to lie down for a few hours. Blood and urine tests will be periodically taken.
CAUTIONS
Children: This drug is either not recommended for children, or is recommended only for children above a certain age.
Pregnancy and breastfeeding: This drug is either not recommended for use by women who are pregnant or breastfeeding, or the precise effects are not known and it should therefore only be used with caution and under medical advice.
Alcohol: Alcohol should not be consumed, or only consumed with caution - after medical advice has been sought— while you are taking this drug.
Driving and operating machinery: This drug may have some effect on your driving ability, so it is advisable not to drive or operate machinery while taking it.

ENOXAPARIN

Brand name: Clexane
Type of drug: Anti-coagulant
Uses: The prevention of deep-vein thrombosis.
How it works: Acts on the clotting mechanism of the blood to stop clots forming.

Possible adverse effects: Nausea, confusion. Any sign of unusual bruising or bleeding should be reported.

Availability: Available only with a prescription from a doctor.

Other information: Administered as an injection, usually in hospital.

CAUTIONS

Children: This drug is either not recommended for children, or is recommended only for children above a certain age.

Pregnancy and breastfeeding: This drug is either not recommended for use by women who are pregnant or breastfeeding, or the precise effects are not known and it should therefore only be used with caution and under medical advice.

Alcohol: No known problems if taken with alcohol.

Driving and operating machinery: There are no commonly reported problems which may impact on the ability to drive or operate machinery. However, many drugs can cause dizziness or drowsiness in a few people, so it is wise to see how the drug affects you before driving or working with dangerous machinery.

ENOXIMONE

Brand name: Perfan

Type of drug: Anti-emetic and anti-psychotic

Uses: Used to treat congestive heart failure.

How it works: Acts on the heart muscle to increase the heart's ability to pump blood around the body. Alleviates the symptoms, but is not a cure for the condition.

Possible adverse effects: Fall in blood pressure, irregular heart rhythm, nausea and vomiting, diarrhoea, headache.

Availability: Available only with a prescription from a doctor.

Other information: Administered as an injection, usually in hospital.

CAUTIONS

Children: There are no commonly reported problems associated with prescribing this medication for children.

Pregnancy and breastfeeding: This drug is either not recommended for use by women who are pregnant or breastfeeding, or the precise effects are not known and it should therefore only be used with caution and under medical advice.

Alcohol: No known problems if taken with alcohol.

Driving and operating machinery: There are no commonly reported problems which may impact on the ability to drive or operate machinery. However, many drugs can cause dizziness or drowsiness in a few people, so it is wise to see how the drug affects you before driving or working with dangerous machinery.

EPHEDRINE

Brand name: CAM

Type of drug: Bronchodilator and decongestant

Uses: To treat the symptoms of respiratory problems.

How it works: It relaxes the muscles surrounding the airways to ease breathing difficulties.

Possible adverse effects: Anxiety and insomnia and restlessness, occasionally palpitations if taken by mouth.

Availability: Available with or without a prescription.

Other information: Prolonged use is not recommended.

CAUTIONS

Children: There are no commonly reported problems associated with prescribing this medication for children.

Pregnancy and breastfeeding: This drug is either not recommended for use by women who are pregnant or breastfeeding, or the precise effects are not known and it should therefore only be used with caution and under medical advice.

Alcohol: No known problems if taken with alcohol.

Driving and operating machinery: This drug may have some effect on your driving ability, so it is advisable not to drive or operate machinery while taking it.

EPINEPHRINE (Adrenaline)

Brand name: Ana-Guard, EpiPen, Eppy, Medihaler-Epi, Mini-I-Jet Epinephrine, Simplene

Type of drug: Stimulant

Uses: Used as an emergency treatment for acute heart failure and anaphylactic shock. Also given as eye drops to treat glaucoma.

How it works: Stimulates part of the nervous system, with the result that it relaxes smooth muscle within the lungs, stimulates the heart to beat more effectively and lowers pressure within the eyeball that is symptomatic of glaucoma.

Possible adverse effects: Dry mouth, nervousness, palpitations, headache and blurred vision.

Availability: Available only with a prescription from a doctor.

Other information: Can be administered as an injection, inhaler and eye drops. If used for glaucoma, soft contact lenses should not be worn.

CAUTIONS

Children: There are no commonly reported problems associated with prescribing this medication for children.

Pregnancy and breastfeeding: This drug is either not recommended for use by women who are pregnant or breastfeeding, or the precise effects are not known and it should therefore only be used with caution and under medical advice.

Alcohol: No known problems if taken with alcohol.

Driving and operating machinery: There are no commonly reported problems which may impact on the ability to drive or operate machinery. However, many drugs can cause dizziness or drowsiness in a few people, so it is wise to see how the drug affects you before driving or working with dangerous machinery.

EPOPROSTENOL

Brand name: Flolan

Type of drug: Anti-coagulant

Uses: During kidney dialysis.

How it works: Used to prevent the blood clotting during kidney dialysis, by stopping platelets from sticking together.

Possible adverse effects: Flushing, headache and a drop in blood pressure.

Availability: Available only with a prescription from a doctor.

Other information: Given as an intravenous drip during dialysis.

CAUTIONS

Children: There are no commonly reported problems associated with prescribing this medication for children.

Pregnancy and breastfeeding: This drug is either not recommended for use by women who are pregnant or breastfeeding, or the precise effects are not known and it should therefore only be used with caution and under medical advice.

Alcohol: No known problems if taken with alcohol.

Driving and operating machinery: There are no commonly reported problems which may impact on the ability to drive or operate machinery. However, many drugs can cause dizziness or drowsiness in a few people, so it is wise to see how the drug affects you before driving or working with dangerous machinery.

ERGOCALCIFEROL

Brand name: Calciferol, Vitamin D2

Type of drug: Vitamin

Uses: Prevention and treatment of certain types of vitamin D deficiency.

How it works: Delivers vitamin D to people who are deficient for a number of reasons, including inadequate diet, malabsorption problems or long-term liver disease.

Possible adverse effects: Loss of appetite, nausea and vomiting, diarrhoea, weight loss, sweating, headache and thirst.

Availability: Some preparations are available over the counter.

Other information: Blood tests will be taken regularly to monitor the impact of the drug.

CAUTIONS

Children: There are no commonly reported problems associated with prescribing this medication for children.

Pregnancy and breastfeeding: This drug is either not recommended for use by women who are pregnant or breastfeeding, or the precise effects are not known and it should therefore only be used with caution and under medical advice.

Alcohol: No known problems if taken with alcohol.

Driving and operating machinery: There are no commonly reported problems which may impact on the ability to drive or operate machinery. However, many drugs can cause dizziness or drowsiness in a few people, so it is wise to see how the drug affects you before driving or working with dangerous machinery.

ERGOMETRINE

Brand name: Syntometrine

Type of drug: Prostaglandin

Uses: Used to prevent bleeding from the uterus after childbirth.

How it works: Causes contractions of the uterus, thus helping the blood vessels to heal and therefore stop bleeding.

Possible adverse effects: Nausea, vomiting, headache, dizziness, palpitations.

Availability: Available only with a prescription from a doctor.

Other information: Given as an injection after childbirth.

CAUTIONS

Children: Unlikely to be prescribed.

Pregnancy and breastfeeding: No specific problems documented, but any medication should be taken with utmost caution by women who are either pregnant or breastfeeding, and only after professional medical or pharmaceutical advice has been sought.

Alcohol: No known problems if taken with alcohol.

Driving and operating machinery: There are no commonly reported problems which may impact on the ability to drive or operate machinery. However, many drugs can cause dizziness or drowsiness in a few people, so it is wise to see how the drug affects you before driving or working with dangerous machinery.

ERGOTAMINE

Brand name: Lingraine, Medihaler-Ergotamine, Cafergot, Migril

Type of drug: Migraine treatment

Uses: To treat migraine in people for whom traditional pain relief is not effective.

How it works: Narrows the blood vessels around the skull and prevents pulsing effect which often accompanies migraine.

Possible adverse effects: Nausea and stomach upset. Can reduce circulation to the hands and feet and should not be taken by people known to have poor circulation.

Availability: Available only with a prescription from a doctor.

Other information: Most effective when taken at the first indication of a migraine attack, when the 'aura' is perceived.

CAUTIONS

Children: This drug is either not recommended for children, or is recommended only for children above a certain age.

Pregnancy and breastfeeding: This drug is either not recommended for

use by women who are pregnant or breastfeeding, or the precise effects are not known and it should therefore only be used with caution and under medical advice.

Alcohol: No known problems if taken with alcohol.

Driving and operating machinery: This drug may have some effect on your driving ability, so it is advisable not to drive or operate machinery while taking it.

ERYTHROMYCIN

Brand name: Arpimycin, Erycen, Erymax, Erythrocin, Erythromid, Erythroped, Ilosone, Rommix, Stiemycin

Type of drug: Antibiotic

Uses: Treatment of a range of bacterial infections, including those of the throat, ear and lungs. Can also be helpful in treating acne.

How it works: Kills the organisms which are causing the infection.

Possible adverse effects: Nausea and vomiting; also abdominal discomfort.

Availability: Available only with a prescription from a doctor.

Other information: Can be administered as tablets, capsules, liquid, injection or as a solution to be applied to the skin.

CAUTIONS

Children: There are no commonly reported problems associated with prescribing this medication for children.

Pregnancy and breastfeeding: This drug is either not recommended for use by women who are pregnant or breastfeeding, or the precise effects are not known and it should therefore only be used with caution and under medical advice.

Alcohol: No known problems if taken with alcohol.

Driving and operating machinery: There are no commonly reported problems which may impact on the ability to drive or operate machinery. However, many drugs can cause dizziness or drowsiness in a few people, so it is wise to see how the drug affects you before driving or working with dangerous machinery.

ERYTHROPOIETIN

Brand name: Eprex, Recormon

Type of drug: Kidney hormone

Uses: To treat anaemia due to kidney failure.

How it works: The drug stimulates the body to produce red blood cells, which people with kidney failure cannot do in the right quantity.

Possible adverse effects: Increased blood pressure, headache, dizziness.

Availability: Available only with a prescription from a doctor.

Other information: Regular blood tests will be required to measure blood composition.

CAUTIONS

Children: There are no commonly reported problems associated with prescribing this medication for children.

Pregnancy and breastfeeding: This drug is either not recommended for use by women who are pregnant or breastfeeding, or the precise effects are not known and it should therefore only be used with caution and under medical advice.

Alcohol: Alcohol should not be consumed, or only consumed with caution - after medical advice has been sought - while you are taking this drug.

Driving and operating machinery: There are no commonly reported problems which may impact on the ability to drive or operate machinery. However, many drugs can cause dizziness or drowsiness in a few people, so it is wise to see how the drug affects you before driving or working with dangerous machinery.

ESTRAMUSTINE

Brand name: Estracyt

Type of drug: Anti-cancer

Uses: To treat cancer of the prostate gland.

How it works: The hormone affects the cancerous cells.

Possible adverse effects: Nausea, vomiting, diarrhoea. Breast tenderness and hair thinning may also occur.

Availability: Available only with a prescription from a doctor.

Other information: Treatment with this drug may continue for up to three months. Milk, milk products and calcium-rich foods can impair the absorption of the drug.

CAUTIONS

Children: There are no commonly reported problems associated with prescribing this medication for children.

Pregnancy and breastfeeding: This drug is either not recommended for use by women who are pregnant or breastfeeding, or the precise effects are not known and it should therefore only be used with caution and under medical advice.

Alcohol: No known problems if taken with alcohol.

Driving and operating machinery: There are no commonly reported problems which may impact on the ability to drive or operate machinery. However, many drugs can cause dizziness or drowsiness in a few people, so it is wise to see how the drug affects you before driving or working with dangerous machinery.

ETHAMBUTOL

Brand name: Myambutol

Type of drug: Anti-tuberculous

Uses: Treatment of tuberculosis.

How it works: Works in conjunction with other drugs to attack the organisms that cause the infection.

Possible adverse effects: Side effects are uncommon, but this drug can occasionally cause eye problems such as temporary colour blindness.

Availability: Available only with a prescription from a doctor.

Other information: Regular eye tests will be conducted.

CAUTIONS

Children: This drug is either not recommended for children, or is recommended only for children above a certain age.

Pregnancy and breastfeeding: This drug is either not recommended for use by women who are pregnant or breastfeeding, or the precise effects are not known and it should therefore only be used with caution and under medical advice.

Alcohol: No known problems if taken with alcohol.

Driving and operating machinery: This drug may have some effect on your driving ability, so it is advisable not to drive or operate machinery while taking it.

ETHAMSYLATE

Brand name: Dicynene

Type of drug: Haemostatic

Uses: To stop heavy menstrual bleeding and to prevent bleeding in premature low birth-weight babies.

How it works: Corrects blood clotting malfunction.

Possible adverse effects: Nausea, headache and rashes.

Availability: Available only with a prescription from a doctor.

Other information: In patients with heavy periods the drug will usually be given as tablets, to be taken during menstruation; for low birth-weight babies, it will be given as an injection.

CAUTIONS

Children: There are no commonly reported problems associated with prescribing this medication for children.

Pregnancy and breastfeeding: This drug is either not recommended for use by women who are pregnant or breastfeeding, or the precise effects are not known and it should therefore only be used with caution and under medical advice.

Alcohol: No known problems if taken with alcohol.

Driving and operating machinery: There are no commonly reported problems which may impact on the ability to drive or operate machinery. However, many drugs can cause dizziness or drowsiness in a few people, so it is wise to see how the drug affects you before driving or working with dangerous machinery.

ETHOSUXIMIDE

Brand name: Emeside, Zarontin

Type of drug: Anti-convulsant

Uses: Treatment of certain types of epilepsy, particularly petit mal (daydreaming type episodes).

How it works: Has an anti-convulsant effect.

Possible adverse effects: Rare except when levels of the drug in the blood become too high.

Availability: Available only with a prescription from a doctor.

Other information: Can reduce the production of blood cells.

CAUTIONS

Children: There are no commonly reported problems associated with prescribing this medication for children.

Pregnancy and breastfeeding: This drug is either not recommended for

use by women who are pregnant or breastfeeding, or the precise effects are not known and it should therefore only be used with caution and under medical advice.

Alcohol: Alcohol should not be consumed, or only consumed with caution - after medical advice has been sought - while you are taking this drug.

Driving and operating machinery: This drug may have some effect on your driving ability, so it is advisable not to drive or operate machinery while taking it.

ETIDRONATE

Brand name: Didronel, Didronel PMO

Type of drug: Bone disorders treatment

Uses: To treat Paget's disease, and in combination with calcium tablets it is also used to treat osteoporosis.

How it works: Reduces the activity of the bone cells, thus stopping the progress of the disease.

Possible adverse effects: Diarrhoea and nausea.

Availability: Available only with a prescription from a doctor.

Other information: Should be taken on an empty stomach.

CAUTIONS

Children: This drug is either not recommended for children, or only for children above a certain age.

Pregnancy and breastfeeding: This drug is either not recommended for use by women who are pregnant or breastfeeding, or the precise effects are not known and it should therefore only be used with caution and under medical advice.

Alcohol: No known problems if taken with alcohol.

Driving and operating machinery: There are no commonly reported problems which may impact on the ability to drive or operate machinery. However, many drugs can cause dizziness or drowsiness in a few people, so it is wise to see how the drug affects you before driving or working with dangerous machinery.

FACTOR VIII FRACTION, FREEZE DRIED

Brand name: Alpha VIII, Monoclate-P, 8SM, 8Y, High Potency Factor VIII Concentrate

Type of drug: Haemophilia treatment

Uses: To control bleeding in people with haemophilia.

How it works: Replaces a chemical vital for blood clotting, which is deficient in people with haemophilia.

Possible adverse effects: Fever, chills, flushing, tingling which may indicate an allergic reaction.

Availability: Available only with a prescription from a doctor.

Other information: Administered via an intravenous infusion (drip) in hospital.

CAUTIONS

Children: There are no commonly reported problems associated with prescribing this medication for children.

Pregnancy and breastfeeding: No specific problems documented, but any medication should be taken with utmost caution by women who are either pregnant or breastfeeding, and only after professional medical or pharmaceutical advice has been sought.

Alcohol: No known problems if taken with alcohol.

Driving and operating machinery: There are no commonly reported problems which may impact on the ability to drive or operate machinery. However, many drugs can cause dizziness or drowsiness in a few people, so it is wise to see how the drug affects you before driving or working with dangerous machinery.

FAMCICLOVIR

Brand name: Famvir

Type of drug: Anti-viral

Uses: Used to treat herpes zoster, shingles, herpes simplex, genital herpes.

How it works: Enters the cells of the virus and acts to prevent them from replicating.

Possible adverse effects: Headache and nausea.

Availability: Available only with a prescription from a doctor.

Other information: Treatment is most effective when started within 48 hours of onset.

CAUTIONS

Children: This drug is either not recommended for children, or is recommended only for children above a certain age.

Pregnancy and breastfeeding: This drug is either not recommended for use by women who are pregnant or breastfeeding, or the precise effects are not known and it should therefore only be used with caution and under medical advice.

Alcohol: No known problems if taken with alcohol.

Driving and operating machinery: There are no commonly reported problems which may impact on the ability to drive or operate machinery. However, many drugs can cause dizziness or drowsiness in a few people, so it is wise to see how the drug affects you before driving or working with dangerous machinery.

FAMOTIDINE

Brand name: Pepcid, Pepcid AC

Type of drug: Anti-ulcer

Uses: Used to treat duodenal and gastric ulcers.

How it works: Inhibits the production of the stomach acids which are causing the lining of the gut to ulcerate.

Possible adverse effects: Headache, dizziness and stomach and bowel upsets.

Availability: Available with or without a prescription.

Other information: Treatment will be more beneficial if the dose is taken at bedtime.

CAUTIONS

Children: This drug is either not recommended for children, or is recommended only for children above a certain age.

Pregnancy and breastfeeding: This drug is either not recommended for use by women who are pregnant or breastfeeding, or the precise effects are not known and it should therefore only be used with caution and under medical advice.

Alcohol: No known problems if taken with alcohol.

Driving and operating machinery: There are no commonly reported problems which may impact on the ability to drive or operate machinery. However, many drugs can cause dizziness or drowsiness in a few people, so it is wise to see how the drug affects you before driving or working with dangerous machinery.

FELODIPINE

Brand name: Plendil

Type of drug: Anti-hypertensive

Uses: Used to treat high blood pressure and angina.

How it works: Causes the blood vessels to relax and dilate - or widen - which means that the pressure inside them is lowered.

Possible adverse effects: Headache, dizziness, palpitations and fatigue. Has also been connected with mild gum problems.

Availability: Available only with a prescription from a doctor.

Other information: Not to be used by patients who have low blood pressure or a fast heart rate. The medication is given in tablet form. The tablets should be swallowed whole and not crushed or chewed. Do not take any other over-the-counter products while taking this medication without first consulting a doctor.

CAUTIONS

Children: There are no commonly reported problems associated with prescribing this medication for children.

Pregnancy and breastfeeding: This drug is either not recommended for use by women who are pregnant or breastfeeding, or the precise effects are not known and it should therefore only be used with caution and under medical advice.

Alcohol: No known problems if taken with alcohol.

Driving and operating machinery: There are no commonly reported problems which may impact on the ability to drive or operate machinery. However, many drugs can cause dizziness or drowsiness in a few people, so it is wise to see how the drug affects you before driving or working with dangerous machinery.

FENBUFEN

Brand name: Lederfen, Fenbuzip

Type of drug: Non-steroidal anti-inflammatory

Uses: The relief of inflammation, pain and stiffness which occurs with rheumatoid arthritis, osteoarthritis and gout.

How it works: Acts to relieve the inflammation which causes the symptoms of inflammatory diseases at the same time as treating the pain which often accompanies them.

Possible adverse effects: Like other non-steroidal anti-inflammatories, Fenbufen can irritate the lining of the stomach and other parts of the intestine. Any sign of blood in the vomit or faeces should be reported immediately, as should episodes of wheezing or breathlessness whilst taking this medication.

Availability: Available only with a prescription from a doctor.

Other information: Prescribed as tablets or capsules. It is important not to take more than the prescribed dose. Do not take aspirin or other anti-inflammatory drugs except under the advice of a doctor.

CAUTIONS

Children: This drug is either not recommended for children, or is recommended only for children above a certain age.

Pregnancy and breastfeeding: This drug is either not recommended for use by women who are pregnant or breastfeeding, or the precise effects are not known and it should therefore only be used with caution and under medical advice.

Alcohol: Alcohol should not be consumed, or only consumed with caution - after medical advice has been sought - while you are taking this drug.

Driving and operating machinery: There are no commonly reported problems which may impact on the ability to drive or operate machinery. However, many drugs can cause dizziness or drowsiness in a few people, so it is wise to see how the drug affects you before driving or working with dangerous machinery.

FENFLURAMINE/DEXFENFLURAMINE

Brand name: [Fenfluramine] Ponderax, [Dexfenfluramine] Adifax

Type of drug: Appetite suppressant

Uses: Used in the treatment of severe obesity.

How it works: The drugs increase the activity of serotonin (a chemical in the brain) with the result that the psychological desire to eat is reduced.

Possible adverse effects: Drowsiness, dizziness, headache, stomach disorders.

Availability: Available only with a prescription from a doctor.

Other information: This drug has to be taken in conjunction with a strict diet, under medical supervision, and should be prescribed for no more than three months.

CAUTIONS

Children: This drug is either not recommended for children, or is recommended only for children above a certain age.

Pregnancy and breastfeeding: This drug is either not recommended for use by women who are pregnant or breastfeeding, or the precise effects are not known and it should therefore only be used with caution and under medical advice.

Alcohol: Alcohol should not be consumed, or only consumed with caution - after medical advice has been sought - while you are taking this drug.

Driving and operating machinery: This drug may have some effect on your driving ability, so it is advisable not to drive or operate machinery while taking it.

FENOFIBRATE

Brand name: Lipantil

Type of drug: Lipid lowering

Uses: To lower the cholesterol and fat levels.

How it works: Action is thought to stimulate the breakdown of part of the proteins contained within the fats which are in the blood.

Possible adverse effects: Nausea and stomach upsets, headache, dizziness. Sometimes it can cause episodes of muscle pain and weakness, which should be reported.

Availability: Available only with a prescription from a doctor.

Other information: Usually prescribed as capsules which should be taken with meals to maximise benefits. Not recommended for patients with kidney or gall bladder problems. Patient must also diet and exercise whilst taking this medication.

CAUTIONS

Children: This drug is either not recommended for children, or is recommended only for children above a certain age.

Pregnancy and breastfeeding: This drug is either not recommended for use by women who are pregnant or breastfeeding, or the precise effects are not known and it should therefore only be used with caution and under medical advice.

Alcohol: No known problems if taken with alcohol.

Driving and operating machinery: There are no commonly reported

problems which may impact on the ability to drive or operate machinery. However, many drugs can cause dizziness or drowsiness in a few people, so it is wise to see how the drug affects you before driving or working with dangerous machinery.

FENTANYL

Brand name: Durogesic, Sublimaze

Type of drug: Opioid analgesic

Uses: Its main use is to relieve pain during surgical operations. However, it can also be used to manage long-term pain in people for whom other painkillers are not sufficient.

How it works: Has a similar action to morphine in that it alters the patient's perception of what pain is, so that it is no longer felt.

Possible adverse effects: Depression of respiration, slowing of pulse rate, and nausea and vomiting. Side effects can occur 12 hours after administration of this medication.

Availability: Available only with a prescription from a doctor.

Other information: Given by injection in hospital or for people with long-term pain problems, by a patch, which is attached to the skin and which delivers the dosage over 72 hours. Patients are taught how to use the patch. Soaps, oils and lotions should be avoided on the patch area.

CAUTIONS

Children: There are no commonly reported problems associated with prescribing this medication for children.

Pregnancy and breastfeeding: This drug is either not recommended for use by women who are pregnant or breastfeeding, or the precise effects are not known and it should therefore only be used with caution and under medical advice.

Alcohol: Alcohol should not be consumed, or only consumed with caution, after medical advice has been sought, while taking this drug.

Driving and operating machinery: This drug may have some effect on your driving ability, so it is advisable not to drive or operate machinery while taking it.

FENTICONAZOLE

Brand name: Lomexin

Type of drug: Anti-fungal

Uses: Used in pessaries for vaginal infections which are caused by the fungus, vaginal candidiasis.

How it works: An anti-infective treatment which attacks the fungus which is the cause of the infection.

Possible adverse effects: Mild skin irritation.

Availability: Available only with a prescription from a doctor.

Other information: Prescribed as pessaries. Care should be taken with contraception as this medication damages latex condoms and diaphragms. Always complete the prescribed course of treatment.

CAUTIONS

Children: This drug is either not recommended for children, or is recommended only for children above a certain age.

Pregnancy and breastfeeding: This drug is either not recommended for use by women who are pregnant or breastfeeding, or the precise effects are not known and it should therefore only be used with caution and under medical advice.

Alcohol: No known problems if taken with alcohol.

Driving and operating machinery: There are no commonly reported problems which may impact on the ability to drive or operate machinery. However, many drugs can cause dizziness or drowsiness in a few people, so it is wise to see how the drug affects you before driving or working with dangerous machinery.

FILGRASTIM

Brand name: Neupogen

Type of drug: Immunity booster

Uses: To reduce the risk of infection in people who have had chemotherapy for certain types of cancer and as part of the treatment for some other blood disorders.

How it works: It stimulates the bone marrow to produce white blood cells, which boosts the body's ability to fight off infection.

Possible adverse effects: Rarely, can affect the heart rhythm. More commonly, can cause skeletal pain, fever, tiredness, nausea and diarrhoea.

Availability: Available only with a prescription from a doctor.

Other information: This medication is usually prescribed as an injection or in vials. Patients taking it are instructed in the techniques of self-administration.

Children: There are no commonly reported problems associated with prescribing this medication for children.

Pregnancy and breastfeeding: This drug is either not recommended for use by women who are pregnant or breastfeeding, or the precise effects are not known and it should therefore only be used with caution and under medical advice.

Alcohol: No known problems if taken with alcohol.

Driving and operating machinery: There are no commonly reported problems which may impact on the ability to drive or operate machinery. However, many drugs can cause dizziness or drowsiness in a few people, so it is wise to see how the drug affects you before driving or working with dangerous machinery.

FINASTERIDE

Brand name: Proscar

Type of drug: Anti-androgens

Uses: Used mainly to treat men with enlarged prostate glands, although is also a treatment for first-stage cancer of the prostate.

How it works: Affects the balance of hormones present in the prostate, with the effect that the prostate does not enlarge.

Possible adverse effects: Impotence, decreased libido, breast tenderness and rash.

Availability: Available only with a prescription from a doctor.

Other information: Women of childbearing age must avoid handling the tablets. The use of condoms is recommended if the sexual partner is pregnant or is likely to become pregnant, as the drug is excreted in semen. The effect of treatment with this drug may not become apparent for several months.

CAUTIONS

Children: This drug is either not recommended for children, or is recommended only for children above a certain age.

Pregnancy and breastfeeding: This drug is either not recommended for use by women who are pregnant or breastfeeding, or the precise effects are not known and it should therefore only be used with caution and under medical advice.

Alcohol: No known problems if taken with alcohol.

Driving and operating machinery: There are no commonly reported problems which may impact on the ability to drive or operate machinery. However, many drugs can cause dizziness or drowsiness in a few people, so it is wise to see how the drug affects you before driving or working with dangerous machinery.

FLAVOXATE

Brand name: Urispas

Type of drug: Anti-cholinergic

Uses: The drug is used as an anti-spasmodic to help incontinence and other urinary tract problems.

How it works: Acts on the smooth muscle in the urinary tract, with the result that the bladder is able to hold more urine and the pain associated with urinary problems is controlled.

Possible adverse effects: Drowsiness and headache, diarrhoea and fatigue.

Availability: Available only with a prescription from a doctor.

Other information: Must not be used if there is a prostate problem.

CAUTIONS

Children: This drug is either not recommended for children, or is recommended only for children above a certain age.

Pregnancy and breastfeeding: No specific problems documented, but any medication should be taken with utmost caution by women who are either pregnant or breastfeeding, and only after professional medical or pharmaceutical advice has been sought.

Alcohol: No known problems if taken with alcohol.

Driving and operating machinery: This drug may have some effect on your driving ability, so it is advisable not to drive or operate machinery while taking it.

FLECAINIDE

Brand name: Tambocor

Type of drug: Anti-arrhythmic

Uses: Used to treat heart rhythm disorders (arrhythmia) such as paroxysmal supraventricular tachycardia and atrial fibrillation.

How it works: Affects the electrical impulses in the heart, with the result that a more regular and normal rhythm is re-established.

Possible adverse effects: Dizziness and visual disturbances, nausea and vomiting. Occasionally difficulty in breathing can occur.

Availability: Available only with a prescription from a doctor.

Other information: Treatment will usually be started in hospital.

CAUTIONS

Children: This drug is either not recommended for children, or is recommended only for children above a certain age.

Pregnancy and breastfeeding: This drug is either not recommended for use by women who are pregnant or breastfeeding, or the precise effects are not known and it should therefore only be used with caution and under medical advice.

Alcohol: No known problems if taken with alcohol.

Driving and operating machinery: There are no commonly reported problems which may impact on the ability to drive or operate machinery. However, many drugs can cause dizziness or drowsiness in a few people, so it is wise to see how the drug affects you before driving or working with dangerous machinery.

FLUCONAZOLE

Brand name: Diflucan

Type of drug: Anti-fungal

Uses: To treat thrush (candidiasis) and other infections such as those which occur in the urinary tract or gut and are caused by a fungus. Is also used to treat some types of meningitis and as a preventative treatment for patients undergoing bone marrow transplants.

How it works: Interferes with the individual cells which make up the fungus, with the result that it can no longer grow.

Possible adverse effects: Irritation of the gastrointestinal tract, resulting in nausea, abdominal pain or diarrhoea.

Availability: Some preparations are available over the counter.

Other information: Usually administered as capsules or liquid, but can also be given as an injection. For patients who may suffer a relapse of meningitis this drug may be administered indefinitely.

CAUTIONS

Children: This drug is either not recommended for children, or is recommended only for children above a certain age.

Pregnancy and breastfeeding: This drug is either not recommended for use by women who are pregnant or breastfeeding, or the precise effects are not known and it should therefore only be used with caution and under medical advice.

Alcohol: No known problems if taken with alcohol.

Driving and operating machinery: There are no commonly reported problems which may impact on the ability to drive or operate machinery. However, many drugs can cause dizziness or drowsiness in a few people, so it is wise to see how the drug affects you before driving or working with dangerous machinery.

FLUCYTOSINE
Brand name: Ancobon

Type of drug: Anti-fungal

Uses: To treat yeast and fungal infections.

How it works: Penetrates the cells which make up the fungus and interferes with their ability to multiply.

Possible adverse effects: Nausea, vomiting, diarrhoea and rashes. Can occasionally cause bleeding in the gut. Any signs of blood in vomit or faeces, or bruising, should be reported straight away.

Availability: Available only with a prescription from a doctor.

Other information: Treatment may need to be maintained over a long period.

CAUTIONS

Children: There are no commonly reported problems associated with prescribing this medication for children.

Pregnancy and breastfeeding: This drug is either not recommended for use by women who are pregnant or breastfeeding, or the precise effects are not known and it should therefore only be used with caution and under medical advice.

Alcohol: No known problems if taken with alcohol.

Driving and operating machinery: There are no commonly reported problems which may impact on the ability to drive or operate machinery. However, many drugs can cause dizziness or drowsiness in a few people, so it is wise to see how the drug affects you before driving or working with dangerous machinery.

FLUDARABINE

Brand name: Fludara

Type of drug: Anti-cancer

Uses: Used in the treatment of chronic leukaemia, and some types of lymphoma in patients who have not responded to other treatments.

How it works: Affects the DNA of the cancer cells, with the result that they are unable to multiply, thus preventing the tumour from growing.

Possible adverse effects: Blood disorders and lowering of immunity are the most common side effects. Fatigue, visual disturbances, nausea, vomiting and fever are also possible.

Availability: Available only with a prescription from a doctor.

Other information: It is advisable to stay away from people with infections whilst on this medication, as your immunity will be reduced.

CAUTIONS

Children: This drug is either not recommended for children, or is recommended only for children above a certain age.

Pregnancy and breastfeeding: No specific problems documented, but any medication should be taken with utmost caution by women who are either pregnant or breastfeeding, and only after professional medical or pharmaceutical advice has been sought.

Alcohol: No known problems if taken with alcohol.

Driving and operating machinery: There are no commonly reported problems which may impact on the ability to drive or operate machinery. However, many drugs can cause dizziness or drowsiness in a few people, so it is wise to see how the drug affects you before driving or working with dangerous machinery.

FLUDROCORTISONE

Brand name: Florinef

Type of drug: Mineralocorticoid

Uses: Treatment of disorders of the adrenal glands, which are situated just above the kidneys and which are crucial in the production of hormones which affect the breakdown of carbohydrates and electrolytes as well as the sex glands.

How it works: The replacement of substances usually produced by the adrenal glands.

Possible adverse effects: Hypertension, sodium and water retention and potassium loss. Muscle weakness, numbness, appetite loss and nausea may be signs of electrolyte imbalance and should be reported. A doctor should also be informed of significant weight gain or headaches.

Availability: Available only with a prescription from a doctor.

Other information: It is important not to miss doses or to double dose if one is forgotten.

CAUTIONS

Children: This drug is either not recommended for children, or is recommended only for children above a certain age.

Pregnancy and breastfeeding: No specific problems documented, but any medication should be taken with utmost caution by women who are either pregnant or breastfeeding, and only after professional medical or pharmaceutical advice has been sought.

Alcohol: No known problems if taken with alcohol.

Driving and operating machinery: There are no commonly reported problems which may impact on the ability to drive or operate machinery. However, many drugs can cause dizziness or drowsiness in a few people, so it is wise to see how the drug affects you before driving or working with dangerous machinery.

FLUMAZENIL

Brand name: Anexate

Type of drug: Benzodiazepine antagonist

Uses: Given following a general anaesthetic.

How it works: Used to reverse the sedative effects of benzodiazepines, used for anaesthesia.

Possible adverse effects: Nausea, vomiting, flushing, rise in blood pressure and heart rate.

Availability: Available only with a prescription from a doctor.

Other information: Usually given as an injection to hospital in-patients.

CAUTIONS

Children: This drug is either not recommended for children, or is recommended only for children above a certain age.

Pregnancy and breastfeeding: This drug is either not recommended for use by women who are pregnant or breastfeeding, or the precise effects are

not known and it should therefore only be used with caution and under medical advice.

Alcohol: No known problems if taken with alcohol.

Driving and operating machinery: This drug may have some effect on your driving ability, so it is advisable not to drive or operate machinery while taking it.

FLUOROURACIL
Brand name: Efudix
Type of drug: Anti-cancer
Uses: To treat various cancers, including those which affect the stomach, breast, bladder and pancreas.
How it works: Prevents the DNA in the cancer cells replicating.
Possible adverse effects: Nausea, vomiting, diarrhoea, rashes and dermatitis. Bleeding from the digestive system can occur, so any signs of blood in vomit or faeces should be reported straight away.
Availability: Available only with a prescription from a doctor.
Other information: Usually given as an injection, in hospital, as it is not absorbed sufficiently if taken by mouth. Patients are advised to wear sunscreens, as the drug increases sensitivity to sunlight. People with infections should also be avoided.

CAUTIONS
Children: There are no commonly reported problems associated with prescribing this medication for children.
Pregnancy and breastfeeding: This drug is either not recommended for use by women who are pregnant or breastfeeding, or the precise effects are not known and it should therefore only be used with caution and under medical advice.
Alcohol: Alcohol should not be consumed, or only consumed with caution - after medical advice has been sought - while you are taking this drug.
Driving and operating machinery: This drug may have some effect on your driving ability, so it is advisable not to drive or operate machinery while taking it.

FLUOXETINE
Brand name: Prozac

Type of drug: Antidepressant

Uses: To treat depression, binge eating (bulimia nervosa), panic disorder, alcohol dependence (rarely) and other psychiatric problems.

How it works: Changes the chemicals in the brain, with the result that patients have an elevated mood and feel more able to take an interest in day-to-day living.

Possible adverse effects: Headache, nausea, restlessness, inability to sleep and stomach upsets. Any sign of a rash or hives should be reported instantly, as should a loss of appetite.

Availability: Available only with a prescription from a doctor.

Other information: Side effects decrease in time.

CAUTIONS

Children: This drug is either not recommended for children, or is recommended only for children above a certain age.

Pregnancy and breastfeeding: This drug is either not recommended for use by women who are pregnant or breastfeeding, or the precise effects are not known and it should therefore only be used with caution and under medical advice.

Alcohol: No known problems if taken with alcohol.

Driving and operating machinery: This drug may have some effect on your driving ability, so it is advisable not to drive or operate machinery while taking it.

FLUPENTHIXOL

Brand name: Depixol, Fluanxol

Type of drug: Anti-psychotic

Uses: To treat schizophrenia and other similar disorders, and mild to moderate depression.

How it works: Tranquillises the patient and reduces hallucinations and other psychotic symptoms without having a sedative effect.

Possible adverse effects: Blurred vision, dizziness, nausea, drowsiness, weight gain, palpitations, tremors, Parkinsonism.

Availability: Available only with a prescription from a doctor.

Other information: This medication should be used with caution by patients with heart disease. The control of severe symptoms may take up to six months.

CAUTIONS

Children: This drug is either not recommended for children, or is recommended only for children above a certain age.

Pregnancy and breastfeeding: This drug is either not recommended for use by women who are pregnant or breastfeeding, or the precise effects are not known and it should therefore only be used with caution and under medical advice.

Alcohol: Alcohol should not be consumed, or only consumed with caution - after medical advice has been sought - while you are taking this drug.

Driving and operating machinery: This drug may have some effect on your driving ability, so it is advisable not to drive or operate machinery while taking it.

FLUPHENAZINE

Brand name: Decazate, Modecate, Moditen, Motipress, Motival

Type of drug: Anti-psychotic

Uses: To treat psychotic disorders - those in which the sufferer loses contact with reality.

How it works: Blocks the production of brain chemicals which contribute to the symptoms of psychosis - hallucinations and delusions.

Possible adverse effects: Dizziness, drowsiness and possible weight gain.

Availability: Available only with a prescription from a doctor.

Other information: Patient must report any rashes that appear while on the medication.

CAUTIONS

Children: This drug is either not recommended for children, or is recommended only for children above a certain age.

Pregnancy and breastfeeding: No specific problems documented, but any medication should be taken with utmost caution by women who are either pregnant or breastfeeding, and only after professional medical or pharmaceutical advice has been sought.

Alcohol: Alcohol should not be consumed, or only consumed with caution - after medical advice has been sought - while you are taking this drug.

Driving and operating machinery: This drug may have some effect on your driving ability, so it is advisable not to drive or operate machinery while taking it.

FLURBIPROFEN
Brand name: Froben SR
Type of drug: Nonsteroidal anti-inflammatory
Uses: Mainly used to treat and relieve pain in rheumatoid arthritis and osteoarthritis. Also used for severe menstrual pain and used in an eye solution to relieve inflammation after eye surgery.
How it works: Has an anti-inflammatory and pain-relieving effect which is useful for the treatment of continuous pain and discomfort.
Possible adverse effects: Headache, dizziness, nausea, oedema.
Availability: Available only with a prescription from a doctor.
Other information: Patient to take drug with food or milk to minimise stomach upset, and to report any unusual side effects.
CAUTIONS
Children: This drug is either not recommended for children, or is recommended only for children above a certain age.
Pregnancy and breastfeeding: This drug is either not recommended for use by women who are pregnant or breastfeeding, or the precise effects are not known and it should therefore only be used with caution and under medical advice.
Alcohol: No known problems if taken with alcohol.
Driving and operating machinery: This drug may have some effect on your driving ability, so it is advisable not to drive or operate machinery while taking it.

FLUTAMIDE
Brand name: Drogenil
Type of drug: Anti-cancer
Uses: The treatment of cancer of the prostate.
How it works: Bombards the tumour with hormones that inhibit its growth.
Possible adverse effects: Tenderness and enlargement of the breasts. Diarrhoea and impotence. Nausea, vomiting, headache, insomnia. Can cause fluid retention, which can aggravate heart disease.
Availability: Available only with a prescription from a doctor.
Other information: Some symptoms of the disease may worsen before the treatment starts to be effective.

CAUTIONS

Children: This drug is either not recommended for children, or is recommended only for children above a certain age.

Pregnancy and breastfeeding: This drug is either not recommended for use by women who are pregnant or breastfeeding, or the precise effects are not known and it should therefore only be used with caution and under medical advice.

Alcohol: No known problems if taken with alcohol.

Driving and operating machinery: There are no commonly reported problems which may impact on the ability to drive or operate machinery. However, many drugs can cause dizziness or drowsiness in a few people, so it is wise to see how the drug affects you before driving or working with dangerous machinery.

FLUTICASONE

Brand name: Cutivate, Flixonase, Flixotide

Type of drug: Corticosteroid

Uses: Treatment of asthma and allergic rhinitis.

How it works: As a corticosteroid drug.

Possible adverse effects: Rare, but can irritate the nasal passages if taken as a spray, or encourage fungal infection of the throat if taken by inhaler. Any burning or irritation should be reported.

Availability: Available only with a prescription from a doctor.

Other information: May be prescribed as an ointment, cream, nasal spray or inhaler. Creams and ointments should be applied sparingly. Keep away from eyes, around genital and rectal area and any skin creases. Rinse mouth after inhaling the steroids. Avoid contact with those infected with chickenpox or measles and consult a doctor if you come into contact with either of these diseases.

CAUTIONS

Children: This drug is either not recommended for children, or is recommended only for children above a certain age.

Pregnancy and breastfeeding: This drug is either not recommended for use by women who are pregnant or breastfeeding, or the precise effects are not known and it should therefore only be used with caution and under medical advice.

Alcohol: No known problems if taken with alcohol.

Driving and operating machinery: There are no commonly reported problems which may impact on the ability to drive or operate machinery. However, many drugs can cause dizziness or drowsiness in a few people, so it is wise to see how the drug affects you before driving or working with dangerous machinery.

FLUVOXAMINE

Brand name: Faverin

Type of drug: Antidepressant

Uses: To treat depression and obsessive-compulsive disorders.

How it works: Affects the balance of chemicals in the brain thought to be connected to the development of obsessive-compulsive problems.

Possible adverse effects: Nausea, vomiting, abdominal pain. Headache, dizziness and insomnia.

Availability: Available only with a prescription from a doctor.

Other information: Smoking may decrease the effectiveness of this drug.

CAUTIONS

Children: This drug is either not recommended for children, or is recommended only for children above a certain age.

Pregnancy and breastfeeding: This drug is either not recommended for use by women who are pregnant or breastfeeding, or the precise effects are not known and it should therefore only be used with caution and under medical advice.

Alcohol: Alcohol should not be consumed, or only consumed with caution - after medical advice has been sought - while you are taking this drug.

Driving and operating machinery: This drug may have some effect on your driving ability, so it is advisable not to drive or operate machinery while taking it.

FOLIC ACID

Brand name: Folic acid (non-proprietary)

Type of drug: Vitamin

Uses: For the treatment of some types of anaemia and the prevention of congenital disorders.

How it works: Stimulates the production of blood cells, which are deficient in anaemia. When taken during the early days of pregnancy it prevents neural tube defects, such as spina bifida, developing in the womb. Also given to people with some types of chronic blood disorders.

Possible adverse effects: Possible allergic rash.

Availability: Available only with a prescription from a doctor.

Other information: Should not be used to treat pernicious anaemia or vitamin B12 deficiencies. Not to be used in cancer patients. Dietary sources of folic acid are available.

CAUTIONS

Children: There are no commonly reported problems associated with prescribing this medication for children.

Pregnancy and breastfeeding: No specific problems documented, but any medication should be taken with utmost caution by women who are either pregnant or breastfeeding, and only after professional medical or pharmaceutical advice has been sought.

Alcohol: No known problems if taken with alcohol.

Driving and operating machinery: There are no commonly reported problems which may impact on the ability to drive or operate machinery. However, many drugs can cause dizziness or drowsiness in a few people, so it is wise to see how the drug affects you before driving or working with dangerous machinery.

FOLLITROPIN ALPHA

Brand name: Gonal-F

Type of drug: Hormone

Uses: In assisted fertility treatments, for women who do not ovulate and who have not responded to other treatments.

How it works: This synthetic hormone stimulates the ovaries to produce eggs.

Possible adverse effects: Rarely, it can lead to an over-stimulation of the ovaries which may result in abdominal swelling and pain, nausea, vomiting and diarrhoea. Multiple pregnancies, pain at the injection site and allergic reactions are also possible.

Availability: Available only with a prescription from a doctor.

Other information: Given by an injection under the surface of the skin.

Should be used with caution by women with ovarian cysts or thyroid disorders.

CAUTIONS

Children: Unlikely to be prescribed.

Pregnancy and breastfeeding: Unlikely to be prescribed.

Alcohol: No known problems if taken with alcohol.

Driving and operating machinery: There are no commonly reported problems which may impact on the ability to drive or operate machinery. However, many drugs can cause dizziness or drowsiness in a few people, so it is wise to see how the drug affects you before driving or working with dangerous machinery.

FORMESTANE

Brand name: Lentaron

Type of drug: Hormone antagonist

Uses: To treat breast cancer in post-menopausal women.

How it works: Starves the tumour of the hormones which are vital to its growth.

Possible adverse effects: Nausea, vomiting, rashes, hot flushes, drowsiness, headache.

Availability: Available only with a prescription from a doctor.

Other information: This medication will usually be given to patients by injection, in hospital. It is not suitable for use in women who have not gone through the menopause.

CAUTIONS

Children: There are no commonly reported problems associated with prescribing this medication for children.

Pregnancy and breastfeeding: This drug is either not recommended for use by women who are pregnant or breastfeeding, or the precise effects are not known and it should therefore only be used with caution and under medical advice.

Alcohol: No known problems if this medication is taken with alcohol, so long as consumption is moderate.

Driving and operating machinery: This drug may have some effect on your driving ability, so it is advisable not to drive or operate machinery while taking it.

FOSCARNET

Brand name: Foscavir

Type of drug: Anti-viral

Uses: Used to treat serious viral infections such as cytomegalovirus, a herpes virus, and retinitis in AIDS patients.

How it works: Affects the DNA to stop the virus from replicating.

Possible adverse effects: Anaemia, nausea, vomiting, diarrhoea, abdominal pain, headache and fatigue.

Availability: Available only with a prescription from a doctor.

Other information: Blood calcium level and kidney function tests need to be carried out every other day. Patient must report any tingling and numbness.

CAUTIONS

Children: This drug is either not recommended for children, or is recommended only for children above a certain age.

Pregnancy and breastfeeding: This drug is either not recommended for use by women who are pregnant or breastfeeding, or the precise effects are not known and it should therefore only be used with caution and under medical advice.

Alcohol: No known problems if taken with alcohol.

Driving and operating machinery: There are no commonly reported problems which may impact on the ability to drive or operate machinery. However, many drugs can cause dizziness or drowsiness in a few people, so it is wise to see how the drug affects you before driving or working with dangerous machinery.

FOSFOMYCIN

Brand name: Monuril

Type of drug: Antibiotic

Uses: To treat urinary tract infections and cystitis which are caused by the E. Coli bacteria.

How it works: Acts on the wall of the bacteria to stop them multiplying.

Possible adverse effects: Headache, nausea, rash.

Availability: Available only with a prescription from a doctor.

Other information: Will usually be prescribed as a sachet of powder which will need to be mixed with water and drunk. The powder should not be taken on its own. Symptoms should improve in two to three days.

CAUTIONS

Children: This drug is either not recommended for children, or is recommended only for children above a certain age.

Pregnancy and breastfeeding: This drug is either not recommended for use by women who are pregnant or breastfeeding, or the precise effects are not known and it should therefore only be used with caution and under medical advice.

Alcohol: No known problems if taken with alcohol.

Driving and operating machinery: There are no commonly reported problems which may impact on the ability to drive or operate machinery. However, many drugs can cause dizziness or drowsiness in a few people, so it is wise to see how the drug affects you before driving or working with dangerous machinery.

FOSINOPRIL

Brand name: Staril

Type of drug: ACE inhibitor

Uses: Used to treat high blood pressure (hypertension) and heart failure.

How it works: Reduces constriction in the arteries and reduces the amount of blood being pumped around the body.

Possible adverse effects: Dizziness, stomach and bowel upsets, palpitations and fatigue. Fever or a sore throat should be reported to a doctor.

Availability: Available only with a prescription from a doctor.

Other information: This medication should be taken one hour before, or two hours after, any food or antacids.

CAUTIONS

Children: This drug is either not recommended for children, or is recommended only for children above a certain age.

Pregnancy and breastfeeding: This drug is either not recommended for use by women who are pregnant or breastfeeding, or the precise effects are not known and it should therefore only be used with caution and under medical advice.

Alcohol: No known problems if taken with alcohol.

Driving and operating machinery: There are no commonly reported problems which may impact on the ability to drive or operate machinery.

However, many drugs can cause dizziness or drowsiness in a few people, so it is wise to see how the drug affects you before driving or working with dangerous machinery.

FRUSEMIDE

Brand name: Dryptal, Froop, Lasix, Rusyde.

Type of drug: Loop diuretic and anti-hypertensive

Uses: Treatment of fluid retention (oedema) which is usually caused by heart failure or lung and kidney disorders.

How it works: Acts on a part of the kidney to promote the excretion of excess fluid and body salts.

Possible adverse effects: Serious problems unlikely, but loss of potassium can lead to muscle cramps and dizziness.

Availability: Available only with a prescription from a doctor.

Other information: You may be advised to wear sunscreens, as some people can develop an increased sensitivity to sunlight which does not occur until 10 days after exposure to the sun.

CAUTIONS

Children: There are no commonly reported problems associated with prescribing this medication for children.

Pregnancy and breastfeeding: This drug is either not recommended for use by women who are pregnant or breastfeeding, or the precise effects are not known and it should therefore only be used with caution.

Alcohol: Alcohol should not be consumed, or only consumed with caution - after medical advice has been sought - while you are taking this drug.

Driving and operating machinery: This drug may have some effect on your driving ability, so it is advisable not to drive or operate machinery while taking it.

GABAPENTIN

Brand name: Neurotin

Type of drug: Anti-epilepsy

Uses: The treatment of epilepsy.

How it works: Acts as an anti-convulsant by damping down the electrical activity which takes place within the brain cells and works to prevent any build-up of electrical activity which could lead to a seizure.

Possible adverse effects: Drowsiness, dizziness, ataxia, fatigue. Headache, nausea, and vomiting.

Availability: Available only with a prescription from a doctor.

Other information: First dose to be taken at bedtime to minimise drowsiness and dizziness. It is not advisable to stop taking this drug suddenly - the dosage should be reduced over at least a week.

CAUTIONS

Children: This drug is either not recommended for children, or is recommended only for children above a certain age.

Pregnancy and breastfeeding: This drug is either not recommended for use by women who are pregnant or breastfeeding, or the precise effects are not known and it should therefore only be used with caution and under medical advice.

Alcohol: No known problems if taken with alcohol.

Driving and operating machinery: This drug may have some effect on your driving ability, so it is advisable not to drive or operate machinery while taking it.

GAMOLENIC ACID

Brand name: Efamast, Epogam, Gamolin, Gamophase

Type of drug: Fatty acid

Uses: Treatment of recurring breast pain which is related to the menstrual cycle.

How it works: Helps with the manufacture of essential cells and chemicals within the body. Relieves breast pain.

Possible adverse effects: Nausea, indigestion, headache.

Availability: Available with or without a prescription (over the counter).

Other information: Available in capsule or liquid form. It may take 8-12 weeks for a beneficial effect to be realised.

CAUTIONS

Children: There are no commonly reported problems associated with prescribing this medication for children.

Pregnancy and breastfeeding: No specific problems documented, but any medication should be taken with utmost caution by women who are either pregnant or breastfeeding, and only after professional medical or pharmaceutical advice has been sought.

Alcohol: No known problems if taken with alcohol.

Driving and operating machinery: There are no commonly reported problems which may impact on the ability to drive or operate machinery. However, many drugs can cause dizziness or drowsiness in a few people so it is wise to see how the drug affects you before driving or working with dangerous machinery.

GANCICLOVIR

Brand name: Cymevene

Type of drug: Anti-viral

Uses: To treat serious infections such as cytomegalovirus, herpes and retinitis.

How it works: Prevents the replication of infected cells.

Possible adverse effects: Blood disorders, rashes, fever, nausea, vomiting, headache, confusion, drowsiness. Any signs of fever, easy bruising or bleeding should be reported immediately.

Availability: Available only with a prescription from a doctor.

Other information: More than one course of this drug may be necessary to keep the infection at bay.

CAUTIONS

Children: This drug is either not recommended for children, or is recommended only for children above a certain age.

Pregnancy and breastfeeding: This drug is either not recommended for use by women who are pregnant or breastfeeding, or the precise effects are not known and it should therefore only be used with caution and under medical advice.

Alcohol: No known problems if taken with alcohol.

Driving and operating machinery: There are no commonly reported problems which may impact on the ability to drive or operate machinery. However, many drugs can cause dizziness or drowsiness in a few people, so it is wise to see how the drug affects you before driving or working with dangerous machinery.

GEMFIBROZIL

Brand name: Lopid

Type of drug: Lipid lowering

Uses: To lower cholesterol and fat levels in the blood in patients for whom a change of diet and other drugs have not worked.

How it works: Reduces the amount of cholesterol in the blood and prevents it from building up again.

Possible adverse effects: Stomach upsets, rash, headache, dizziness.

Availability: Available only with a prescription from a doctor.

Other information: Must not be taken by people with alcohol problems, gallstones or kidney impairment. A fat-lowering diet and exercise regime should be maintained whilst on medication. Take with food to minimise the risk of gastric problems.

CAUTIONS

Children: This drug is either not recommended for children, or is recommended only for children above a certain age.

Pregnancy and breastfeeding: This drug is either not recommended for use by women who are pregnant or breastfeeding, or the precise effects are not known and it should therefore only be used with caution and under medical advice.

Alcohol: Alcohol should not be consumed, or only consumed with caution - after medical advice has been sought - while you are taking this drug.

Driving and operating machinery: There are no commonly reported problems which may impact on the ability to drive or operate machinery. However, many drugs can cause dizziness or drowsiness in a few people, so it is wise to see how the drug affects you before driving or working with dangerous machinery.

GENTAMICIN

Brand name: Cidomycin, Garamycin, Genticin, Minims gentamicin

Type of drug: Antibiotic

Uses: Available as an injection for the treatment of serious infections such as those which affect the lungs, urinary tract, brain (meningitis) and female reproductive system. It is also available as drops and ointment for the treatment of ear and eye infections.

How it works: Binds on to the bacteria and prevents them from replicating.

Possible adverse effects: Seizures, nausea and vomiting, sweatiness and dizziness. The most common side effect of using the creams is a skin irritation, which should be reported.

Availability: Available only with a prescription from a doctor.

Other information: Injections are not recommended if pregnant or breastfeeding. Tests will be taken regularly to monitor the effect of the drug.

CAUTIONS

Children: There are no commonly reported problems associated with prescribing this medication for children.

Pregnancy and breastfeeding: This drug is either not recommended for use by women who are pregnant or breastfeeding, or the precise effects are not known and it should therefore only be used with caution and under medical advice.

Alcohol: No known problems if taken with alcohol.

Driving and operating machinery: There are no commonly reported problems which may impact on the ability to drive or operate machinery. However, many drugs can cause dizziness or drowsiness in a few people, so it is wise to see how the drug affects you before driving or working with dangerous machinery.

GESTRINONE

Brand name: Dimetriose

Type of drug: Endometriosis treatment

Uses: To treat endometriosis.

How it works: Affects the production of hormones in a way that causes the unwanted deposits of endometrial tissue responsible for the symptoms of the condition to shrink.

Possible adverse effects: Fluid retention, weight gain, acne. Stomach and bowel upsets, voice change, change in breast size.

Availability: Available only with a prescription from a doctor.

Other information: Menstruation will stop while you are taking this medication. A barrier method of contraception should be used.

CAUTIONS

Children: This drug is either not recommended for children, or is recommended only for children above a certain age.

Pregnancy and breastfeeding: This drug is either not recommended for use by women who are pregnant or breastfeeding, or the precise effects are

not known and it should therefore only be used with caution and under medical advice.

Alcohol: No known problems if taken with alcohol.

Driving and operating machinery: There are no commonly reported problems which may impact on the ability to drive or operate machinery. However, many drugs can cause dizziness or drowsiness in a few people, so it is wise to see how the drug affects you before driving or working with dangerous machinery.

GESTRONOL

Brand name: Depostat, Gestronol Hexanoate
Type of drug: Progestogens
Uses: To treat cancer of the womb. Also used in males to shrink cancer of the prostate gland.
How it works: As a hormone, affects the ability of the cancer to grow.
Possible adverse effects: Fluid retention, acne, rash, weight gain, breast discomfort, stomach upsets, insomnia depression.
Availability: Available only with a prescription from a doctor.
Other information: Given as an injection.

CAUTIONS

Children: There are no commonly reported problems associated with prescribing this medication for children.

Pregnancy and breastfeeding: No specific problems documented, but any medication should be taken with utmost caution by women who are either pregnant or breastfeeding, and only after professional medical or pharmaceutical advice has been sought.

Alcohol: No known problems if taken with alcohol.

Driving and operating machinery: There are no commonly reported problems which may impact on the ability to drive or operate machinery. However, many drugs can cause dizziness or drowsiness in a few people, so it is wise to see how the drug affects you before driving or working with dangerous machinery.

GLIBENCLAMIDE

Brand name: Calabren, Daonil, Diabetamide, Euglucon, Libanil, Malix, Semi-Daonil

171

Type of drug: Oral anti-diabetic

Uses: Used as treatment and maintenance therapy for people with late (maturity) onset diabetes.

How it works: Stimulates the production of insulin by cells in the pancreas and encourages the body to take up sugar, thereby reducing the amount of sugar in the blood.

Possible adverse effects: These are rare and are usually linked to the level of sugar present in the blood. Feeling faint, weak, confused and sweaty. May have stomach upset and headaches.

Availability: Available only with a prescription from a doctor.

Other information: A low fat, low carbohydrate diet should be adhered to whilst taking this drug. Blood and urine tests will be taken regularly to monitor the effectiveness of the medication regime. The effectiveness of this medication may be reduced at times of severe stress or other injury and so may need to be supplemented with insulin.

CAUTIONS

Children: This drug is either not recommended for children, or is recommended only for children above a certain age.

Pregnancy and breastfeeding: This drug is either not recommended for use by women who are pregnant or breastfeeding, or the precise effects are not known and it should therefore only be used with caution.

Alcohol: Alcohol should not be consumed, or only consumed with caution - after medical advice has been sought - while you are taking this drug.

Driving and operating machinery: This drug may have some effect on your driving ability, so it is advisable not to drive or operate machinery while taking it.

GLICLAZIDE

Brand name: Diamicron

Type of drug: Oral anti-diabetic

Uses: Used as treatment and maintenance therapy for people with late (maturity) onset diabetes.

How it works: Stimulates the production of insulin by cells in the pancreas and encourages the body to take up sugar, thereby reducing the amount of sugar in the blood.

Possible adverse effects: Rare, but include weakness, confusion, sweating and headache.

Availability: Available only with a prescription from a doctor.

Other information: As well as adhering to a low carbohydrate and low fat diet, it is important to exercise regularly while being treated for diabetes. The effectiveness of this medication may be reduced at times of severe stress or injury and so may need to be supplemented with insulin.

CAUTIONS

Children: This drug is either not recommended for children, or is recommended only for children above a certain age.

Pregnancy and breastfeeding: This drug is either not recommended for use by women who are pregnant or breastfeeding, or the precise effects are not known and it should therefore only be used with caution and under medical advice.

Alcohol: Alcohol should not be consumed, or only consumed with caution - after medical advice has been sought - while you are taking this drug.

Driving and operating machinery: This drug may have some effect on your driving ability, so it is advisable not to drive or operate machinery while taking it.

GLUTARALDEHYDE

Brand name: Glutarol, Verucasep

Type of drug: Salicylic acid

Uses: Available as a gel or a liquid to aid the removal of warts.

How it works: Contains a caustic substance which removes the hard layer and underlying layer of the skin where the wart virus has rooted.

Possible adverse effects: May irritate and stain the skin brown.

Availability: Available with or without a prescription (over-the-counter).

Other information: Avoid contact with mouth and eyes. Not to be used on facial or ano-genital warts.

CAUTIONS

Children: This drug is either not recommended for children, or is recommended only for children above a certain age.

Pregnancy and breastfeeding: No specific problems documented, but any medication should be taken with utmost caution by women who are either pregnant or breastfeeding, and only after professional medical or pharmaceutical advice has been sought.

Alcohol: No known problems if taken with alcohol.

Driving and operating machinery: There are no commonly reported problems which may impact on the ability to drive or operate machinery. However, many drugs can cause dizziness or drowsiness in a few people, so it is wise to see how the drug affects you before driving or working with dangerous machinery.

GLYCERYL TRINITRATE (GTN)

Brand name: Coro-nitro, Deponit, Minitran, Nitro-Dur, Nitrolingual, Suscard, Sustac, Transiderm-Nitro

Type of drug: Anti-angina

Uses: To relieve the symptoms of angina. It is not a cure.

How it works: Dilates the blood vessels and enables more blood to reach the heart. It relieves the pain which occurs as the heart muscle is starved of oxygen which is carried by the blood.

Possible adverse effects: Flushing, headache, fainting after first dose.

Availability: Available only with a prescription from a doctor.

Other information: Regular checks on the blood pressure are required with this medication. The drug can be taken in tablet form (slow release), which is placed under the tongue, or as a skin patch, capsule, spray or ointment.

CAUTIONS

Children: This drug is either not recommended for children, or is recommended only for children above a certain age.

Pregnancy and breastfeeding: This drug is either not recommended for use by women who are pregnant or breastfeeding, or the precise effects are not known and it should therefore only be used with caution and under medical advice.

Alcohol: Alcohol should not be consumed, or only consumed with caution - after medical advice has been sought - while you are taking this drug.

Driving and operating machinery: This drug may have some effect on your driving ability, so it is advisable not to drive or operate machinery while taking it.

GONADORELIN

Brand name: GnRH, LH-RH, Fertiral, HRF

Type of drug: Hormone

Uses: Used for treating the absence of periods and infertility problems.

How it works: It increases the levels of certain types of hormones in the blood, with the result that ovulation is stimulated.

Possible adverse effects: Possible nausea, headache, abdominal pain, increased menstrual bleeding.

Availability: Available only with a prescription from a doctor.

Other information: Women taking this drug should be warned that multiple pregnancies are a possibility.

CAUTIONS

Children: This drug is either not recommended for children, or is recommended only for children above a certain age.

Pregnancy and breastfeeding: This drug is either not recommended for use by women who are pregnant or breastfeeding, or the precise effects are not known and it should therefore only be used with caution and under medical advice.

Alcohol: No known problems if taken with alcohol.

Driving and operating machinery: There are no commonly reported problems which may impact on the ability to drive or operate machinery. However, many drugs can cause dizziness or drowsiness in a few people, so it is wise to see how the drug affects you before driving or working with dangerous machinery.

GONADOTROPHIN – See Human Menopausal Gonadotrophins and Chorionic Gonadotrophin

GOSERELIN

Brand name: Zoladex

Type of drug: Gonadorelin analogues

Uses: To treat hormone-related cancers such as those which occur in the prostate and breast. Is also used to treat endometriosis.

How it works: Stimulates changes to hormone levels, thus starving cancerous tumours and preventing the growths which are symptomatic of endometriosis from growing.

Possible adverse effects: Menopause-like symptoms, headache. On rare occasions a rash may appear, which should be reported to a doctor. In both men and women it can lead to a loss of libido.

Availability: Available only with a prescription from a doctor.

Other information: Use a non-hormonal contraceptive whilst on a course of this medication.

CAUTIONS

Children: There are no commonly reported problems associated with prescribing this medication for children.

Pregnancy and breastfeeding: This drug is either not recommended for use by women who are pregnant or breastfeeding, or the precise effects are not known and it should therefore only be used with caution and under medical advice.

Alcohol: No known problems if taken with alcohol.

Driving and operating machinery: There are no commonly reported problems which may impact on the ability to drive or operate machinery. However, many drugs can cause dizziness or drowsiness in a few people, so it is wise to see how the drug affects you before driving or working with dangerous machinery.

GRANISETRON

Brand name: Kytril

Type of drug: Anti-emetic

Uses: To treat nausea and vomiting induced by anti-cancers (chemotherapy) and radiotherapy.

How it works: Blocks the messages to the brain which stimulate the feelings of nausea and instinct to vomit.

Possible adverse effects: Constipation, diarrhoea, headache and rash.

Availability: Available only with a prescription from a doctor.

Other information: Report to a doctor any sign of an anaphylactic reaction such as swelling around the lips and face, difficulty in breathing and a rash.

CAUTIONS

Children: There are no commonly reported problems associated with prescribing this medication for children.

Pregnancy and breastfeeding: This drug is either not recommended for

use by women who are pregnant or breastfeeding, or the precise effects are not known and it should therefore only be used with caution and under medical advice.

Alcohol: No known problems if taken with alcohol.

Driving and operating machinery: There are no commonly reported problems which may impact on the ability to drive or operate machinery. However, many drugs can cause dizziness or drowsiness in a few people, so it is wise to see how the drug affects you before driving or working with dangerous machinery.

GRISEOFULVIN

Brand name: Fulcin, Grisovin

Type of drug: Anti-fungal

Uses: To treat fungal infections of the nails, hair and skin.

How it works: Disrupts the ability of the fungal cell to divide and therefore grow. Also helps the skin to resist the fungus.

Possible adverse effects: Headache, nausea, vomiting, rashes and dizziness. Can alter the taste sensation.

Availability: Available only with a prescription from a doctor.

Other information: Supplied as tablets or capsules. Pregnancy must be avoided until after one month of stopping treatment. Men must not father a child within six months of stopping the treatment. Should be taken around meal times to minimise stomach upset.

CAUTIONS

Children: There are no commonly reported problems associated with prescribing this medication for children.

Pregnancy and breastfeeding: This drug is either not recommended for use by women who are pregnant or breastfeeding, or the precise effects are not known and it should therefore only be used with caution and under medical advice.

Alcohol: Alcohol should not be consumed, or only consumed with caution - after medical advice has been sought - while you are taking this drug.

Driving and operating machinery: This drug may have some effect on your driving ability, so it is advisable not to drive or operate machinery while taking it.

GUANETHIDINE MONOSULPHATE
Brand name: Ismelin
Type of drug: Anti-hypertensive
Uses: To treat moderate to severe high blood pressure and the signs and symptoms of an overactive thyroid gland (thyrotoxicosis).
How it works: Acts on the peripheral parts of the body to prevent the walls of blood vessels constricting, thereby easing the flow of blood through them.
Possible adverse effects: Most common is diarrhoea and a drop in blood pressure which leads to dizziness and faintness. Hot showers and sudden changes of position should be avoided to minimise the possibility of side effects occurring.
Availability: Available only with a prescription from a doctor.
Other information: Take medical advice before taking other over-the-counter preparations. Do not double up on doses if you forget to take one.
CAUTIONS
Children: This drug is either not recommended for children, or is recommended only for children above a certain age.
Pregnancy and breastfeeding: This drug is either not recommended for use by women who are pregnant or breastfeeding, or the precise effects are not known and it should therefore only be used with caution and under medical advice.
Alcohol: No known problems if taken with alcohol.
Driving and operating machinery: This drug may have some effect on your driving ability, so it is advisable not to drive or operate machinery while taking it.

GUAR GUM
Brand name: Guarem
Type of drug: Anti-diabetic
Uses: To help in the treatment of diabetes mellitus.
How it works: Retards carbohydrate absorption, with the result that blood sugar is lowered.
Possible adverse effects: Abdominal discomfort, including flatulence and swelling.
Availability: Available with or without a prescription (over the counter).

Other information: It is important to maintain an adequate fluid intake whilst taking this medication. As this preparation swells when it comes into contact with liquid it should be carefully swallowed with water and not taken immediately before bedtime.

CAUTIONS

Children: There are no commonly reported problems associated with prescribing this medication for children.

Pregnancy and breastfeeding: No specific problems documented, but any medication should be taken with utmost caution by women who are either pregnant or breastfeeding, and only after professional medical or pharmaceutical advice has been sought.

Alcohol: No known problems if taken with alcohol.

Driving and operating machinery: There are no commonly reported problems which may impact on the ability to drive or operate machinery. However, many drugs can cause dizziness or drowsiness in a few people, so it is wise to see how the drug affects you before driving or working with dangerous machinery.

HALOFANTRINE

Brand name: Halfan

Type of drug: Anti-malarial

Uses: To treat some types of malarial infections - P.Falciparum and P.Vivax. It is not an effective protection against malarial infection.

How it works: Interrupts the cycle of the disease.

Possible adverse effects: Possible heart rhythm disturbances, diarrhoea, abdominal pain, nausea and vomiting.

Availability: Available only with a prescription from a doctor.

Other information: Stop drug immediately if sore throat, itching and skin rash occur.

CAUTIONS

Children: There are no commonly reported problems associated with prescribing this medication for children.

Pregnancy and breastfeeding: This drug is either not recommended for use by women who are pregnant or breastfeeding, or the precise effects are not known and it should therefore only be used with caution and under medical advice.

Alcohol: No known problems if taken with alcohol.

Driving and operating machinery: There are no commonly reported problems which may impact on the ability to drive or operate machinery. However, many drugs can cause dizziness or drowsiness in a few people, so it is wise to see how the drug affects you before driving or working with dangerous machinery.

HALOPERIDOL

Brand name: Dozic, Haldol, Serenace

Type of drug: Anti-psychotic

Uses: To treat schizophrenia, manias and dementia. Also a short-term treatment for severe anxiety.

How it works: Reduces the violent and aggressive symptoms of schizophrenia and other illnesses where delusions and hallucinations occur. It controls the symptoms rather than curing the disease.

Possible adverse effects: Side effects experienced are abnormal involuntary movements and stiffness of face and limbs, headaches, confusion, dizziness and drowsiness.

Availability: Available only with a prescription from a doctor.

Other information: This drug should not be used at the same time as other anti-depressants.

CAUTIONS

Children: This drug is either not recommended for children, or is recommended only for children above a certain age.

Pregnancy and breastfeeding: This drug is either not recommended for use by women who are pregnant or breastfeeding, or the precise effects are not known and it should therefore only be used with caution and under medical advice.

Alcohol: Alcohol should not be consumed, or only consumed with caution - after medical advice has been sought - while you are taking this drug.

Driving and operating machinery: This drug may have some effect on your driving ability, so it is advisable not to drive or operate machinery while taking it.

HEPARIN

Brand name: Calciparine, Minihep, Monoparin, Multiparin, Uniparin; LMWH Clexane, Fragmin, Innohep

Type of drug: Anti-coagulant

Uses: Prevents formation of blood clots and assists in their breakdown.

How it works: Dissolves existing blood clots before they can reach vital organs such as the brain. It can also be used to prevent blood clots forming during procedures such as surgery and dialysis.

Possible adverse effects: Excessive bleeding is a risk, so the dosage will be monitored carefully. Bruising may appear around the site of the injection.

Availability: Available only with a prescription from a doctor.

Other information: Heparin will usually only be given in hospital, by injection. Patient must avoid aspirin and aspirin derivatives.

CAUTIONS

Children: There are no commonly reported problems associated with prescribing this medication for children.

Pregnancy and breastfeeding: This drug is either not recommended for use by women who are pregnant or breastfeeding, or the precise effects are not known and it should therefore only be used with caution and under medical advice.

Alcohol: No known problems if taken with alcohol.

Driving and operating machinery: This drug may have some effect on your driving ability, so it is advisable not to drive or operate machinery while taking it.

HEXAMINE HIPPURATE

Brand name: Hiprex

Type of drug: Anti-fungal

Uses: To treat recurrent infections of the urinary system.

How it works: Forms formaldehyde in the urine, in which the infected organisms cannot survive.

Possible adverse effects: Stomach and bowel upsets, bladder irritation and rash.

Availability: Available only with a prescription from a doctor.

Other information: Administered in tablet form. This drug is now only used rarely.

CAUTIONS

Children: There are no commonly reported problems associated with prescribing this medication for children.

Pregnancy and breastfeeding: This drug is either not recommended for use by women who are pregnant or breastfeeding, or the precise effects are not known and it should therefore only be used with caution and under medical advice.

Alcohol: No known problems if taken with alcohol.

Driving and operating machinery: There are no commonly reported problems which may impact on the ability to drive or operate machinery. However, many drugs can cause dizziness or drowsiness in a few people, so it is wise to see how the drug affects you before driving or working with dangerous machinery.

HOMATROPINE

Brand name: Minims homatropine

Type of drug: Anti-cholinergic

Uses: Preparation for eye surgery.

How it works: Affects the muscles within the eye, with the result that the pupil is dilated and remains so for around 12 hours.

Possible adverse effects: Local irritation and stinging

Availability: Available only with a prescription from a doctor.

Other information: Not to be used for patients with closed-angle glaucoma.

CAUTIONS

Children: This drug is either not recommended for children, or is recommended only for children above a certain age.

Pregnancy and breastfeeding: This drug is either not recommended for use by women who are pregnant or breastfeeding, or the precise effects are not known and it should therefore only be used with caution and under medical advice.

Alcohol: No known problems if taken with alcohol.

Driving and operating machinery: This drug may have some effect on your driving ability, so it is advisable not to drive or operate machinery while taking it.

HUMAN MENOPAUSAL GONADOTROPHINS

Brand name: Humegon, Normegon, Pergonal, Menogon

Type of drug: Gonadotrophin

Uses: To treat infertility due to an insufficiency of the pituitary gland; also given to women who have not responded to other infertility treatments.

How it works: Stimulates the ovaries. The preparation is produced from purified extracts of urine from women who have passed the menopause.

Possible adverse effects: Headache, fatigue, irritability, depression.

Availability: Available only with a prescription from a doctor.

Other information: Patient must be told about possibility of multiple pregnancy.

CAUTIONS

Children: There are no commonly reported problems associated with prescribing this medication for children.

Pregnancy and breastfeeding: No specific problems documented, but any medication should be taken with utmost caution by women who are either pregnant or breastfeeding, and only after professional medical or pharmaceutical advice has been sought.

Alcohol: No known problems if taken with alcohol.

Driving and operating machinery: There are no commonly reported problems which may impact on the ability to drive or operate machinery. However, many drugs can cause dizziness or drowsiness in a few people, so it is wise to see how the drug affects you before driving or working with dangerous machinery.

HYDRALAZINE

Brand name: Apresoline

Type of drug: Anti-hypertensive

Uses: To treat moderate to severe high blood pressure.

How it works: Acts on the smooth muscle of the veins and has a relaxant effect which causes the blood pressure to fall.

Possible adverse effects: Increase in heart rate, fluid retention, nausea, vomiting, headache.

Availability: Available only with a prescription from a doctor.

Other information: Take medication with meals to enhance drug absorption and minimise gastric irritation.

CAUTIONS

Children: This drug is either not recommended for children, or is recommended only for children above a certain age.

Pregnancy and breastfeeding: This drug is either not recommended for use by women who are pregnant or breastfeeding, or the precise effects are not known and it should therefore only be used with caution and under medical advice.

Alcohol: No known problems if taken with alcohol.

Driving and operating machinery: This drug may have some effect on your driving ability, so it is advisable not to drive or operate machinery while taking it.

HYDROCHLOROTHIAZIDE

Brand name: HydroSaluric
Type of drug: Diuretic
Uses: Used to treat fluid retention (oedema) in people who have heart failure, kidney, liver or pre-menstrual problems. Is also used as a treatment for high blood pressure.
How it works: Affects the kidneys, with the result that the excretion of sodium and water is increased and the excess passed out.
Possible adverse effects: Rare, except if associated with an excess loss of potassium. Possible stomach and bowel upsets.
Availability: Available only with a prescription from a doctor.
Other information: Take medication with food to avoid gastric upset. To avoid having to pass water during the night, do not take at bedtime. Do not take any over-the-counter medication without first discussing it with your doctor.
CAUTIONS
Children: There are no commonly reported problems associated with prescribing this medication for children.
Pregnancy and breastfeeding: This drug is either not recommended for use by women who are pregnant or breastfeeding, or the precise effects are not known and it should therefore only be used with caution and under medical advice.
Alcohol: Alcohol should not be consumed, or only consumed with caution - after medical advice has been sought - while you are taking this drug.
Driving and operating machinery: This drug may have some effect on your driving ability, so it is advisable not to drive or operate machinery while taking it.

HYDROCORTISONE

Brand name: Colifoam, Corlan, Dioderm, Efcortelan, Efcortesol, Hydrocortistab, Hydrocortisyl, Hydrocortone, Solu-Cortef

Type of drug: Corticosteroid

Uses: Used to suppress allergies and severe inflammations.

How it works: Replaces natural hormones where the adrenal glands are not producing sufficient quantities. Suppresses inflammatory reaction in other conditions.

Possible adverse effects: Indigestion, abdominal discomfort, weight gain, acne. Prolonged high dosage of this medication can produce serious side effects such as diabetes and glaucoma, so is avoided where possible.

Availability: Prescription needed except for preparations.

Other information: People on long-term treatment are advised to carry a treatment card in case of emergency. Regular checks will be made on blood pressure if hydrocortisone is being given by mouth.

CAUTIONS

Children: There are no commonly reported problems associated with prescribing this medication for children.

Pregnancy and breastfeeding: No specific problems documented, but any medication should be taken with utmost caution by women who are either pregnant or breastfeeding, and only after professional medical or pharmaceutical advice has been sought.

Alcohol: Alcohol should not be consumed, or only consumed with caution - after medical advice has been sought - while you are taking this drug.

Driving and operating machinery: There are no commonly reported problems which may impact on the ability to drive or operate machinery. However, many drugs can cause dizziness or drowsiness in a few people, so it is wise to see how the drug affects you before driving or working with dangerous machinery.

HYDROXOCOBALAMIN

Brand name: Cobalin-H, Neo-Cytamen

Type of drug: Vitamin

Uses: Used to treat pernicious anaemia and other vitamin B12 deficient anaemias.

How it works: Replaces the vitamin B12, which is deficient in people suffering with anaemia.

Possible adverse effects: Itching, hot flushes, nausea and dizziness. Rarely, allergic reactions may occur.

Availability: Available only with a prescription from a doctor.

Other information: Administered as an injection. Treatment will usually be for life.

CAUTIONS

Children: There are no commonly reported problems associated with prescribing this medication for children.

Pregnancy and breastfeeding: No specific problems documented, but any medication should be taken with utmost caution by women who are either pregnant or breastfeeding, and only after professional medical or pharmaceutical advice has been sought.

Alcohol: No known problems if taken with alcohol.

Driving and operating machinery: There are no commonly reported problems which may impact on the ability to drive or operate machinery. However, many drugs can cause dizziness or drowsiness in a few people, so it is wise to see how the drug affects you before driving or working with dangerous machinery.

HYDROXYAPATITE

Brand name: Ossopan

Type of drug: Calcium and phosphorous supplement

Uses: To treat calcium deficiency.

How it works: Replaces calcium which is lost through disorders such as osteoporosis, rickets and osteomalacia and through inadequate intake in the diet. It may also be used during breastfeeding.

Possible adverse effects: Mild gastro-intestinal disturbances, changes to the heart rhythm.

Availability: Available with or without a prescription (over the counter).

Other information: Can be given in tablet or injection form. This drug will not be used for people who have a history of kidney problems.

CAUTIONS

Children: There are no commonly reported problems associated with prescribing this medication for children.

Pregnancy and breastfeeding: No specific problems documented, but any medication should be taken with utmost caution by women who are either pregnant or breastfeeding, and only after professional medical or pharmaceutical advice has been sought.

Alcohol: No known problems if taken with alcohol.

Driving and operating machinery: There are no commonly reported problems which may impact on the ability to drive or operate machinery. However, many drugs can cause dizziness or drowsiness in a few people, so it is wise to see how the drug affects you before driving or working with dangerous machinery.

HYDROXYPROGESTERONE

Brand name: Proluton Depot

Type of drug: Female sex hormone

Uses: To treat problems such as amenorrhoea (absence of periods), uterine bleeding and recurrent miscarriages.

How it works: Replaces hormones, the lack of which is thought to be contributing to the problem.

Possible adverse effects: Fluid retention and weight gain. May rarely cause coughing and difficulty in breathing.

Availability: Available only with a prescription from a doctor.

Other information: Must not become pregnant during therapy. There is some debate as to the effectiveness of this kind of treatment.

CAUTIONS

Children: There are no commonly reported problems associated with prescribing this medication for children.

Pregnancy and breastfeeding: This drug is either not recommended for use by women who are pregnant or breastfeeding, or the precise effects are not known and it should therefore only be used with caution and under medical advice.

Alcohol: No known problems if taken with alcohol.

Driving and operating machinery: There are no commonly reported problems which may impact on the ability to drive or operate machinery. However, many drugs can cause dizziness or drowsiness in a few people, so it is wise to see how the drug affects you before driving or working with dangerous machinery.

HYOSCINE

Brand name: Buscopan, Joy-Rides, Kwells, Scopoderm TTS, Travel Calm

Type of drug: Anti-cholinergic

Uses: To treat irritable bowel spasms and motion sickness. Also an ingredient in eye drops.

How it works: Slows down the gut and reduces the secretion of gastric acid.

Possible adverse effects: Drowsiness, dry mouth.

Availability: Available without a prescription (over the counter).

Other information: Can cause constipation, so the intake of fluid should be kept high whilst taking this medication.

CAUTIONS

Children: This drug is either not recommended for children, or is recommended only for children above a certain age.

Pregnancy and breastfeeding: This drug is either not recommended for use by women who are pregnant or breastfeeding, or the precise effects are not known and it should therefore only be used with caution and under medical advice.

Alcohol: Alcohol should not be consumed, or only consumed with caution - after medical advice has been sought - while you are taking this drug.

Driving and operating machinery: This drug may have some effect on your driving ability, so it is advisable not to drive or operate machinery while taking it.

IBUPROFEN

Brand name: Arthrofen, Brufen, Ebufac, Fenbid, Ibufac, Ibugel, Ibuleve, Inoven, Motrin, Nurofen

Type of drug: Non-steroidal anti-inflammatory

Uses: Treatment of the symptoms of conditions such as osteo- and rheumatoid arthritis, back pain and gout. Also effective for headaches, menstrual pain, soft tissue injuries and backache,

How it works: Relieves pain, inflammation and stiffness.

Possible adverse effects: Heartburn and indigestion, which can be minimised by taking it with food or milk. Rarely, Ibuprofen can cause nausea and vomiting.

Availability: Available with or without a prescription (over the counter).

Other information: Available as tablets, slow release tablets, capsules, liquid, granules or cream.

CAUTIONS

Children: There are no commonly reported problems associated with prescribing this medication for children.

Pregnancy and breastfeeding: This drug is either not recommended for use by women who are pregnant or breastfeeding, or the precise effects are not known and it should therefore only be used with caution and under medical advice.

Alcohol: Alcohol should not be consumed, or only consumed with caution - after medical advice has been sought - while you are taking this drug.

Driving and operating machinery: There are no commonly reported problems which may impact on the ability to drive or operate machinery. However, many drugs can cause dizziness or drowsiness in a few people, so it is wise to see how the drug affects you before driving or working with dangerous machinery.

IDARUBICIN

Brand name: Zavedos

Type of drug: Anti-cancer

Uses: To part-treat some types of leukaemia; used with other medications.

How it works: Inhibits part of the chemical process which takes place as the disease progresses.

Possible adverse effects: Headache, nausea, vomiting, cramps, diarrhoea, hair loss, fever, rash on palms and soles. Patients are at an increased risk of infection whilst on this treatment, so symptoms such as a sore throat or fever should be reported immediately. Increased risk of bleeding.

Availability: Available only with a prescription from a doctor.

Other information: Administered as an intravenous infusion (drip).

CAUTIONS

Children: This drug is either not recommended for children, or is recommended only for children above a certain age.

Pregnancy and breastfeeding: This drug is either not recommended for use by women who are pregnant or breastfeeding, or the precise effects are not known and it should therefore only be used with caution and under medical advice.

Alcohol: Alcohol should not be consumed, or only consumed with caution - after medical advice has been sought - while you are taking this drug.

Driving and operating machinery: There are no commonly reported problems which may impact on the ability to drive or operate machinery. However, many drugs can cause dizziness or drowsiness in a few people, so it is wise to see how the drug affects you before driving or working with dangerous machinery.

IDOXURIDINE

Brand name: Herpid, Iduridin

Type of drug: Anti-viral

Uses: Treatment of herpes infections of the eye.

How it works: Blocks the ability of the virus to reproduce.

Possible adverse effects: These occur rarely, but adverse effects include irritation, burning and pain in the eye. A mild swelling of the eyelid may also be experienced. Any signs of an adverse reaction should be reported immediately.

Availability: Available only with a prescription from a doctor.

Other information: Administered as eye drops. Not recommended for long-term use because of the risk of eye damage. Do not mix with any other solutions or medication. Avoid sharing towels and flannels with others to prevent the infection from spreading. Always wash hands before and after application.

CAUTIONS

Children: This drug is either not recommended for children, or is recommended only for children above a certain age.

Pregnancy and breastfeeding: This drug is either not recommended for use by women who are pregnant or breastfeeding, or the precise effects are not known and it should therefore only be used with caution and under medical advice.

Alcohol: No known problems if taken with alcohol.

Driving and operating machinery: There are no commonly reported problems which may impact on the ability to drive or operate machinery. However, many drugs can cause dizziness or drowsiness in a few people, so it is wise to see how the drug affects you before driving or working with dangerous machinery.

IMIPRAMINE

Brand name: Tofranil

Type of drug: Tricyclic anti-depressant

Uses: Prescribed for the long-term treatment of depression. It is also sometimes prescribed to treat children who have a night-time bedwetting problem.

How it works: A tricyclic anti-depressant which helps to improve mood and appetite at the same time as stimulating an interest in everyday activities which usually diminishes with depression.

Possible adverse effects: Sweating, dry mouth, blurred vision and constipation. Should be taken with milk or food if it appears to upset the stomach.

Availability: Available only with a prescription from a doctor.

Other information: The full effects of the drug may not be experienced for up to four weeks after starting treatment. Less sedating than many anti-depressants. An overdose should be treated as a medical emergency.

CAUTIONS

Children: There are no commonly reported problems associated with prescribing this medication for children.

Pregnancy and breastfeeding: This drug is either not recommended for use by women who are pregnant or breastfeeding, or the precise effects are not known and it should therefore only be used with caution and under medical advice.

Alcohol: Alcohol should not be consumed, or only consumed with caution - after medical advice has been sought - while you are taking this drug.

Driving and operating machinery: There are no commonly reported problems which may impact on the ability to drive or operate machinery. However, many drugs can cause dizziness or drowsiness in a few people, so it is wise to see how the drug affects you before driving or working with dangerous machinery.

INDAPAMIDE

Brand name: Natrilix

Type of drug: Diuretic

Uses: For the treatment of high blood pressure and oedema due to heart failure.

How it works: Affects the kidneys and encourages excess water to be expelled from the body.

Possible adverse effects: Headache, dizziness and vertigo, particularly on standing up. Occasionally a rash may appear.

Availability: Available only with a prescription from a doctor.

Other information: Will be dispensed as tablets.

CAUTIONS

Children: This drug is either not recommended for children, or is recommended only for children above a certain age.

Pregnancy and breastfeeding: This drug is either not recommended for use by women who are pregnant or breastfeeding, or the precise effects are not known and it should therefore only be used with caution and under medical advice.

Alcohol: No known problems if taken with alcohol.

Driving and operating machinery: There are no commonly reported problems which may impact on the ability to drive or operate machinery. However, many drugs can cause dizziness or drowsiness in a few people, so it is wise to see how the drug affects you before driving or working with dangerous machinery.

INDOMETHACIN

Brand name: Artracin, Flexin Continus, Imbrilon, Indocid, Indolar, Maximet, Mobilan, Rheumacin LA , Slo-Indo

Type of drug: Non-steroidal anti-inflammatory, gout treatment

Uses: Treatment of conditions such as rheumatoid arthritis, osteoarthritis, ankylosing spondylitis, gout and bursitis.

How it works: Has an anti-inflammatory effect.

Possible adverse effects: As with all non-steroidal anti-inflammatories, there is a risk of irritation of the gut. Also, headaches, dizziness and nausea.

Availability: Available only with a prescription from a doctor.

Other information: Do not take aspirin or similar medication without consulting a doctor first.

CAUTIONS

Children: This drug is either not recommended for children, or is recommended only for children above a certain age.

Pregnancy and breastfeeding: This drug is either not recommended for

use by women who are pregnant or breastfeeding, or the precise effects are not known and it should therefore only be used with caution and under medical advice.

Alcohol: Alcohol should not be consumed, or only consumed with caution - after medical advice has been sought - while you are taking this drug.

Driving and operating machinery: This drug may have some effect on your driving ability, so it is advisable not to drive or operate machinery while taking it.

INOSINE PRANOBEX
Brand name: Imunovir
Type of drug: Anti-viral
Uses: Given by mouth to treat infections caused by the herpes virus, including herpes simplex and genital herpes. Can also be used to treat some brain infections caused by the virus.
How it works: Attacks the virus, but does not eradicate it.
Possible adverse effects: Nausea, vomiting, headache, dizziness.
Availability: Available only with a prescription from a doctor.
Other information: The course of treatment is likely to last for up to a month for genital herpes infections and for 14 days for other infections.
CAUTIONS
Children: This drug is either not recommended for children, or is recommended only for children above a certain age.
Pregnancy and breastfeeding: This drug is either not recommended for use by women who are pregnant or breastfeeding, or the precise effects are not known and it should therefore only be used with caution.
Alcohol: No known problems if taken with alcohol.
Driving and operating machinery: There are no commonly reported problems which may impact on the ability to drive or operate machinery. However, many drugs can cause dizziness or drowsiness in a few people, so it is wise to see how the drug affects you before driving or working with dangerous machinery.

INSULIN
Brand name: Humalog, Human Actrapid, Human Insulatard, Human

Mixtard, Human Monotard, Human Ultratard, Human Velosulin, Humulin, Hypurin, Lentard MC, Pork Insulatard, Pork Mixtard, Pork Velosulin, Rapitard MC, Semitard MC

Type of drug: Anti-diabetic

Uses: Treatment of diabetes mellitus. It is the only effective treatment for juvenile onset diabetes.

How it works: Provides the body with the hormone insulin, which is made in the pancreas and which is lacking in diabetics. Insulin is crucial if the body is to be able to metabolise and use sugar.

Possible adverse effects: Most of the adverse effects are associated with a low blood sugar level (hypoglycaemia), and include light-headedness, confusion, sweating and dizziness. These can usually be prevented by a correction to the dose. Serious allergic reactions are rare.

Availability: Available only with a prescription from a doctor.

Other information: An overdose should be reported to a doctor immediately. People prescribed insulin should carry some kind of warning card. Do not take any other medication without consulting a doctor, as it may contain sugar.

CAUTIONS

Children: There are no commonly reported problems associated with prescribing this medication for children.

Pregnancy and breastfeeding: No specific problems documented, but any medication should be taken with utmost caution by women who are either pregnant or breastfeeding, and only after professional medical or pharmaceutical advice has been sought.

Alcohol: Alcohol should not be consumed, or only consumed with caution - after medical advice has been sought - while you are taking this drug.

Driving and operating machinery: There are no commonly reported problems which may impact on the ability to drive or operate machinery. However, many drugs can cause dizziness or drowsiness in a few people, so it is wise to see how the drug affects you before driving or working with dangerous machinery.

INTERFERON

Brand name: Betaferon, Immukin, Intron-A, Roferon-A, Viraferon, Wellferon

Type of drug: Anti-viral and anticancer

Uses: There are three types of Interferon. Interferon Alpha is used to treat leukaemias, some cancers and active hepatitis. Interferon Beta is used for multiple sclerosis. Interferon gamma is used with antibiotics for people with granulomatous disease.

How it works: Interferon are substances which have been infected by viruses and are effective at resisting other types of infections.

Possible adverse effects: Headache, listlessness, dizziness and sleepiness, digestive upsets and fever are relatively common.

Availability: Available only with a prescription from a doctor.

Other information: Administered as an injection in hospital. Frequent blood tests will be taken to monitor the impact of this medication.

CAUTIONS

Children: This drug is either not recommended for children, or is recommended only for children above a certain age.

Pregnancy and breastfeeding: This drug is either not recommended for use by women who are pregnant or breastfeeding, or the precise effects are not known and it should therefore only be used with caution and under medical advice.

Alcohol: No known problems if taken with alcohol.

Driving and operating machinery: There are no commonly reported problems which may impact on the ability to drive or operate machinery. However, many drugs can cause dizziness or drowsiness in a few people, so it is wise to see how the drug affects you before driving or working with dangerous machinery.

IPECACUANHA

Brand name: Ipecacuanha Emetic Mixture, Paediatric

Type of drug: Emetic

Uses: Used to induce vomiting in people who have either deliberately or accidentally swallowed poisonous substances.

How it works: Irritates the lining of the gut to the point where vomiting occurs. It usually results in the stomach being completely empty within 30 minutes of ingesting dose.

Possible adverse effects: Irritates the digestive system, so can lead to vomiting and diarrhoea.

Availability: Available with or without a prescription (over-the-counter).

Other information: This drug will only be used with caution and should never be used in people who are not conscious. Should be taken with water, with a dose repeated after 20 minutes if necessary.

CAUTIONS

Children: There are no commonly reported problems associated with prescribing this medication for children.

Pregnancy and breastfeeding: No specific problems documented, but any medication should be taken with utmost caution by women who are either pregnant or breastfeeding, and only after professional medical or pharmaceutical advice has been sought.

Alcohol: No known problems if taken with alcohol.

Driving and operating machinery: There are no commonly reported problems which may impact on the ability to drive or operate machinery. However, many drugs can cause dizziness or drowsiness in a few people, so it is wise to see how the drug affects you before driving or working with dangerous machinery.

IPRATROPIUM BROMIDE

Brand name: Atrovent, Rinatec

Type of drug: Bronchodilator

Uses: Treatment of lung problems such as chronic bronchitis.

How it works: Usually given by nebuliser or inhaler to relax the muscles of the airways to aid easier breathing. Also prescribed as a nasal spray for the treatment of a persistent runny nose due to an allergic reaction.

Possible adverse effects: Rare, except for dry mouth and throat.

Availability: Available only with a prescription from a doctor.

Other information: Should be used with caution by people with glaucoma.

CAUTIONS

Children: There are no commonly reported problems associated with prescribing this medication for children.

Pregnancy and breastfeeding: No specific problems documented, but any medication should be taken with utmost caution by women who are either pregnant or breastfeeding, and only after professional medical or pharmaceutical advice has been sought.

Alcohol: No known problems if taken with alcohol.

Driving and operating machinery: There are no commonly reported problems which may impact on the ability to drive or operate machinery. However, many drugs can cause dizziness or drowsiness in a few people, so it is wise to see how the drug affects you before driving or working with dangerous machinery.

ISOCARBOXAZID

Brand name: Isocarboxazid
Type of drug: Anti-depressant
Uses: To treat depressive illness.
How it works: Enables people with depressive illnesses to lead more normal lives.
Possible adverse effects: Can interact with certain types of food such as cheese, pickled herring, broad beans, Bovril, Oxo and Marmite to cause a headache and high blood pressure. These foods should therefore be avoided. Hypotension (low blood pressure) leading to feelings of dizziness. Also drowsiness, dryness of the mouth.
Availability: Available only with a prescription from a doctor.
Other information: Do not eat any food which you do not believe to be fresh whilst on this medication.
CAUTIONS
Children: This drug is either not recommended for children, or is recommended only for children above a certain age.
Pregnancy and breastfeeding: No specific problems documented, but any medication should be taken with utmost caution by women who are either pregnant or breastfeeding, and only after professional medical or pharmaceutical advice has been sought.
Alcohol: Alcohol should not be consumed, or only consumed with caution - after medical advice has been sought - while you are taking this drug.
Driving and operating machinery: This drug may have some effect on your driving ability, so it is advisable not to drive or operate machinery while taking it.

ISONIAZID

Brand name: Rimifon
Type of drug: Anti-tuberculous drug

Uses: Used on its own to prevent tuberculosis and in conjunction with other drugs as a treatment for the disease.

How it works: Interferes with the cell wall of the bacteria to stop them reproducing.

Possible adverse effects: Problems are rare but should be reported because of the risk of liver damage.

Availability: Available only with a prescription from a doctor.

Other information: Therapy is likely to continue for at least 18 months. Should be taken on an empty stomach. Medical advice should always be sought if an overdose is taken.

CAUTIONS

Children: There are no commonly reported problems associated with prescribing this medication for children.

Pregnancy and breastfeeding: This drug is either not recommended for use by women who are pregnant or breastfeeding, or the precise effects are not known and it should therefore only be used with caution.

Alcohol: Alcohol should not be consumed, or only consumed with caution - after medical advice has been sought - while you are taking this drug.

Driving and operating machinery: There are no commonly reported problems which may impact on the ability to drive or operate machinery. However, many drugs can cause dizziness or drowsiness in a few people, so it is wise to see how the drug affects you before driving or working with dangerous machinery.

ISOPRENALINE

Brand name: Medihaler-iso, Saventrine

Type of drug: Bronchodilator

Uses: To treat the symptoms of lung conditions such as asthma, bronchitis and emphysema. It also improves the transmission of electrical signals that take place in the heart.

How it works: Expands the small air passages in the lungs and relieves bronchospasm. If given as an injection, can treat some heart conditions.

Possible adverse effects: Side effects such as dry mouth, tremor and agitation usually disappear once the body has become used to the drug. Palpitations should be reported to a doctor.

Availability: Available only with a prescription from a doctor.

Other information: Seek medical attentions in all cases of overdose.

CAUTIONS

Children: There are no commonly reported problems associated with prescribing this medication for children.

Pregnancy and breastfeeding: This drug is either not recommended for use by women who are pregnant or breastfeeding, or the precise effects are not known and it should therefore only be used with caution and under medical advice.

Alcohol: No known problems if taken with alcohol.

Driving and operating machinery: This drug may have some effect on your driving ability, so it is advisable not to drive or operate machinery while taking it.

ISOSORBIDE DINITRATE/MONONITRATE

Brand name: Dinitrate Cedocard, Imtack, Isoket, Isordil, Soni-slo, Sorbichew, Sorbid SA, Sorbitrate; Mononitrate Elantan, Imdur, Ismo, Isotrate, MCR-50, Monit, Mono-Cedocard

Type of drug: Nitrate vasodilator and anti-angina

Uses: Treatment of angina and occasionally heart failure.

How it works: Acts to dilate the blood vessels around the heart, enabling the blood to flow more freely and oxygen to reach the heart.

Possible adverse effects: Headache, dizziness and flushing are relatively common, but usually pass off. Occasionally a sudden drop in blood pressure occurs.

Availability: Available only with a prescription from a doctor.

Other information: Blood pressure will be regularly monitored.

CAUTIONS

Children: This drug is either not recommended for children, or is recommended only for children above a certain age.

Pregnancy and breastfeeding: This drug is either not recommended for use by women who are pregnant or breastfeeding, or the precise effects are not known and it should therefore only be used with caution and under medical advice.

Alcohol: Alcohol should not be consumed, or only consumed with caution - after advice has been sought from a medical practitioner - while you are taking this drug.

Driving and operating machinery: There are no commonly reported problems which may impact on the ability to drive or operate machinery. However, many drugs can cause dizziness or drowsiness in a few people, so it is wise to see how the drug affects you before driving or working with dangerous machinery.

ISOTRETINOIN

Brand name: Isotrex, Roaccutane

Type of drug: Acne treatment

Uses: Treatment of severe acne which has not responded to other types of treatment.

How it works: Reduces the production of skin oils by the sebaceous glands. Also has an anti-inflammatory action.

Possible adverse effects: Most people experience dryness of the eye, nose and mouth, together with flaking skin. Any episodes of abdominal pain and diarrhoea or bloody faeces should be reported immediately.

Availability: Available only with a prescription from a doctor.

Other information: A course of treatment usually lasts for 16-20 weeks. Should be taken with, or shortly after, meals, to minimise gastric discomfort. Women should take extra care to avoid pregnancy whilst on this medication.

CAUTIONS

Children: This drug is either not recommended for children, or is recommended only for children above a certain age.

Pregnancy and breastfeeding: This drug is either not recommended for use by women who are pregnant or breastfeeding, or the precise effects are not known and it should therefore only be used with caution and under medical advice.

Alcohol: Alcohol should not be consumed, or only consumed with caution - after medical advice has been sought - while you are taking this drug.

Driving and operating machinery: There are no commonly reported problems which may impact on the ability to drive or operate machinery. However, many drugs can cause dizziness or drowsiness in a few people, so it is wise to see how the drug affects you before driving or working with dangerous machinery.

ISPAGHULA HUSK

Brand name: Fybogel, Fybozest, Isogel, Manevac, Regulan, Konsyl

Type of drug: Laxative

Uses: To relieve the constipation associated with conditions such as haemorrhoids, colostomy, ileostomy, diverticular disease and irritable bowel syndrome.

How it works: Increases the bulk passing through the gut, thus accelerating the rate at which food is digested and making stools easier to pass.

Possible adverse effects: Wind, abdominal swelling.

Availability: Available with or without a prescription (over-the-counter).

Other information: Large amounts of fluid should be taken to prevent blockage. Do not take just before bedtime.

CAUTIONS

Children: There are no commonly reported problems associated with prescribing this medication for children.

Pregnancy and breastfeeding: No specific problems documented, but any medication should be taken with utmost caution by women who are either pregnant or breastfeeding, and only after professional medical or pharmaceutical advice has been sought.

Alcohol: No known problems if taken with alcohol.

Driving and operating machinery: There are no commonly reported problems which may impact on the ability to drive or operate machinery. However, many drugs can cause dizziness or drowsiness in a few people, so it is wise to see how the drug affects you before driving or working with dangerous machinery.

ISRADIPINE

Brand name: Prescal

Type of drug: Anti-emetic and anti-psychotic

Uses: The long-term treatment of high blood pressure.

How it works: Changes the chemicals in the heart muscle with the result that the blood vessels around the heart increase in size and the blood can flow more easily.

Possible adverse effects: Dizziness, headache.

Availability: Available only with a prescription from a doctor.

Other information: Any episodes of palpitations or irregular heart beat should be reported.

CAUTIONS

Children: This drug is either not recommended for children, or is recommended only for children above a certain age.

Pregnancy and breastfeeding: This drug is either not recommended for use by women who are pregnant or breastfeeding, or the precise effects are not known and it should therefore only be used with caution and under medical advice.

Alcohol: No known problems if taken with alcohol.

Driving and operating machinery: There are no commonly reported problems which may impact on the ability to drive or operate machinery. However, many drugs can cause dizziness or drowsiness in a few people, so it is wise to see how the drug affects you before driving or working with dangerous machinery.

ITRACONAZOLE

Brand name: Sporanox

Type of drug: Anti-fungal

Uses: The treatment of severe fungal infections.

How it works: Attaches itself to the fungal cells and prevents them replicating.

Possible adverse effects: Nausea is the most common. Liver problems can sometimes occur, so any sign of jaundice, unusually dark urine or nausea should be reported.

Availability: Available only with a prescription from a doctor.

Other information: The capsules should be taken with food to maximise absorption and therefore effectiveness.

CAUTIONS

Children: This drug is either not recommended for children, or is recommended only for children above a certain age.

Pregnancy and breastfeeding: This drug is either not recommended for use by women who are pregnant or breastfeeding, or the precise effects are not known and it should therefore only be used with caution and under medical advice.

Alcohol: No known problems if taken with alcohol.

Driving and operating machinery: There are no commonly reported

problems which may impact on the ability to drive or operate machinery. However, many drugs can cause dizziness or drowsiness in a few people, so it is wise to see how the drug affects you before driving or working with dangerous machinery.

KETOCONAZOLE
Brand name: Nizoral
Type of drug: Anti-fungal
Uses: Treatment of severe fungal infections which have spread through the body. It is also given to treat skin infections caused by the candida yeast.
How it works: Kills the organisms that are causing the symptoms.
Possible adverse effects: Nausea is common but can be controlled if the drug is taken with meals.
Availability: Available only with a prescription from a doctor.
Other information: Do not take over-the-counter preparations to try and dispel nausea.
CAUTIONS
Children: There are no commonly reported problems associated with prescribing this medication for children.
Pregnancy and breastfeeding: This drug is either not recommended for use by women who are pregnant or breastfeeding, or the precise effects are not known and it should therefore only be used with caution and under medical advice.
Alcohol: Alcohol should not be consumed, or only consumed with caution - after medical advice has been sought - while you are taking this drug.
Driving and operating machinery: There are no commonly reported problems which may impact on the ability to drive or operate machinery. However, many drugs can cause dizziness or drowsiness in a few people, so it is wise to see how the drug affects you before driving or working with dangerous machinery.

KETOPROFEN
Brand name: Alrheumat, Fenoket, Ketocid, Ketovail, Ketozip, Larafen, Orudis, Oruvail
Type of drug: Non-steroidal anti-inflammatory
Uses: To relieve the symptoms of rheumatoid arthritis, osteoarthritis and

ankylosing spondylitis. This medication is also used to relieve pain associated with menstruation or injury.

How it works: The anti-inflammatory action of this drug relieves the pain and stiffness which are characteristic features of the above-mentioned conditions.

Possible adverse effects: Gastro-intestinal irritation leading to nausea, heartburn or abdominal pain. Black or bloodstained faeces should be reported immediately.

Availability: Available with or without a prescription (over-the-counter).

Other information: Do not take over-the-counter medication whilst on this drug without discussing it with your doctor first. It is advisable to wear a sunscreen whilst on this drug, as it can increase sensitivity to sunlight.

CAUTIONS

Children: This drug is either not recommended for children, or is recommended only for children above a certain age.

Pregnancy and breastfeeding: No specific problems documented, but any medication should be taken with utmost caution by women who are either pregnant or breastfeeding, and only after professional medical or pharmaceutical advice has been sought.

Alcohol: Alcohol should not be consumed, or only consumed with caution - after medical advice has been sought - while you are taking this drug.

Driving and operating machinery: This drug may have some effect on your driving ability, so it is advisable not to drive or operate machinery while taking it.

KETOROLAC TROMETAMOL

Brand name: Toradol

Type of drug: Painkiller

Uses: The short-term treatment of moderately severe, acute pain.

How it works: Acts as a non-steroidal anti-inflammatory to alleviate pain.

Possible adverse effects: Drowsiness, sedative effect, pain at injection site. Can irritate the stomach and gut leading to indigestion and abdominal discomfort which should be reported.

Availability: Available only with a prescription from a doctor.

Other information: Supplied as either tablets or injection. Aspirin and products containing aspirin should be avoided.

CAUTIONS

Children: This drug is either not recommended for children, or is recommended only for children above a certain age.

Pregnancy and breastfeeding: This drug is either not recommended for use by women who are pregnant or breastfeeding, or the precise effects are not known and it should therefore only be used with caution and under medical advice.

Alcohol: Alcohol should not be consumed, or only consumed with caution - after medical advice has been sought - while you are taking this drug.

Driving and operating machinery: There are no commonly reported problems which may impact on the ability to drive or operate machinery. However, many drugs can cause dizziness or drowsiness in a few people, so it is wise to see how the drug affects you before driving or working with dangerous machinery.

KETOTIFEN

Brand name: Zaditen

Type of drug: Anti-allergy

Uses: The prevention of asthma and hay fever.

How it works: Inhibits the production of histamine, a naturally occurring substance which gives rise to the symptoms of allergic conditions.

Possible adverse effects: Drowsiness, dry mouth, weight gain and dizziness.

Availability: Available only with a prescription from a doctor.

Other information: Tablets should be taken with food.

CAUTIONS

Children: There are no commonly reported problems associated with prescribing this medication for children.

Pregnancy and breastfeeding: This drug is either not recommended for use by women who are pregnant or breastfeeding, or the precise effects are not known and it should therefore only be used with caution and under medical advice.

Alcohol: No known problems if taken with alcohol.

Driving and operating machinery: This drug may have some effect on your driving ability, so it is advisable not to drive or operate machinery while taking it.

LABETALOL

Brand name: Trandate

Type of drug: Beta-blocker

Uses: The treatment of high blood pressure.

How it works: Has a relaxant effect by slowing and steadying the heart rate. It also allows the blood vessels to dilate, easing the flow of blood.

Possible adverse effects: Dizziness - particularly on standing up. Scalp tingling may be experienced during the early days of therapy.

Availability: Available only with a prescription from a doctor.

Other information: Supplied as tablets or injection.

CAUTIONS

Children: This drug is either not recommended for children, or is recommended only for children above a certain age.

Pregnancy and breastfeeding: No specific problems documented, but any medication should be taken with utmost caution by women who are either pregnant or breastfeeding, and only after professional medical or pharmaceutical advice has been sought.

Alcohol: No known problems if taken with alcohol.

Driving and operating machinery: There are no commonly reported problems which may impact on the ability to drive or operate machinery. However, many drugs can cause dizziness or drowsiness in a few people, so it is wise to see how the drug affects you before driving or working with dangerous machinery.

LACTITOL

Brand name: Lactitol monohydrate

Type of drug: Laxative

Uses: The treatment or prevention of constipation.

How it works: Acts by retaining fluid in the bowel and keeping the stool moist and thus easier to pass. It is not absorbed.

Possible adverse effects: Wind, bloatedness, itchy anus and gastric discomfort.

Availability: Available with or without a prescription (over the counter).

Other information: Take plenty of fluids whilst on this medication. It is supplied as a powder which should be mixed with food or liquid and taken with one to two glasses of liquid.

CAUTIONS

Children: There are no commonly reported problems associated with prescribing this medication for children.

Pregnancy and breastfeeding: No specific problems documented, but any medication should be taken with utmost caution by women who are either pregnant or breastfeeding, and only after professional medical or pharmaceutical advice has been sought.

Alcohol: No known problems if taken with alcohol.

Driving and operating machinery: There are no commonly reported problems which may impact on the ability to drive or operate machinery. However, many drugs can cause dizziness or drowsiness in a few people, so it is wise to see how the drug affects you before driving or working with dangerous machinery.

LACTULOSE

Brand name: Duphalac, Lactugal, Laxose, Osmolax, Regulose
Type of drug: Laxative
Uses: The treatment of constipation.
How it works: Softens the faeces by increasing the amount of water in the bowel.
Possible adverse effects: Stomach cramps and wind may occur during the early days of treatment but they usually pass off. Discuss with your doctor if diarrhoea occurs.
Availability: Available without a prescription (over-the-counter).
Other information: Available in liquid or powder form.

CAUTIONS

Children: There are no commonly reported problems associated with prescribing this medication for children.

Pregnancy and breastfeeding: No specific problems documented, but any medication should be taken with utmost caution by women who are either pregnant or breastfeeding, and only after professional medical or pharmaceutical advice has been sought.

Alcohol: No known problems if taken with alcohol.

Driving and operating machinery: There are no commonly reported problems which may impact on the ability to drive or operate machinery. However, many drugs can cause dizziness or drowsiness in a few people,

so it is wise to see how the drug affects you before driving or working with dangerous machinery.

LAMIVUDINE

Brand name: Epivir

Type of drug: Anti-viral

Uses: Used at the same time as other drugs to treat infection with the HIV virus.

How it works: Acts on the DNA to prevent the virus from replicating. When used in conjunction with other drugs it can suppress or delay the emergence of resistant strains of the virus.

Possible adverse effects: Headache, tiredness, dizziness, sleeplessness, fever, chills, bone and muscle pain, nausea, diarrhoea and vomiting. Can cause pancreatitis in children.

Availability: Available only with a prescription from a doctor.

Other information: The long-term effects of this drug are unknown but the benefits of it are thought to outweigh the risks that come with this uncertainty. It is crucial to take this drug exactly as prescribed.

CAUTIONS

Children: There are no commonly reported problems associated with prescribing this medication for children.

Pregnancy and breastfeeding: This drug is either not recommended for use by women who are pregnant or breastfeeding, or the precise effects are not known and it should therefore only be used with caution and under medical advice.

Alcohol: No known problems if taken with alcohol.

Driving and operating machinery: There are no commonly reported problems which may impact on the ability to drive or operate machinery. However, many drugs can cause dizziness or drowsiness in a few people, so it is wise to see how the drug affects you before driving or working with dangerous machinery.

LAMOTRIGINE

Brand name: Lamictal

Type of drug: Anti-convulsant

Uses: The treatment of epilepsy.

How it works: Restores the balance of chemicals in the brain, with the result that epileptic seizures are reduced.

Possible adverse effects: Rare, but include rash, visual disturbances, headache and a lack of co-ordination. A rash may occur during the early days of treatment which will usually resolve itself but should be reported.

Availability: Available only with a prescription from a doctor.

Other information: Supplied as tablets. Blood tests will be taken regularly to assess the effect of the drug.

CAUTIONS

Children: This drug is either not recommended for children, or is recommended only for children above a certain age.

Pregnancy and breastfeeding: This drug is either not recommended for use by women who are pregnant or breastfeeding, or the precise effects are not known and it should therefore only be used with caution.

Alcohol: Alcohol should not be consumed, or only consumed with caution - after medical advice has been sought - while you are taking this drug.

Driving and operating machinery: This drug may have some effect on your driving ability, so it is advisable not to drive or operate machinery while taking it.

LANSOPRAZOLE

Brand name: Zoton

Type of drug: Proton pump inhibitor

Uses: The treatment of duodenal ulcers, stomach ulcers and reflux oesophagitis.

How it works: Reduces the production of gastric acid which causes the symptoms of the problems.

Possible adverse effects: Gastric disturbances, headache and skin irritation.

Availability: Available only with a prescription from a doctor.

Other information: Supplied as capsules which should be taken before meals. Capsules should not be chewed, but swallowed whole.

CAUTIONS

Children: This drug is either not recommended for children, or is recommended only for children above a certain age.

Pregnancy and breastfeeding: This drug is either not recommended for

use by women who are pregnant or breastfeeding, or the precise effects are not known and it should therefore only be used with caution and under medical advice.

Alcohol: No known problems if taken with alcohol.

Driving and operating machinery: There are no commonly reported problems which may impact on the ability to drive or operate machinery. However, many drugs can cause dizziness or drowsiness in a few people, so it is wise to see how the drug affects you before driving or working with dangerous machinery.

LEUPRORELIN

Brand name: Prostap SR, Prostap 3

Type of drug: Anti-cancer

Uses: The treatment of serious cancer of the prostate. Sometimes also used to treat endometriosis.

How it works: Prevents the production of male hormones to produce an effect similar to castration, with the result that the cancer cells can no longer reproduce.

Possible adverse effects: Similar for both men and women. Decreased libido, hot flushes, sweating, tiredness and nausea.

Availability: Available only with a prescription from a doctor.

Other information: Do not use an oral contraceptive whilst on this medication.

CAUTIONS

Children: This drug is either not recommended for children, or is recommended only for children above a certain age.

Pregnancy and breastfeeding: This drug is either not recommended for use by women who are pregnant or breastfeeding, or the precise effects are not known and it should therefore only be used with caution and under medical advice.

Alcohol: No known problems if taken with alcohol.

Driving and operating machinery: There are no commonly reported problems which may impact on the ability to drive or operate machinery. However, many drugs can cause dizziness or drowsiness in a few people, so it is wise to see how the drug affects you before driving or working with dangerous machinery.

LEVOCABASTINE

Brand name: Livostin

Type of drug: Anti-allergy

Uses: To reduce the symptoms which occur with hay fever.

How it works: Acts rapidly to alleviate the runny nose and eyes which are symptomatic of hay fever.

Possible adverse effects: Headache, tiredness, sleeplessness.

Availability: Available only with a prescription from a doctor.

Other information: Available as nasal spray and eye drops. Do not use the eye drops at the same time as wearing soft contact lenses.

CAUTIONS

Children: This drug is either not recommended for children, or is recommended only for children above a certain age.

Pregnancy and breastfeeding: No specific problems documented, but any medication should be taken with utmost caution by women who are either pregnant or breastfeeding, and only after professional medical or pharmaceutical advice has been sought.

Alcohol: No known problems if taken with alcohol.

Driving and operating machinery: There are no commonly reported problems which may impact on the ability to drive or operate machinery. However, many drugs can cause dizziness or drowsiness in a few people, so it is wise to see how the drug affects you before driving or working with dangerous machinery.

LEVODOPA

Brand name: Brocadopa, Larodopa

Type of drug: Parkinsonism treatment

Uses: To treat the symptoms of Parkinson's disease.

How it works: Becomes transformed into dopamine, a chemical which is deficient in people with Parkinson's disease. Although it can effectively relieve many of the symptoms of Parkinson's disease, it is not a cure for the condition.

Possible adverse effects: These can be severe and include nausea, dizziness, palpitations, digestive disturbance, nervousness, dark-coloured urine.

Availability: Available only with a prescription from a doctor.

Other information: Levodopa is usually prescribed with other drugs which help minimise its side effects. Its benefits usually diminish with time.

CAUTIONS

Children: This drug is either not recommended for children, or is recommended only for children above a certain age.

Pregnancy and breastfeeding: This drug is either not recommended for use by women who are pregnant or breastfeeding, or the precise effects are not known and it should therefore only be used with caution and under medical advice.

Alcohol: No known problems if taken with alcohol.

Driving and operating machinery: This drug may have some effect on your driving ability, so it is advisable not to drive or operate machinery while taking it.

LIOTHYRONINE

Brand name: Tetroxin

Type of drug: Thyroid hormone

Uses: The treatment of thyroid deficiency conditions.

How it works: Replaces the hormone produced by the thyroid gland which is deficient in conditions such as cretinism and myxoedema.

Possible adverse effects: Insomnia, tremor, heart rhythm disturbances. Any sign of a headache or diarrhoea should be reported.

Availability: Available only with a prescription from a doctor.

Other information: The drug should be stored in a warm place to prevent it from deteriorating. The drug should be taken at the same time each day.

CAUTIONS

Children: There are no commonly reported problems associated with prescribing this medication for children.

Pregnancy and breastfeeding: No specific problems documented, but any medication should be taken with utmost caution by women who are either pregnant or breastfeeding, and only after professional medical or pharmaceutical advice has been sought.

Alcohol: No known problems if taken with alcohol.

Driving and operating machinery: There are no commonly reported

problems which may impact on the ability to drive or operate machinery. However, many drugs can cause dizziness or drowsiness in a few people, so it is wise to see how the drug affects you before driving or working with dangerous machinery.

LISINOPRIL
Brand name: Carace, Zestril, Zestoretic
Type of drug: ACE inhibitor
Uses: Most commonly used as a treatment for mild to severe high blood pressure. Can also be used for people with heart failure and those who have had a heart attack.
How it works: Reduces the body's ability to retain sodium and water, which is one of the main causes of high blood pressure.
Possible adverse effects: Dizziness, headache, fatigue, nasal congestion and a dry cough. Any signs of light-headedness or infection should be reported.
Availability: Available only with a prescription from a doctor.
Other information: Do not take any over-the-counter products - especially to treat a cold - without checking with your doctor first. Do not use salt substitutes which contain potassium.
CAUTIONS
Children: This drug is either not recommended for children, or is recommended only for children above a certain age.
Pregnancy and breastfeeding: No specific problems documented, but any medication should be taken with utmost caution by women who are either pregnant or breastfeeding, and only after professional medical or pharmaceutical advice has been sought.
Alcohol: No known problems if taken with alcohol.
Driving and operating machinery: There are no commonly reported problems which may impact on the ability to drive or operate machinery. However, many drugs can cause dizziness or drowsiness in a few people, so it is wise to see how the drug affects you before driving or working with dangerous machinery.

LITHIUM
Brand name: Camcolit, Li-liquid, Liskonum, Litarex, Priadel
Type of drug: Anti-manic

Uses: Treatment of mania associated with manic depression. It is also occasionally used for the treatment of severe depression.

How it works: Prevents the intensity of mood swings between the manic and depressive stages of the disorder.

Possible adverse effects: Nausea, vomiting and tremor. These side-effects are usually caused by high levels of the drug circulating in the body and should be reported to your doctor, because it may be necessary to reduce the dosage.

Availability: Available only with a prescription from a doctor.

Other information: It may take two to three weeks for this drug to take effect. An overdose should be treated as an emergency. Long-term treatment (more than five years) can lead to kidney problems.

CAUTIONS

Children: This drug is either not recommended for children, or is recommended only for children above a certain age.

Pregnancy and breastfeeding: This drug is either not recommended for use by women who are pregnant or breastfeeding, or the precise effects are not known and it should therefore only be used with caution and under medical advice.

Alcohol: Alcohol should not be consumed, or only consumed with caution - after medical advice has been sought - while you are taking this drug.

Driving and operating machinery: This drug may have some effect on your driving ability, so it is advisable not to drive or operate machinery while taking it.

LOFEPRAMINE

Brand name: Gamanil

Type of drug: Tricyclic anti-depressant

Uses: The long-term treatment of depression.

How it works: It improves the mood, energy levels and interest in day-to-day living without the sedative effects of many similar drugs.

Possible adverse effects: These are relatively uncommon but include sweating and flushing.

Availability: Available only with a prescription from a doctor.

Other information: Smoking while taking this drug may reduce its beneficial effects. Do not stop taking this drug suddenly.

CAUTIONS

Children: This drug is either not recommended for children, or is recommended only for children above a certain age.

Pregnancy and breastfeeding: This drug is either not recommended for use by women who are pregnant or breastfeeding, or the precise effects are not known and it should therefore only be used with caution and under medical advice.

Alcohol: Alcohol should not be consumed, or only consumed with caution - after medical advice has been sought - while you are taking this drug.

Driving and operating machinery: This drug may have some effect on your driving ability, so it is advisable not to drive or operate machinery while taking it.

LOFEXIDINE

Brand name: BritLofex

Type of drug: Anti-emetic and anti-psychotic

Uses: The management of symptoms which addicts experience during withdrawal from heroin or other opium-based drugs.

How it works: Acts on the central nervous system to produce a relaxant effect without the corresponding fall in blood pressure which can occur with similar drugs.

Possible adverse effects: Drowsiness, dry mouth, throat and nose, slow pulse.

Availability: Available only with a prescription from a doctor.

Other information: Will be supplied as tablets.

CAUTIONS

Children: This drug is either not recommended for children, or is recommended only for children above a certain age.

Pregnancy and breastfeeding: This drug is either not recommended for use by women who are pregnant or breastfeeding, or the precise effects are not known and it should therefore only be used with caution and under medical advice.

Alcohol: Alcohol should not be consumed, or only consumed with caution - after medical advice has been sought - while you are taking this drug.

Driving and operating machinery: This drug may have some effect on

your driving ability, so it is advisable not to drive or operate machinery while taking it.

LOPERAMIDE

Brand name: Arret, Diasorb, Diocalm Ultra, Imodium

Type of drug: Antidiarrhoeal drug

Uses: To treat diarrhoea.

How it works: Acts on the muscles of the intestinal wall, with the result that the movements of the gut are slowed down.

Possible adverse effects: Bloating, abdominal cramps and occasionally rashes.

Availability: Available with or without a prescription (over-the-counter).

Other information: Usually taken as an over the counter preparation. Consult a doctor if the problem does not abate within 48 hours of onset. Should not be used by people who have existing bowel problems such as ulcerative colitis.

CAUTIONS

Children: There are no commonly reported problems associated with prescribing this medication for children.

Pregnancy and breastfeeding: This drug is either not recommended for use by women who are pregnant or breastfeeding, or the precise effects are not known and it should therefore only be used with caution and under medical advice.

Alcohol: No known problems if taken with alcohol.

Driving and operating machinery: There are no commonly reported problems which may impact on the ability to drive or operate machinery. However, many drugs can cause dizziness or drowsiness in a few people, so it is wise to see how the drug affects you before driving or working with dangerous machinery.

LORATADINE

Brand name: Clarityn

Type of drug: Antihistamine

Uses: The treatment of hay fever and other allergic conditions such as recurrent urticaria (itching).

How it works: Treats the symptoms of allergic conditions (eg, runny nose, sneezing and itchy eyes) without the sedative effects of many similar drugs.

Possible adverse effects: Headache, nausea, tiredness and heart rhythm disturbances.

Availability: Available with or without a prescription (over-the-counter).

Other information: Should be taken on an empty stomach, at least two hours after a meal.

CAUTIONS

Children: There are no commonly reported problems associated with prescribing this medication for children.

Pregnancy and breastfeeding: This drug is either not recommended for use by women who are pregnant or breastfeeding, or the precise effects are not known and it should therefore only be used with caution and under medical advice.

Alcohol: No known problems if taken with alcohol.

Driving and operating machinery: There are no commonly reported problems which may impact on the ability to drive or operate machinery. However, many drugs can cause dizziness or drowsiness in a few people, so it is wise to see how the drug affects you before driving or working with dangerous machinery.

LOSARTAN POTASSIUM

Brand name: Cozaar

Type of drug: Anti-hypertensive

Uses: The treatment of high blood pressure.

How it works: Blocks the production of chemicals which cause the blood vessels to constrict.

Possible adverse effects: Dizziness, fall in blood pressure on standing after sitting or lying down. Diarrhoea and insomnia.

Availability: Available only with a prescription from a doctor.

Other information: Patient should avoid sodium substitutes.

CAUTIONS

Children: This drug is either not recommended for children, or is recommended only for children above a certain age.

Pregnancy and breastfeeding: This drug is either not recommended for use by women who are pregnant or breastfeeding, or the precise effects are not known and it should therefore only be used with caution and under medical advice.

Alcohol: No known problems if taken with alcohol.

Driving and operating machinery: There are no commonly reported problems which may impact on the ability to drive or operate machinery. However, many drugs can cause dizziness or drowsiness in a few people, so it is wise to see how the drug affects you before driving or working with dangerous machinery.

LOXAPINE

Brand name: Loxapac

Type of drug: Anti-psychotic

Uses: The treatment of long-term psychosis, such as that which occurs with schizophrenia.

How it works: Has a sedating effect without causing drowsiness.

Possible adverse effects: Nausea and vomiting, weakness, drowsiness, dizziness, dry mouth and headache.

Availability: Available only with a prescription from a doctor.

Other information: Patient should avoid other depressants and sedatives.

CAUTIONS

Children: This drug is either not recommended for children, or is recommended only for children above a certain age.

Pregnancy and breastfeeding: This drug is either not recommended for use by women who are pregnant or breastfeeding, or the precise effects are not known and it should therefore only be used with caution and under medical advice.

Alcohol: Alcohol should not be consumed, or only consumed with caution - after medical advice has been sought - while you are taking this drug.

Driving and operating machinery: This drug may have some effect on your driving ability, so it is advisable not to drive or operate machinery while taking it.

MAPROTILINE

Brand name: Ludiomil

Type of drug: Anti-depressant

Uses: The treatment of depression when there is also a need for a sedative effect.

How it works: Has a sedative effect at the same time as raising the patient's mood, stimulates appetite and generally enables the patient to lead a more normal daily life.

Possible adverse effects: Dry mouth, blurred vision, drowsiness, rapid beating of the heart, constipation.

Availability: Available only with a prescription from a doctor.

Other information: Not for patients who have heart problems or for those with suicidal tendencies.

CAUTIONS

Children: This drug is either not recommended for children, or is recommended only for children above a certain age.

Pregnancy and breastfeeding: This drug is either not recommended for use by women who are pregnant or breastfeeding, or the precise effects are not known and it should therefore only be used with caution and under medical advice.

Alcohol: Alcohol should not be consumed, or only consumed with caution - after medical advice has been sought - while you are taking this drug.

Driving and operating machinery: This drug may have some effect on your driving ability, so it is advisable not to drive or operate machinery while taking it.

MEBEVERINE

Brand name: Colofac

Type of drug: Anti-spasmodic

Uses: The alleviation of episodes of painful spasms in the bowel which often occur with conditions such as irritable bowel syndrome.

How it works: Acts on the muscles in the bowel wall and on the nerves which send messages to it, with the result that the bowel wall muscles relax and the spasms are halted.

Possible adverse effects: Side effects are rare, but constipation can occur.

Availability: Available only with a prescription from a doctor.

Other information: Take medication with plenty of water. Should not be taken just before bedtime.

CAUTIONS

Children: There are no commonly reported problems associated with prescribing this medication for children.

Pregnancy and breastfeeding: This drug is either not recommended for use by women who are pregnant or breastfeeding, or the precise effects are not known and it should therefore only be used with caution and under medical advice.

Alcohol: No known problems if taken with alcohol.

Driving and operating machinery: There are no commonly reported problems which may impact on the ability to drive or operate machinery. However, many drugs can cause dizziness or drowsiness in a few people, so it is wise to see how the drug affects you before driving or working with dangerous machinery.

MEDROXYPROGESTERONE

Brand name: Depo-Provera, Farlutal, Provera

Type of drug: Female sex hormone

Uses: Used to treat a range of disorders related to the menstrual cycle, including endometriosis. It is also used in conjunction with other drugs to treat cancer of the breast, uterus and prostate.

How it works: Mimics the action of the female sex hormone, progesterone, the lack of which is thought to be a key factor in disorders of this type.

Possible adverse effects: Rare, but include weight gain, swollen ankles and sore breasts.

Availability: Available only with a prescription from a doctor.

Other information: Long-term use of this drug may increase the risk of blood clots in the leg veins.

CAUTIONS

Children: This drug is either not recommended for children, or is recommended only for children above a certain age.

Pregnancy and breastfeeding: This drug is either not recommended for use by women who are pregnant or breastfeeding, or the precise effects are not known and it should therefore only be used with caution and under medical advice.

Alcohol: No known problems if taken with alcohol.

Driving and operating machinery: There are no commonly reported problems which may impact on the ability to drive or operate machinery.

However, many drugs can cause dizziness or drowsiness in a few people, so it is wise to see how the drug affects you before driving or working with dangerous machinery.

MEFENAMIC ACID

Brand name: Dysman, Ponstan

Type of drug: Non-steroidal anti-inflammatory

Uses: To treat headache, toothache, menstruation pains, rheumatoid arthritis and osteoarthritis.

How it works: Relieves the pain and inflammation associated with the above conditions.

Possible adverse effects: Drowsiness, indigestion, nausea and diarrhoea. The most common side effect is an irritation of the stomach and gut. A rash, or black or bloodstained faeces should be reported to a doctor.

Availability: Available only with a prescription from a doctor.

Other information: Blood tests will be taken at regular intervals to monitor the effect of this medication.

CAUTIONS

Children: There are no commonly reported problems associated with prescribing this medication for children.

Pregnancy and breastfeeding: This drug is either not recommended for use by women who are pregnant or breastfeeding, or the precise effects are not known and it should therefore only be used with caution and under medical advice.

Alcohol: Alcohol should not be consumed, or only consumed with caution - after medical advice has been sought - while you are taking this drug.

Driving and operating machinery: This drug may have some effect on your driving ability, so it is advisable not to drive or operate machinery while taking it.

MEFLOQUINE

Brand name: Lariam

Type of drug: Anti-malarial

Uses: To prevent and treat malaria.

How it works: It is effective against all human types of malaria, including choloroquine-resistant and other persistent strains.

Possible adverse effects: Side effects can be serious in some patients. Dizziness, headache, confusion, hallucinations, nausea, vomiting and diarrhoea. Also sleep disorders. Any signs of depression or confusion may indicate a toxic effect and the drug should be discontinued.

Availability: Available only with a prescription from a doctor.

Other information: This drug should not be taken on an empty stomach and always taken with a large glass of water.

CAUTIONS

Children: This drug is either not recommended for children, or is recommended only for children above a certain age.

Pregnancy and breastfeeding: This drug is either not recommended for use by women who are pregnant or breastfeeding, or the precise effects are not known and it should therefore only be used with caution and under medical advice.

Alcohol: Alcohol should not be consumed, or only consumed with caution - after medical advice has been sought - while you are taking this drug.

Driving and operating machinery: This drug may have some effect on your driving ability, so it is advisable not to drive or operate machinery while taking it.

MEGESTROL

Brand name: Megace

Type of drug: Female sex hormone and anti-cancer

Uses: The treatment of cancer of the breast and uterus.

How it works: Helps to inhibit growth and therefore reduces the size of the tumour.

Possible adverse effects: Weight gain. Also nausea, vomiting and diarrhoea.

Availability: Available only with a prescription from a doctor.

Other information: Could increase risk of blood clots in leg veins.

CAUTIONS

Children: This drug is either not recommended for children, or is recommended only for children above a certain age.

Pregnancy and breastfeeding: This drug is either not recommended for

use by women who are pregnant or breastfeeding, or the precise effects are not known and it should therefore only be used with caution and under medical advice.

Alcohol: No known problems if taken with alcohol.

Driving and operating machinery: There are no commonly reported problems which may impact on the ability to drive or operate machinery. However, many drugs can cause dizziness or drowsiness in a few people, so it is wise to see how the drug affects you before driving or working with dangerous machinery.

MELATONIN

Brand name: Melatonin

Type of drug: Hormone

Uses: To induce sleep and help the body re-adjust to its normal circadian (day-night) rhythm. Useful to treat jet lag and for blind people and for shift workers to alter the body clock.

How it works: It is a natural hormone which affects the pineal gland which controls the natural sleep/wake rhythms of the body.

Possible adverse effects: Drowsiness.

Availability: Available only with a prescription from a doctor.

Other information: Not commercially available in the United Kingdom.

CAUTIONS

Children: This drug is either not recommended for children, or is recommended only for children above a certain age.

Pregnancy and breastfeeding: This drug is either not recommended for use by women who are pregnant or breastfeeding, or the precise effects are not known and it should therefore only be used with caution and under medical advice.

Alcohol: Alcohol should not be consumed, or only consumed with caution - after medical advice has been sought - while you are taking this drug.

Driving and operating machinery: This drug may have some effect on your driving ability, so it is advisable not to drive or operate machinery while taking it.

MERCAPTOPURINE

Brand name: Puri-Nethol

Type of drug: Anti-cancer

Uses: The treatment of lymphoblastic and myeloblastic leukaemias.

How it works: Affects the DNA and RNA of cancer cells and kills them.

Possible adverse effects: Nausea, vomiting, mouth ulcers and diarrhoea.

Availability: Available only with a prescription from a doctor.

Other information: Regular blood counts are required, as drug can interfere with blood cell production. Anaemia and other blood disorders could result.

CAUTIONS

Children: There are no commonly reported problems associated with prescribing this medication for children.

Pregnancy and breastfeeding: This drug is either not recommended for use by women who are pregnant or breastfeeding, or the precise effects are not known and it should therefore only be used with caution and under medical advice.

Alcohol: Alcohol should not be consumed, or only consumed with caution - after medical advice has been sought - while you are taking this drug.

Driving and operating machinery: There are no commonly reported problems which may impact on the ability to drive or operate machinery. However, many drugs can cause dizziness or drowsiness in a few people, so it is wise to see how the drug affects you before driving or working with dangerous machinery.

MESALAZINE

Brand name: Asacol, Pentasa, Salofalk

Type of drug: Chronic diarrhoea treatment

Uses: Treatment of mild to moderate cases of inflammatory bowel diseases such as ulcerative colitis and Crohn's disease.

How it works: Inhibits the production of chemicals which are key factors in the development of the disease, with the result that the inflammation of the bowel which is associated with an attack is relieved. It also has a role in preventing acute attacks.

Possible adverse effects: Nausea, abdominal pain and diarrhoea.

Availability: Available only with a prescription from a doctor.

Other information: If medication is in the form of tablets patients are advised to swallow them whole, not chew or crush them. If given as a suppository, it should be retained for as long as possible.

CAUTIONS

Children: This drug is either not recommended for children, or is recommended only for children above a certain age.

Pregnancy and breastfeeding: This drug is either not recommended for use by women who are pregnant or breastfeeding, or the precise effects are not known and it should therefore only be used with caution and under medical advice.

Alcohol: No known problems if taken with alcohol.

Driving and operating machinery: There are no commonly reported problems which may impact on the ability to drive or operate machinery. However, many drugs can cause dizziness or drowsiness in a few people, so it is wise to see how the drug affects you before driving or working with dangerous machinery.

METARAMINOL

Brand name: Aramine

Type of drug: Anti-hypotensive

Uses: Used to treat a fall in blood pressure.

How it works: Increases the resistance of blood vessels and constricts them, with the result that the pressure within them is increased.

Possible adverse effects: Dizziness, headache, rapid beating of the heart or a prolonged rise in blood pressure.

Availability: Available only with a prescription from a doctor.

Other information: Patient should report any adverse reaction quickly.

CAUTIONS

Children: This drug is either not recommended for children, or is recommended only for children above a certain age.

Pregnancy and breastfeeding: This drug is either not recommended for use by women who are pregnant or breastfeeding, or the precise effects are not known and it should therefore only be used with caution and under medical advice.

Alcohol: No known problems if taken with alcohol.

Driving and operating machinery: There are no commonly reported problems which may impact on the ability to drive or operate machinery.

However, many drugs can cause dizziness or drowsiness in a few people, so it is wise to see how the drug affects you before driving or working with dangerous machinery.

METFORMIN
Brand name: Glucophage, Glucamet, Orabet
Type of drug: Anti-diabetic
Uses: Used in the management of late onset diabetes in cases where the pancreas is still producing some insulin.
How it works: Reduces the production of sugar and lowers the amount of glucose which is absorbed from the gut into the bloodstream.
Possible adverse effects: Appetite loss, nausea, abdominal discomfort. Dizziness, sweatiness and confusion could indicate that the blood sugar level has dropped too far.
Availability: Available only with a prescription from a doctor.
Other information: Should be taken in conjunction with a low sugar, low fat, diabetic diet. Do not take any over-the-counter products without prior consultation with your doctor.
CAUTIONS
Children: This drug is either not recommended for children, or is recommended only for children above a certain age.
Pregnancy and breastfeeding: This drug is either not recommended for use by women who are pregnant or breastfeeding, or the precise effects are not known and it should therefore only be used with caution and under medical advice.
Alcohol: Alcohol should not be consumed, or only consumed with caution - after medical advice has been sought - while you are taking this drug.
Driving and operating machinery: There are no commonly reported problems which may impact on the ability to drive or operate machinery. However, many drugs can cause dizziness or drowsiness in a few people, so it is wise to see how the drug affects you before driving or working with dangerous machinery.

METHADONE
Brand name: Methadose, Physeptone
Type of drug: Opioid analgesic

Uses: For the treatment of severe pain and for heroin addiction.

How it works: Its chemical similarity to morphine makes methadone an effective painkiller. It is also used as a substitute for morphine during the detoxification process of people who are addicted to heroin.

Possible adverse effects: Constipation, drowsiness, nausea and vomiting.

Availability: Available only with a prescription from a doctor.

Other information: Not suitable for patients with respiratory problems.

CAUTIONS

Children: This drug is either not recommended for children, or is recommended only for children above a certain age.

Pregnancy and breastfeeding: This drug is either not recommended for use by women who are pregnant or breastfeeding, or the precise effects are not known and it should therefore only be used with caution and under medical advice.

Alcohol: No known problems if taken with alcohol.

Driving and operating machinery: This drug may have some effect on your driving ability, so it is advisable not to drive or operate machinery while taking it.

METHOCARBAMOL

Brand name: Robaxin, Robaxisal forte

Type of drug: Muscle relaxant

Uses: To treat muscular pain and spasms.

How it works: Acts on the brain and spinal cord to relieve painful spasms in skeletal muscles.

Possible adverse effects: Drowsiness, dizziness, confusion and nausea.

Availability: Available only with a prescription from a doctor.

Other information: Urine may change colour. Patient should change position slowly to avoid dizziness. Beware of over-the-counter preparations that contain alcohol.

CAUTIONS

Children: This drug is either not recommended for children, or is recommended only for children above a certain age.

Pregnancy and breastfeeding: This drug is either not recommended for use by women who are pregnant or breastfeeding, or the precise effects are

not known and it should therefore only be used with caution and under medical advice.

Alcohol: Alcohol should not be consumed, or only consumed with caution - after medical advice has been sought - while you are taking this drug.

Driving and operating machinery: This drug may have some effect on your driving ability, so it is advisable not to drive or operate machinery while taking it.

METHYLCELLULOSE

Brand name: Celevac

Type of drug: Laxative and antidiarrhoeal

Uses: To treat chronic constipation, particularly that associated with diverticular disease and irritable bowel syndrome.

How it works: It works by absorbing up to 25 times its volume of water, with the result that faeces are softened and easier to pass through the gut. It also bulks out diarrhoea. It is not absorbed into the intestine.

Possible adverse effects: Flatulence, abdominal discomfort.

Availability: Available with or without a prescription (over the counter).

Other information: Take medication with plenty of water. Should not take dosage just before bedtime.

CAUTIONS

Children: There are no commonly reported problems associated with prescribing this medication for children.

Pregnancy and breastfeeding: No specific problems documented, but any medication should be taken with utmost caution by women who are either pregnant or breastfeeding, and only after professional medical or pharmaceutical advice has been sought.

Alcohol: No known problems if taken with alcohol.

Driving and operating machinery: There are no commonly reported problems which may impact on the ability to drive or operate machinery. However, many drugs can cause dizziness or drowsiness in a few people, so it is wise to see how the drug affects you before driving or working with dangerous machinery.

METHYLDOPA

Brand name: Aldomet, Dopamet

Type of drug: Anti-hypertensive

Uses: To treat high blood pressure.

How it works: Decreases peripheral resistance of the circulatory system, thus reducing the pressure of blood within the blood vessels.

Possible adverse effects: Drowsiness, dry mouth, depression, headaches, diarrhoea and fluid retention.

Availability: Available only with a prescription from a doctor.

Other information: Will usually be prescribed together with a diuretic. Taking drug at bedtime minimises its effects. Do not take other over-the-counter preparations unless checked with a doctor first.

CAUTIONS

Children: There are no commonly reported problems associated with prescribing this medication for children.

Pregnancy and breastfeeding: No specific problems documented, but any medication should be taken with utmost caution by women who are either pregnant or breastfeeding, and only after professional medical or pharmaceutical advice has been sought.

Alcohol: Alcohol should not be consumed or only consumed with caution (after medical advice has been sought) while you are taking this drug.

Driving and operating machinery: This drug may have some effect on your driving ability, so it is advisable not to drive or operate machinery while taking it.

METHYLPHENIDATE

Brand name: Ritalin

Type of drug: Stimulant

Uses: Controversial medication used to treat children who have been diagnosed as having attention deficit hyperactivity disorder.

How it works: Although a stimulant, the drug has the effect of calming hyperactive children.

Possible adverse effects: Stomach and bowel upsets, nervousness and insomnia. Drug has been associated with growth suppression.

Availability: Available only with a prescription from a doctor.

Other information: Tablets must not be chewed or crushed. Not recommended for children under six years of age. Caffeine should be avoided.

CAUTIONS

Children: There are no commonly reported problems associated with prescribing this medication for children.

Pregnancy and breastfeeding: This drug is either not recommended for use by women who are pregnant or breastfeeding, or the precise effects are not known and it should therefore only be used with caution and under medical advice.

Alcohol: Alcohol should not be consumed or only consumed with caution - after medical advice has been sought - while you are taking this drug.

Driving and operating machinery: This drug may have some effect on your driving ability, so it is advisable not to drive or operate machinery while taking it.

METHYSERGIDE

Brand name: Deseril

Type of drug: Anti-migraine

Uses: To help prevent recurrent migraine, cluster and other vascular headaches.

How it works: Constricts the blood vessels around the brain. Its pain-killing properties are thought to result from the impact the drug has on the patient's perception of pain.

Possible adverse effects: Nausea, drowsiness and dizziness, vomiting, abdominal discomfort and weight gain.

Availability: Available only with a prescription from a doctor.

Other information: Patient to take drug with food. Report any tingling or numbness in hands or feet.

CAUTIONS

Children: This drug is either not recommended for children, or is recommended only for children above a certain age.

Pregnancy and breastfeeding: This drug is either not recommended for use by women who are pregnant or breastfeeding, or the precise effects are not known and it should therefore only be used with caution and under medical advice.

Alcohol: Alcohol should not be consumed, or only consumed with caution - after medical advice has been sought - while you are taking this drug.

Driving and operating machinery: This drug may have some effect on your driving ability, so it is advisable not to drive or operate machinery while taking it.

METOCLOPRAMIDE
Brand name: Gastrobid Continus, Gastroflux, Gastromax, Maxolon, Metramid, Parmid, Primperan
Type of drug: Anti-emetic
Uses: To relieve the nausea and vomiting associated with chemotherapy and to alleviate the symptoms of a hiatus hernia.
How it works: Acts directly on the gut to increase the speed at which food is propelled through the stomach and intestine.
Possible adverse effects: Drowsiness, headache, dizziness, restlessness and bowel upsets. Report any involuntary movements.
Availability: Available only with a prescription from a doctor.
Other information: This medication should be taken 30 minutes before eating.
CAUTIONS
Children: There are no commonly reported problems associated with prescribing this medication for children.
Pregnancy and breastfeeding: This drug is either not recommended for use by women who are pregnant or breastfeeding, or the precise effects are not known and it should therefore only be used with caution and under medical advice.
Alcohol: Alcohol should not be consumed or only consumed with caution - after medical advice has been sought - while you are taking this drug.
Driving and operating machinery: This drug may have some effect on your driving ability, so it is advisable not to drive or operate machinery while taking it.

METRONIDAZOLE
Brand name: Anabact, Flagyl, Metrogel, Metrolyl, Metrotop, Metrozol, Rozex, Vaginyl, Zadstat
Type of drug: Anti-bacterial and anti-protozoal
Uses: Treatment of a variety of infections, particularly those affecting the abdomen, pelvis and mouth, pressure sores and leg ulcers.

How it works: Invades the infecting organisms - protozoa and bacteria - and prevents them from replicating.

Possible adverse effects: Nausea, loss of appetite and dark urine.

Availability: Available only with a prescription from a doctor.

Other information: The importance of maintaining good hygiene is necessary to prevent re-infection.

CAUTIONS

Children: There are no commonly reported problems associated with prescribing this medication for children.

Pregnancy and breastfeeding: This drug is either not recommended for use by women who are pregnant or breastfeeding, or the precise effects are not known and it should therefore only be used with caution and under medical advice.

Alcohol: Alcohol should not be consumed, or only consumed with caution - after medical advice has been sought - while you are taking this drug.

Driving and operating machinery: This drug may have some effect on your driving ability, so it is advisable not to drive or operate machinery while taking it.

MIANSERIN

Brand name: Mianserin hydrochloride

Type of drug: Anti-depressant

Uses: Treatment of severe depression, particularly that associated with insomnia.

How it works: Improves mood, energy levels and appetite and generally stimulates a renewed interest in day-to-day activities. The accompanying sedative effect means it is particularly useful for depressed patients who also have trouble sleeping.

Possible adverse effects: Drowsiness, tremor, sweating and light-headedness when standing from a sitting or lying down position.

Availability: Available only with a prescription from a doctor.

Other information: It may take up to four weeks before the full beneficial effects of the medication are felt. A full blood count is required every month. The patient should report signs of sore throat or infection immediately.

CAUTIONS

Children: This drug is either not recommended for children, or is recommended only for children above a certain age.

Pregnancy and breastfeeding: This drug is either not recommended for use by women who are pregnant or breastfeeding, or the precise effects are not known and it should therefore only be used with caution and under medical advice.

Alcohol: Alcohol should not be consumed, or only consumed with caution - after medical advice has been sought - while you are taking this drug.

Driving and operating machinery: This drug may have some effect on your driving ability, so it is advisable not to drive or operate machinery while taking it.

MICONAZOLE

Brand name: Acnidazil, Daktacort, Daktarin, Dumicoat, Gyno-Daktarin
Type of drug: Anti-fungal
Uses: To treat fungal infections particularly those affecting the mouth and intestine.
How it works: Thickens the fungal cell wall, with the result that the fungus can no longer replicate. It also directly attacks and kills the organisms.
Possible adverse effects: Nausea and diarrhoea, bowel upsets and skin rashes.
Availability: Available with or without a prescription (over-the-counter).
Other information: Supplied as an injection, cream, powder, spray, vaginal cream and suppositories. Hygiene is important to prevent re-infection, particularly of the vaginal area.
CAUTIONS
Children: There are no commonly reported problems associated with prescribing this medication for children.
Pregnancy and breastfeeding: This drug is either not recommended for use by women who are pregnant or breastfeeding, or the precise effects are not known and it should therefore only be used with caution and under medical advice.
Alcohol: No known problems if taken with alcohol.
Driving and operating machinery: There are no commonly reported

problems which may impact on the ability to drive or operate machinery. However, many drugs can cause dizziness or drowsiness in a few people, so it is wise to see how the drug affects you before driving or working with dangerous machinery.

MIFEPRISTONE
Brand name: Mifegyne
Type of drug: Hormone
Uses: To induce an abortion up to 63 days of gestation.
How it works: This drug reversibly competes with progesterone (which protects the embryo) and so causes the death of the embryo.
Possible adverse effects: Malaise, fainting, nausea, headache. Vomiting, rashes and sometimes severe vaginal bleeding.
Availability: Available only with a prescription from a doctor.
Other information: Aspirin or similar medication must not be taken for at least 8-12 days after taking this drug.
CAUTIONS
Children: Unlikely to be prescribed.
Alcohol: No known problems if taken with alcohol.
Driving and operating machinery: There are no commonly reported problems which may impact on the ability to drive or operate machinery. However, many drugs can cause dizziness or drowsiness in a few people, so it is wise to see how the drug affects you before driving or working with dangerous machinery.

MILRINONE
Brand name: Primacor
Type of drug: Phosphodiesterase inhibitor
Uses: Used in treatment of severe congestive heart failure.
How it works: Acts on the chemicals which control the cardiac muscle to increase the pumping effectiveness of the heart muscle.
Possible adverse effects: Headache and hypotension, angina and disorders of the heart rhythm.
Availability: Available only with a prescription from a doctor.
Other information: Will usually be administered in hospital as an injection.

CAUTIONS
Children: This drug is either not recommended for children, or is recommended only for children above a certain age.
Pregnancy and breastfeeding: This drug is either not recommended for use by women who are pregnant or breastfeeding, or the precise effects are not known and it should therefore only be used with caution and under medical advice.
Alcohol: No known problems if taken with alcohol.
Driving and operating machinery: There are no commonly reported problems which may impact on the ability to drive or operate machinery. However, many drugs can cause dizziness or drowsiness in a few people, so it is wise to see how the drug affects you before driving or working with dangerous machinery.

MINOCYCLINE

Brand name: Aknemin, Blemix, Cyclomin, Minocin MR, Minogal
Type of drug: Tetracycline antibiotic
Uses: To treat infections such as pneumonia, gonorrhoea and other sexually transmitted diseases. Also given to people with chronic bronchitis to prevent infection.
How it works: The drug is widely distributed throughout the body and binds to the bacterial cell wall, preventing the organisms from multiplying.
Possible adverse effects: Nausea and dizziness.
Availability: Available only with a prescription from a doctor.
Other information: A glass of water should be taken after each dose to wash it through the oesophagus.

CAUTIONS
Children: This drug is either not recommended for children, or is recommended only for children above a certain age.
Pregnancy and breastfeeding: This drug is either not recommended for use by women who are pregnant or breastfeeding, or the precise effects are not known and it should therefore only be used with caution.
Alcohol: No known problems if taken with alcohol.
Driving and operating machinery: This drug may have some effect on your driving ability, so it is advisable not to drive or operate machinery while taking it.

MINOXIDIL

Brand name: Loniten, Regaine

Type of drug: Anti-hypertensive

Uses: Treatment of high blood pressure and a treatment for hair loss.

How it works: Increases the size of the blood vessels to reduce blood pressure. Increases hair growth, an effect which is now being put to use as Monixidil is increasingly prescribed as a treatment for baldness.

Possible adverse effects: Fluid retention and increased heart rate, for which a diuretic and beta-blocker will usually be prescribed. Prolonged use may lead to ankle swelling.

Availability: Prescription needed except for scalp lotions.

Other information: Usually supplied as tablets, but a solution will be used for baldness treatment.

CAUTIONS

Children: There are no commonly reported problems associated with prescribing this medication for children.

Pregnancy and breastfeeding: This drug is either not recommended for use by women who are pregnant or breastfeeding, or the precise effects are not known and it should therefore only be used with caution and under medical advice.

Alcohol: Alcohol should not be consumed, or only consumed with caution - after medical advice has been sought - while you are taking this drug.

Driving and operating machinery: This drug may have some effect on your driving ability, so it is advisable not to drive or operate machinery while taking it.

MISOPROSTOL

Brand name: Cytotec

Type of drug: Anti-ulcer

Uses: Treatment and prevention of gastric and duodenal ulcers.

How it works: Reduces the amount of acid produced in the stomach with the result that the ulcerated areas have a chance to heal.

Possible adverse effects: Diarrhoea and indigestion. These can be minimised if preparations containing magnesium are avoided.

Availability: Available only with a prescription from a doctor.

Other information: Side effects may be reduced if each dose is taken with

food. Ulcers will usually heal after a few weeks of treatment.

CAUTIONS

Children: This drug is either not recommended for children, or is recommended only for children above a certain age.

Pregnancy and breastfeeding: This drug is either not recommended for use by women who are pregnant or breastfeeding, or the precise effects are not known and it should therefore only be used with caution and under medical advice.

Alcohol: No known problems if taken with alcohol.

Driving and operating machinery: There are no commonly reported problems which may impact on the ability to drive or operate machinery. However, many drugs can cause dizziness or drowsiness in a few people, so it is wise to see how the drug affects you before driving or working with dangerous machinery.

MITOMYCIN

Brand name: Mitomycin C Kyowa

Type of drug: Anti-cancer

Uses: To treat upper gastro-intestinal cancers, including those of the stomach and pancreas.

How it works: Acts as a cytotoxic (poisonous to cancer) antibiotic. Acts on the DNA in the cancer cells to promote their death.

Possible adverse effects: Headache, drowsiness, fatigue, nausea. Ability to fight off infections will be impaired, so any sign of a fever should be reported.

Availability: Available only with a prescription from a doctor.

Other information: Prolonged use causes delayed bone marrow damage. Patient should avoid exposure to people with infections.

CAUTIONS

Children: There are no commonly reported problems associated with prescribing this medication for children.

Pregnancy and breastfeeding: No specific problems documented, but any medication should be taken with utmost caution by women who are either pregnant or breastfeeding, and only after professional medical or pharmaceutical advice has been sought.

Alcohol: No known problems if taken with alcohol.

237

Driving and operating machinery: There are no commonly reported problems which may impact on the ability to drive or operate machinery. However, many drugs can cause dizziness or drowsiness in a few people, so it is wise to see how the drug affects you before driving or working with dangerous machinery.

MOCLOBEMIDE
Brand name: Manerix
Type of drug: Anti-depressant
Uses: Treatment of depression.
How it works: Acts as a Monoamine Oxidase Inhibitor Antidepressant. Heightens mood, improves energy levels, and restores interest in life.
Possible adverse effects: Side effects such as sleep disturbances, headache and dizziness are usually only temporary. Because of unpleasant interactions, certain types of food should be avoided, including those containing large amounts of caffeine, yeast extract, and pickled herring, liver, dry sausages, game, bean pods and textured vegetable proteins.
Availability: Available only with a prescription from a doctor.
Other information: Can take up to two weeks to lift depression.
CAUTIONS
Children: This drug is either not recommended for children, or is recommended only for children above a certain age.
Pregnancy and breastfeeding: This drug is either not recommended for use by women who are pregnant or breastfeeding, or the precise effects are not known and it should therefore only be used with caution and under medical advice.
Alcohol: Alcohol should not be consumed, or only consumed with caution - after medical advice has been sought - while you are taking this drug.
Driving and operating machinery: This drug may have some effect on your driving ability, so it is advisable not to drive or operate machinery while taking it.

MOEXIPRIL
Brand name: Perdix
Type of drug: Anti-hypertensive
Uses: To treat raised blood pressure.

How it works: Inhibits the production of a chemical which constricts the blood vessels, with the result that the vessels dilate and the pressure within them is reduced.

Possible adverse effects: Dizziness, headache, fatigue, disorders of the heart rhythm and angina.

Availability: Available only with a prescription from a doctor.

Other information: Patients should take dose on an empty stomach. Avoid products that contain potassium. Report any fevers or a sore throat immediately.

CAUTIONS

Children: There are no commonly reported problems associated with prescribing this medication for children.

Pregnancy and breastfeeding: This drug is either not recommended for use by women who are pregnant or breastfeeding, or the precise effects are not known and it should therefore only be used with caution and under medical advice.

Alcohol: No known problems if taken with alcohol.

Driving and operating machinery: There are no commonly reported problems which may impact on the ability to drive or operate machinery. However, many drugs can cause dizziness or drowsiness in a few people, so it is wise to see how the drug affects you before driving or working with dangerous machinery.

MORACIZINE

Brand name: Ethmozine

Type of drug: Anti-arrhythmic

Uses: For treatment of life-threatening ventricular arrhythmias.

How it works: Affects the electrical currents which control the heart beat, with the result that the heart rate is normalised.

Possible adverse effects: Dizziness, headache, fatigue, gastro-intestinal disturbances. Chest pain and palpitations.

Availability: Available only with a prescription from a doctor.

Other information: Supplied as tablets.

CAUTIONS

Children: This drug is either not recommended for children, or is recommended only for children above a certain age.

Pregnancy and breastfeeding: This drug is either not recommended for use by women who are pregnant or breastfeeding, or the precise effects are not known and it should therefore only be used with caution and under medical advice.

Alcohol: No known problems if taken with alcohol.

Driving and operating machinery: There are no commonly reported problems which may impact on the ability to drive or operate machinery. However, many drugs can cause dizziness or drowsiness in a few people, so it is wise to see how the drug affects you before driving or working with dangerous machinery.

MORPHINE

Brand name: MST Continus, MXL, Oramorph, Sevredol

Type of drug: Opioid analgesic

Uses: The relief of severe pain such as that caused by cancer, heart attack or injury.

How it works: Acts rapidly to alter the patient's perception of pain, with the result that it is no longer perceived.

Possible adverse effects: Nausea, vomiting and constipation are common.

Availability: Available only with a prescription from a doctor.

Other information: Dependence may occur if the medication is taken for extended periods. Tablets should be swallowed whole and not broken or crushed.

CAUTIONS

Children: There are no commonly reported problems associated with prescribing this medication for children.

Pregnancy and breastfeeding: No specific problems documented, but any medication should be taken with utmost caution by women who are either pregnant or breastfeeding, and only after professional medical or pharmaceutical advice has been sought.

Alcohol: Alcohol should not be consumed, or only consumed with caution, and in moderation - after medical advice has been sought - while you are taking this drug.

Driving and operating machinery: This drug may have some effect on your driving ability, so it is advisable not to drive or operate machinery while taking it.

MOXONIDINE

Brand name: Physiotens

Type of drug: Anti-hypertensive

Uses: To treat mild to moderate hypertension.

How it works: Stimulates certain receptors on the blood pressure centres in the brain, causing blood vessels to dilate and blood pressure to fall.

Possible adverse effects: Headache, dry mouth, dizziness, nausea, drowsiness.

Availability: Available only with a prescription from a doctor.

Other information: Do not stop taking this drug suddenly.

CAUTIONS

Children: There are no commonly reported problems associated with prescribing this medication for children.

Pregnancy and breastfeeding: This drug is either not recommended for use by women who are pregnant or breastfeeding, or the precise effects are not known and it should therefore only be used with caution and under medical advice.

Alcohol: Alcohol should not be consumed, or only consumed with caution - after medical advice has been sought - while you are taking this drug.

Driving and operating machinery: There are no commonly reported problems which may impact on the ability to drive or operate machinery. However, many drugs can cause dizziness or drowsiness in a few people, so it is wise to see how the drug affects you before driving or working with dangerous machinery.

MYCOPHENOLATE MOFETIL

Brand name: CellCept

Type of drug: Immuno-suppressant

Uses: Given to prevent rejection of a kidney following a transplant operation.

How it works: Acts on the immune system to prevent it perceiving the kidney as a foreign body and attacking it.

Possible adverse effects: Vomiting, diarrhoea, headache, dizziness.

Availability: Available only with a prescription from a doctor.

Other information: Capsules are to be swallowed whole, not chewed or crushed.

CAUTIONS

Children: There are no commonly reported problems associated with prescribing this medication for children.

Pregnancy and breastfeeding: This drug is either not recommended for use by women who are pregnant or breastfeeding, or the precise effects are not known and it should therefore only be used with caution and under medical advice.

Alcohol: No known problems if taken with alcohol.

Driving and operating machinery: There are no commonly reported problems which may impact on the ability to drive or operate machinery. However, many drugs can cause dizziness or drowsiness in a few people, so it is wise to see how the drug affects you before driving or working with dangerous machinery.

NABILONE

Brand name: Cesamet

Type of drug: Anti-emetic

Uses: To treat nausea and vomiting in patients undergoing cancer treatment.

How it works: Closely related - chemically - to cannabis, its precise actions are unknown but it is thought to act on the part of the brain which controls nausea and vomiting to alter the patient's perception of pain.

Possible adverse effects: Drowsiness, vertigo, dry mouth, depression and euphoria.

Availability: Available only with a prescription from a doctor.

Other information: Patients should be made aware that this drug can cause mood and behavioural changes.

CAUTIONS

Children: There are no commonly reported problems associated with prescribing this medication for children.

Pregnancy and breastfeeding: This drug is either not recommended for use by women who are pregnant or breastfeeding, or the precise effects are not known and it should therefore only be used with caution and under medical advice.

Alcohol: Alcohol should not be consumed, or only consumed with caution - after medical advice has been sought - while you are taking this drug.

Driving and operating machinery: This drug may have some effect on your driving ability, so it is advisable not to drive or operate machinery while taking it.

NAFARELIN

Brand name: Synarel

Type of drug: Gonadorelin analogues

Uses: To treat endometriosis.

How it works: It stimulates the release of pituitary hormones which reduce the levels of female hormones and relieve the symptoms of endometriosis.

Possible adverse effects: Irregular bleeding, nausea, vomiting and constipation.

Availability: Available only with a prescription from a doctor.

Other information: Sexual intercourse is best avoided or a form of barrier contraception should be used. Avoid use of nasal decongestants for at least 30 minutes after treatment.

CAUTIONS

Children: There are no commonly reported problems associated with prescribing this medication for children.

Pregnancy and breastfeeding: This drug is either not recommended for use by women who are pregnant or breastfeeding, or the precise effects are not known and it should therefore only be used with caution and under medical advice.

Alcohol: No known problems if taken with alcohol.

Driving and operating machinery: There are no commonly reported problems which may impact on the ability to drive or operate machinery. However, many drugs can cause dizziness or drowsiness in a few people, so it is wise to see how the drug affects you before driving or working with dangerous machinery.

NAPROXEN

Brand name: Arthrosin, Arthroxen, Laraflex, Naprosyn, Nycopren, Prosaid, Synflex, Timpron, Valrox

Type of drug: Non-steroidal anti-inflammatory.

Uses: To treat the symptoms of conditions such as rheumatoid arthritis, ankylosing spondylitis and osteoarthritis. Also useful in the treatment of gout, migraine and pain following surgery.

How it works: Non-steroidal, anti-inflammatory action which reduces pain, stiffness and inflammation associated with the above conditions.

Possible adverse effects: Gastrointestinal problems such as indigestion and nausea should soon diminish.

Availability: Available only with a prescription from a doctor.

Other information: Any sign of blood in the faeces should be reported immediately. Can take up to two weeks to work effectively.

CAUTIONS

Children: There are no commonly reported problems associated with prescribing this medication for children.

Pregnancy and breastfeeding: This drug is either not recommended for use by women who are pregnant or breastfeeding, or the precise effects are not known and it should therefore only be used with caution and under medical advice.

Alcohol: No known problems if taken with alcohol.

Driving and operating machinery: This drug may have some effect on your driving ability, so it is advisable not to drive or operate machinery while taking it.

NEDOCROMIL SODIUM

Brand name: Tilade aerosol

Type of drug: Anti-inflammatory

Uses: To treat mild to moderate bronchial asthma.

How it works: Has an anti-inflammatory and anti-allergic action on the cells in the airways within the lungs.

Possible adverse effects: Unpleasant taste in the mouth, coughing, throat irritation, nausea, stomach and bowel upsets.

Availability: Available only with a prescription from a doctor.

Other information: Should not be used instead of drugs which have a bronchodilator drug. Benefits may not be apparent until after a week of use.

CAUTIONS

Children: There are no commonly reported problems associated with prescribing this medication for children.

Pregnancy and breastfeeding: This drug is either not recommended for use by women who are pregnant or breastfeeding, or the precise effects are not known and it should therefore only be used with caution and under medical advice.

Alcohol: No known problems if taken with alcohol.

Driving and operating machinery: There are no commonly reported problems which may impact on the ability to drive or operate machinery. However, many drugs can cause dizziness or drowsiness in a few people, so it is wise to see how the drug affects you before driving or working with dangerous machinery.

NEFAZODONE
Brand name: Dutonin
Type of drug: Anti-depressant
Uses: To treat depression
How it works: Action of the drug affects the balance of chemicals in the brain which are thought to control mood in individuals, with the result that the mood is lifted and patients are more able to lead normal day-to-day lives.
Possible adverse effects: Dry mouth, nausea, dizziness and drowsiness.
Availability: Available only with a prescription from a doctor.
Other information: It may take several weeks treatment before the full effect of the drug is felt.
CAUTIONS
Children: This drug is either not recommended for children, or is recommended only for children above a certain age.
Pregnancy and breastfeeding: This drug is either not recommended for use by women who are pregnant or breastfeeding, or the precise effects are not known and it should therefore only be used with caution and under medical advice.
Alcohol: Alcohol should not be consumed, or only consumed with caution - after medical advice has been sought - while you are taking this drug.
Driving and operating machinery: This drug may have some effect on your driving ability, so it is advisable not to drive or operate machinery while taking it.

NEFOPAM

Brand name: Acupan

Type of drug: Non-opioid analgesic

Uses: To relieve pain associated with surgery, injury or cancer.

How it works: Acts quickly to reduce the brain's perception of pain without interfering with breathing or leading to dependence, as is the case with many drugs which have a similar effect.

Possible adverse effects: Nausea and dry mouth, which can often be alleviated by a change to the dosage regime.

Availability: Available only with a prescription from a doctor.

Other information: Supplied in tablet or injection form. A harmless pink discoloration of the urine may occur.

CAUTIONS

Children: This drug is either not recommended for children, or is recommended only for children above a certain age.

Pregnancy and breastfeeding: This drug is either not recommended for use by women who are pregnant or breastfeeding, or the precise effects are not known and it should therefore only be used with caution and under medical advice.

Alcohol: Alcohol should not be consumed, or only consumed with caution - after medical advice has been sought - while you are taking this drug.

Driving and operating machinery: This drug may have some effect on your driving ability, so it is advisable not to drive or operate machinery while taking it.

NEOMYCIN

Brand name: Nivemycin, Mycifradin

Type of drug: Antibiotic

Uses: Treatment of infections of the skin and mucous membranes. Also used to sterilise the bowel in preparation for surgery.

How it works: Binds to the bacteria, thus preventing them from replicating.

Possible adverse effects: Possible skin reactions to creams. Do not apply to sore or open wounds.

Availability: Available only with a prescription from a doctor.

Other information: Supplied as tablets.

CAUTIONS

Children: There are no commonly reported problems associated with prescribing this medication for children.

Pregnancy and breastfeeding: This drug is either not recommended for use by women who are pregnant or breastfeeding, or the precise effects are not known and it should therefore only be used with caution and under medical advice.

Alcohol: No known problems if taken with alcohol.

Driving and operating machinery: There are no commonly reported problems which may impact on the ability to drive or operate machinery. However, many drugs can cause dizziness or drowsiness in a few people, so it is wise to see how the drug affects you before driving or working with dangerous machinery.

NEOSTIGMINE

Brand name: Prostigmin

Type of drug: Muscle stimulant

Uses: To treat myasthenia gravis, a rare autoimmune condition. Can also relieve urinary retention and temporary paralysis of the bowel.

How it works: Enhances the transmission of nerve messages to the muscles, which are weakened by the disease to the point of being unable to work.

Possible adverse effects: Abdominal cramps, excessive saliva, dizziness, drowsiness, nausea, headache, sweating, blurred vision, diarrhoea.

Availability: Available only with a prescription from a doctor.

Other information: It is recommended taking the drug with food or milk to minimise side effects.

CAUTIONS

Children: There are no commonly reported problems associated with prescribing this medication for children.

Pregnancy and breastfeeding: This drug is either not recommended for use by women who are pregnant or breastfeeding, or the precise effects are not known and it should therefore only be used with caution and under medical advice.

Alcohol: No known problems if taken with alcohol.

Driving and operating machinery: This drug may have some effect on

your driving ability, so it is advisable not to drive or operate machinery while taking it.

NICARDIPINE

Brand name: Cardene
Type of drug: Anti-hypertensive
Uses: To treat angina and raised blood pressure.
How it works: Alters the electrical activity in the heart, with the result that the blood vessels dilate, increasing the blood flow through the heart.
Possible adverse effects: Dizziness, headache, palpitations, nausea, abdominal discomfort.
Availability: Available only with a prescription from a doctor.
Other information: Avoid grapefruit juice. Supplied as capsules or given as an injection.
CAUTIONS
Children: This drug is either not recommended for children, or is recommended only for children above a certain age.
Pregnancy and breastfeeding: This drug is either not recommended for use by women who are pregnant or breastfeeding, or the precise effects are not known and it should therefore only be used with caution and under medical advice.
Alcohol: No known problems if taken with alcohol.
Driving and operating machinery: There are no commonly reported problems which may impact on the ability to drive or operate machinery. However, many drugs can cause dizziness or drowsiness in a few people, so it is wise to see how the drug affects you before driving or working with dangerous machinery.

NICORANDIL

Brand name: Ikorel
Type of drug: Anti-angina
Uses: To alleviate the symptoms of angina.
How it works: Widens both veins and arteries, with the result that more oxygenated blood can reach the heart muscle and the heart's workload is lessened.
Possible adverse effects: Headache, nausea, flushing and palpitations.

Availability: Available only with a prescription from a doctor.

Other information: Supplied as tablets.

CAUTIONS

Children: This drug is either not recommended for children, or is recommended only for children above a certain age.

Pregnancy and breastfeeding: This drug is either not recommended for use by women who are pregnant or breastfeeding, or the precise effects are not known and it should therefore only be used with caution and under medical advice.

Alcohol: Alcohol should not be consumed, or only consumed with caution - after medical advice has been sought - while you are taking this drug.

Driving and operating machinery: This drug may have some effect on your driving ability, so it is advisable not to drive or operate machinery while taking it.

NICOTINIC ACID

Brand name: Nicotinic acid

Type of drug: Lipid lowering

Uses: Used to treat high levels of fat in the blood. Helps to improve circulatory problems such as Raynaud's disease and chilblains.

How it works: Has a vasodilator effect, meaning that the drug widens blood vessels and increases blood flow. Lowers blood cholesterol and fat levels.

Possible adverse effects: Flushing and headaches, dizziness and palpitations.

Availability: Available with or without a prescription (over-the-counter).

Other information: A low fat diet is recommended if drug is taken to help reduce fat levels.

CAUTIONS

Children: There are no commonly reported problems associated with prescribing this medication for children.

Pregnancy and breastfeeding: This drug is either not recommended for use by women who are pregnant or breastfeeding, or the precise effects are not known and it should therefore only be used with caution and under medical advice.

Alcohol: No known problems if taken with alcohol.

Driving and operating machinery: This drug may have some effect on your driving ability, so it is advisable not to drive or operate machinery while taking it.

NIFEDIPINE

Brand name: Adalat, Adalat Retard, Adipine, Angiopine, Calcilat, Coracten, Nifensar XL, Tensipine MR

Type of drug: Anti-angina and anti-hypertensive

Uses: Treatment of angina and high blood pressure.

How it works: Affects electrical conduction of the heart with the result that the blood vessels are widened, causing the blood pressure to fall. It also makes the pumping action of the heart more effective.

Possible adverse effects: Headache, dizziness, ankle swelling. Can cause blood pressure to drop too low and to cause ankle swelling.

Availability: Available only with a prescription from a doctor.

Other information: Patient should swallow medication whole, not chew or crush the capsules.

CAUTIONS

Children: This drug is either not recommended for children, or is recommended only for children above a certain age.

Pregnancy and breastfeeding: This drug is either not recommended for use by women who are pregnant or breastfeeding, or the precise effects are not known and it should therefore only be used with caution.

Alcohol: Alcohol should not be consumed, or only consumed with caution - after medical advice has been sought - while you are taking this drug.

Driving and operating machinery: This drug may have some effect on your driving ability, so it is advisable not to drive or operate machinery while taking it.

NITROFURANTOIN

Brand name: Furadantin, Macrobid, Macrodantin

Type of drug: Anti-bacterial

Uses: To treat initial and recurrent urinary-tract infections.

How it works: At lower doses it prevents the organisms causing the infection from replicating. At higher doses it kills them.

Possible adverse effects: Side effects are common and include stomach irritation and upset, nausea and vomiting, anorexia, diarrhoea. Urine may be discoloured.

Availability: Available only with a prescription from a doctor.

Other information: Take with milk or food to minimise side effects.

CAUTIONS

Children: There are no commonly reported problems associated with prescribing this medication for children.

Pregnancy and breastfeeding: This drug is either not recommended for use by women who are pregnant or breastfeeding, or the precise effects are not known and it should therefore only be used with caution.

Alcohol: No known problems if taken with alcohol.

Driving and operating machinery: There are no commonly reported problems which may impact on the ability to drive or operate machinery. However, many drugs can cause dizziness or drowsiness in a few people, so it is wise to see how the drug affects you before driving or working with dangerous machinery.

NIZATIDINE

Brand name: Axid, Zinga

Type of drug: H2-receptor antagonist

Uses: To treat gastric and duodenal ulcers, gastro-oesophageal reflux and heartburn.

How it works: Reduces the production of gastric acid, the main factor in causing the problems.

Possible adverse effects: Diarrhoea and other gastrointestinal disturbances, headaches and dizziness.

Availability: Available with or without a prescription (over-the-counter).

Other information: Do not smoke whilst taking this medication, as it increases the production of gastric acid and therefore lessens the effectiveness of the treatment.

CAUTIONS

Children: This drug is either not recommended for children, or is recommended only for children above a certain age.

Pregnancy and breastfeeding: This drug is either not recommended for use by women who are pregnant or breastfeeding, or the precise effects are not known and it should therefore only be used with caution and under medical advice.

Alcohol: No known problems if taken with alcohol.

Driving and operating machinery: There are no commonly reported problems which may impact on the ability to drive or operate machinery. However, many drugs can cause dizziness or drowsiness in a few people, so it is wise to see how the drug affects you before driving or working with dangerous machinery.

NORADRENALINE

Brand name: Levophed

Type of drug: Sympathomimetic

Uses: Used as an emergency treatment for a sudden fall in blood pressure and/or cardiac arrest.

How it works: Causes the blood vessels to constrict, thus raising the pressure within them.

Possible adverse effects: Hypertension, headache, palpitations, disorders of heart rhythm.

Availability: Available only with a prescription from a doctor.

Other information: Must not be given to patients with raised blood pressure. Usually administered as an injection or intravenous infusion (drip) in hospital.

CAUTIONS

Children: This drug is either not recommended for children, or is recommended only for children above a certain age.

Pregnancy and breastfeeding: This drug is either not recommended for use by women who are pregnant or breastfeeding, or the precise effects are not known and it should therefore only be used with caution and under medical advice.

Alcohol: Alcohol should not be consumed, or only consumed with caution - after medical advice has been sought - while you are taking this drug.

Driving and operating machinery: This drug may have some effect on your driving ability, so it is advisable not to drive or operate machinery while taking it.

NORETHISTERONE

Brand name: Menzol, Micronor, Noriday, Noristerat, Primolut N, Utovlan

Type of drug: Female sex hormone

Uses: To treat a range of menstrual disorders, including endometriosis. Is also an ingredient of the contraceptive pill. Can be used to treat certain types of breast cancer.

How it works: Acts in a similar way to the female hormone progesterone.

Possible adverse effects: Breakthrough bleeding in between normal periods.

Availability: Available only with a prescription from a doctor.

Other information: Given as an injection or in tablet form. Blood tests to check liver function may be conducted at intervals during treatment.

CAUTIONS

Children: This drug is either not recommended for children, or is recommended only for children above a certain age.

Pregnancy and breastfeeding: This drug is either not recommended for use by women who are pregnant or breastfeeding, or the precise effects are not known and it should therefore only be used with caution and under medical advice.

Alcohol: No known problems if taken with alcohol.

Driving and operating machinery: There are no commonly reported problems which may impact on the ability to drive or operate machinery. However, many drugs can cause dizziness or drowsiness in a few people, so it is wise to see how the drug affects you before driving or working with dangerous machinery.

NORFLOXACIN

Brand name: Utinor

Type of drug: Antibiotic

Uses: To treat infections of the urinary tract.

How it works: Acts on the DNA in the infected organism to prevent it replicating.

Possible adverse effects: Nausea, heartburn, abdominal cramps, diarrhoea, headache, dizziness, anxiety.

Availability: Available only with a prescription from a doctor.

Other information: The patient is advised to take this medication one hour before - or two hours after - meals or antacids.

CAUTIONS

Children: There are no commonly reported problems associated with prescribing this medication for children.

Pregnancy and breastfeeding: This drug is either not recommended for use by women who are pregnant or breastfeeding, or the precise effects are not known and it should therefore only be used with caution and under medical advice.

Alcohol: No known problems if taken with alcohol.

Driving and operating machinery: This drug may have some effect on your driving ability, so it is advisable not to drive or operate machinery while taking it.

NYSTATIN

Brand name: Nystamont, Nystan

Type of drug: Anti-fungal

Uses: To treat yeast infections such as thrush, and other infections of the skin, mouth, throat, gut and vagina.

How it works: Acts against infections caused by fungi, by either preventing them from replicating or killing them.

Possible adverse effects: These are uncommon and usually pass off quickly.

Availability: Available only with a prescription from a doctor.

Other information: Good hygiene is essential to prevent re-infection. Vaginal tablets can be used by pregnant women up to six weeks before the due date. Always finish the course prescribed in order to minimise the risk of re-infection.

CAUTIONS

Children: There are no commonly reported problems associated with prescribing this medication for children.

Pregnancy and breastfeeding: No specific problems documented, but any medication should be taken with utmost caution by women who are either pregnant or breastfeeding, and only after medical advice.

Alcohol: No known problems if taken with alcohol.

Driving and operating machinery: There are no commonly reported problems which may impact on the ability to drive or operate machinery. However, many drugs can cause dizziness or drowsiness in a few people, so it is wise to see how the drug affects you before driving or working with dangerous machinery.

OCTREOTIDE

Brand name: Sandostatin

Type of drug: Hormone

Uses: To treat acromegaly - abnormal growth of the hands, feet and face due to excessive pituitary gland activity caused by a tumour.

How it works: Mimics the action of naturally occurring chemicals, with the result that the symptoms are decreased. It is not known if the drug affects the tumour directly.

Possible adverse effects: Gastrointestinal disturbances, abdominal pain, nausea, vomiting, diarrhoea.

Availability: Available only with a prescription from a doctor.

Other information: This drug can cause gallstones, so patient is advised to report serious abdominal discomfort promptly.

CAUTIONS

Children: There are no commonly reported problems associated with prescribing this medication for children.

Pregnancy and breastfeeding: This drug is either not recommended for use by women who are pregnant or breastfeeding, or the precise effects are not known and it should therefore only be used with caution and under medical advice.

Alcohol: No known problems if taken with alcohol.

Driving and operating machinery: There are no commonly reported problems which may impact on the ability to drive or operate machinery. However, many drugs can cause dizziness or drowsiness in a few people, so it is wise to see how the drug affects you before driving or working with dangerous machinery.

OESTRADIOL

Brand name: Climaval, Estraderm, Estrapak, FemSeven, Menorest, Oestrogel, Progynova, Vagifem, Zumenon

Type of drug: Female sex hormone

Uses: Treatment of the symptoms of the menopause and post-menopausal period.

How it works: Replaces hormones lost during the menopause, with the result that symptoms such as hot flushes, night sweats and vaginal dryness are lessened.

Possible adverse effects: Symptoms similar to those experienced during the early stages of pregnancy, including nausea, sore breasts and weight gain. Skin patches sometimes can cause a local rash.

Availability: Available only with a prescription from a doctor.

Other information: Available as tablets, pessaries, skin gel, skin patches, implants and vaginal ring. Often given with a progestogen.

CAUTIONS

Children: This drug is either not recommended for children, or is recommended only for children above a certain age.

Pregnancy and breastfeeding: This drug is either not recommended for use by women who are pregnant or breastfeeding, or the precise effects are not known and it should therefore only be used with caution and after medical advice.

Alcohol: No known problems if taken with alcohol.

Driving and operating machinery: There are no commonly reported problems which may impact on the ability to drive or operate machinery. However, many drugs can cause dizziness or drowsiness in a few people so it is wise to see how the drug affects you before driving or working with dangerous machinery.

OESTROGEN - See under Conjugated Oestrogen

OFLOXACIN

Brand name: Tarivid

Type of drug: Anti-bacterial

Uses: To treat infections of the urinary tract, the lower respiratory tract, the genital tract and infections of the eyes such as conjunctivitis.

How it works: Interferes with the DNA of the infected organism, preventing it from replicating.

Possible adverse effects: Dizziness, sleep disorders, headache, nervousness, visual disturbances. Stinging and irritation of the eye.

Availability: Available only with a prescription from a doctor.

Other information: Patient should be advised to drink plenty of fluids. Also must discontinue drug if a rash or similar allergic reaction occurs. Prolonged exposure to the sun should be avoided. If being treated for eye infection, do not wear soft contact lenses.

CAUTIONS

Children: This drug is either not recommended for children, or is recommended only for children above a certain age.

Pregnancy and breastfeeding: This drug is either not recommended for use by women who are pregnant or breastfeeding, or the precise effects are not known and it should therefore only be used with caution and under medical advice.

Alcohol: Alcohol should not be consumed, or only consumed with caution - after medical advice has been sought - while you are taking this drug.

Driving and operating machinery: This drug may have some effect on your driving ability, so it is advisable not to drive or operate machinery while taking it.

OLANZAPINE

Brand name: Zyprexa

Type of drug: Anti-psychotic

Uses: The management of manifestations of psychotic disorders such as schizophrenia.

How it works: Alters the chemicals in the brain, with the result that paranoia and hallucinations are lessened and speech, thought and mood are improved.

Possible adverse effects: Dizziness, drowsiness, increased appetite, weight gain, dry mouth and blurred vision.

Availability: Available only with a prescription from a doctor.

Other information: Patient is not to have any over-the-counter preparations unless advised by a doctor.

CAUTIONS

Children: This drug is either not recommended for children, or is recommended only for children above a certain age.

Pregnancy and breastfeeding: This drug is either not recommended for use by women who are pregnant or breastfeeding, or the precise effects are not known and it should therefore only be used with caution and under medical advice.

Alcohol: Alcohol should not be consumed, or only consumed with caution - after medical advice has been sought - while you are taking this drug.

Driving and operating machinery: This drug may have some effect on

your driving ability, so it is advisable not to drive or operate machinery while taking it.

OMEPRAZOLE

Brand name: Losec

Type of drug: Anti-ulcer

Uses: Treatment of stomach ulcers, reflux oesophagitis and, in conjunction with other drugs, of the Helicobacter pylori bacteria.

How it works: Reduces the amount of acid that the stomach produces by about 70 per cent. When given in conjunction with antibiotics it is effective at eradicating the Helicobacter pylori bacteria that are known to cause many gastric ulcers.

Possible adverse effects: Headache, dizziness, nausea, flatulence, constipation and diarrhoea.

Availability: Available only with a prescription from a doctor.

Other information: Patients are advised to take the drug exactly as prescribed; also to take it before meals and not to crush the capsules, but to swallow them whole.

CAUTIONS

Children: This drug is either not recommended for children, or is recommended only for children above a certain age.

Pregnancy and breastfeeding: This drug is either not recommended for use by women who are pregnant or breastfeeding, or the precise effects are not known and it should therefore only be used with caution and under medical advice.

Alcohol: Alcohol should not be consumed, or only consumed with caution - after medical advice has been sought - while you are taking this drug.

Driving and operating machinery: There are no commonly reported problems which may impact on the ability to drive or operate machinery. However, many drugs can cause dizziness or drowsiness in a few people, so it is wise to see how the drug affects you before driving or working with dangerous machinery.

ONDANSETRON

Brand name: Zofran

Type of drug: Anti-emetic

Uses: To treat post-operative nausea and vomiting and nausea resulting from chemotherapy treatment.

How it works: Precise action is not known, but it is most effective if given prior to the dose of chemotherapy that causes nausea and vomiting.

Possible adverse effects: Headache, fatigue, constipation, flushing.

Availability: Available only with a prescription from a doctor.

Other information: Administered either as tablets or as an injection.

CAUTIONS

Children: There are no commonly reported problems associated with prescribing this medication for children.

Pregnancy and breastfeeding: This drug is either not recommended for use by women who are pregnant or breastfeeding, or the precise effects are not known and it should therefore only be used with caution and under medical advice.

Alcohol: No known problems if taken with alcohol.

Driving and operating machinery: There are no commonly reported problems which may impact on the ability to drive or operate machinery. However, many drugs can cause dizziness or drowsiness in a few people, so it is wise to see how the drug affects you before driving or working with dangerous machinery.

ORPHENADRINE

Brand name: Biorphen, Disipal, Norflex

Type of drug: Muscle relaxant

Uses: Treatment of symptoms of Parkinson's disease.

How it works: Acts on the part of the brain which controls muscle tone, with the result that muscle stiffness and spasm, which are characteristic of Parkinsonism, are relieved.

Possible adverse effects: Dry mouth, blurred vision, insomnia, confusion, headache, difficulty in passing water.

Availability: Available only with a prescription from a doctor.

Other information: Patient should be warned that some over-the-counter preparations contain alcohol and so should be used cautiously.

CAUTIONS

Children: This drug is either not recommended for children, or is recommended only for children above a certain age.

Pregnancy and breastfeeding: This drug is either not recommended for use by women who are pregnant or breastfeeding, or the precise effects are not known and it should therefore only be used with caution and under medical advice.

Alcohol: Alcohol should not be consumed or only consumed with caution - after medical advice has been sought - while you are taking this drug.

Driving and operating machinery: This drug may have some effect on your driving ability, so it is advisable not to drive or operate machinery while taking it.

OXITROPIUM

Brand name: Oxivent

Type of drug: Bronchodilator

Uses: The alleviation of the symptoms of respiratory disease such as chronic bronchitis and asthma.

How it works: Relieves the constriction of the airways which is characteristic of chronic obstructive pulmonary disease.

Possible adverse effects: Rarely, dry mouth and irritation of the throat.

Availability: Available only with a prescription from a doctor.

Other information: The medication is delivered through an inhaler. Patient is advised not to exceed prescribed dose. Should not be used by people with glaucoma.

CAUTIONS

Children: This drug is either not recommended for children, or is recommended only for children above a certain age.

Pregnancy and breastfeeding: This drug is either not recommended for use by women who are pregnant or breastfeeding, or the precise effects are not known and it should therefore only be used with caution and under medical advice.

Alcohol: No known problems if taken with alcohol.

Driving and operating machinery: There are no commonly reported problems which may impact on the ability to drive or operate machinery. However, many drugs can cause dizziness or drowsiness in a few people, so it is wise to see how the drug affects you before driving or working with dangerous machinery.

OXYBUTYNIN
Brand name: Cystrin, Ditropan
Type of drug: Anti-spasmodic
Uses: To treat the frequency and urgency to pass urine which is associated with incontinence.
How it works: Increases bladder capacity by diminishing the unwanted muscle contractions which cause the problem.
Possible adverse effects: Dizziness, blurred vision, dry mouth, abdominal discomfort.
Availability: Available only with a prescription from a doctor.
Other information: Drug will be discontinued periodically to see if the patient still requires it.
CAUTIONS
Children: There are no commonly reported problems associated with prescribing this medication for children.
Pregnancy and breastfeeding: This drug is either not recommended for use by women who are pregnant or breastfeeding, or the precise effects are not known and it should therefore only be used with caution and under medical advice.
Alcohol: No known problems if taken with alcohol.
Driving and operating machinery: This drug may have some effect on your driving ability, so it is advisable not to drive or operate machinery while taking it.

PANTOPRAZOLE
Brand name: Protium
Type of drug: Protein pump inhibitor
Uses: For treating stomach ulcers.
How it works: Blocks the production of stomach acid, excessive amounts of which cause gastric ulcers.
Possible adverse effects: Headache, abdominal pain, diarrhoea, dizziness, itching and rash.
Availability: Available only with a prescription from a doctor.
Other information: Administered either as an injection or as tablets.
CAUTIONS
Children: This drug is either not recommended for children, or is recommended only for children above a certain age.

Pregnancy and breastfeeding: This drug is either not recommended for use by women who are pregnant or breastfeeding, or the precise effects are not known and it should therefore only be used with caution and under medical advice.

Alcohol: No known problems if taken with alcohol.

Driving and operating machinery: There are no commonly reported problems which may impact on the ability to drive or operate machinery. However, many drugs can cause dizziness or drowsiness in a few people, so it is wise to see how the drug affects you before driving or working with dangerous machinery.

PAROXETINE

Brand name: Seroxat

Type of drug: Anti-depressant

Uses: Treatment of mild to moderate depression, panic disorders and obsessive-compulsive disorders.

How it works: Has an anti-depressant action which results in a heightening of mood and an improved ability to lead a normal daily life.

Possible adverse effects: Nausea and sweating, weakness, inability to sleep and shaking.

Availability: Available only with a prescription from a doctor.

Other information: Some symptoms of withdrawal may be experienced if the drug is stopped suddenly.

CAUTIONS

Children: This drug is either not recommended for children, or is recommended only for children above a certain age.

Pregnancy and breastfeeding: This drug is either not recommended for use by women who are pregnant or breastfeeding, or the precise effects are not known and it should therefore only be used with caution and under medical advice.

Alcohol: Alcohol should not be consumed, or only consumed with caution - after medical advice has been sought - while you are taking this drug.

Driving and operating machinery: This drug may have some effect on your driving ability, so it is advisable not to drive or operate machinery while taking it.

PENICILLAMINE
Brand name: Distamine, Pendramine
Type of drug: Anti-rheumatic drug
Uses: To treat rheumatic disease; also used as an antidote to treat copper and lead poisoning.
How it works: Slows or halts the progression of rheumatoid arthritis.
Possible adverse effects: Nausea, anorexia, vomiting, mouth ulcers. Kidney problems.
Availability: Available only with a prescription from a doctor.
Other information: The patient taking this drug should drink large quantities of water. It may be a few weeks before the benefits are felt. Sore throat or unexplained rashes or fevers must be reported immediately.
CAUTIONS
Children: There are no commonly reported problems associated with prescribing this medication for children.
Pregnancy and breastfeeding: This drug is either not recommended for use by women who are pregnant or breastfeeding, or the precise effects are not known and it should therefore only be used with caution and under medical advice.
Alcohol: No known problems if taken with alcohol.
Driving and operating machinery: There are no commonly reported problems which may impact on the ability to drive or operate machinery. However, many drugs can cause dizziness or drowsiness in a few people, so it is wise to see how the drug affects you before driving or working with dangerous machinery.

PENTAMIDINE
Brand name: Pentacarinat
Type of drug: Anti-protazoal
Uses: To treat pneumonia caused by pneumocystis carinii, in HIV, AIDS, chemotherapy and other immunosuppressed patients.
How it works: Precise action unknown, but is thought to affect the DNA of the infective organism and parts of the organism's metabolic process.
Possible adverse effects: Can cause severe side effects, hypotension, hypoglycaemia, rapid heart beat. Other effects are dizziness, headache, confusion.

Availability: Available only with a prescription from a doctor.

Other information: This treatment will be delivered in hospital under close supervision.

CAUTIONS

Children: This drug is either not recommended for children, or is recommended only for children above a certain age.

Pregnancy and breastfeeding: This drug is either not recommended for use by women who are pregnant or breastfeeding, or the precise effects are not known and it should therefore only be used with caution and under medical advice.

Alcohol: Alcohol should not be consumed, or only consumed with caution - after medical advice has been sought - while you are taking this drug.

Driving and operating machinery: This drug may have some effect on your driving ability, so it is advisable not to drive or operate machinery while taking it.

PENTAZOCINE

Brand name: Fortagesic, Fortral

Type of drug: Opioid analgesic

Uses: To treat moderate to severe pain.

How it works: Exact mechanism of action is unknown.

Possible adverse effects: Dizziness, nausea, vomiting. Respiratory depression is possible. Patient should report rash, confusion or any other serious side effect immediately.

Availability: Available only with a prescription from a doctor.

Other information: Physical dependence is possible.

CAUTIONS

Children: There are no commonly reported problems associated with prescribing this medication for children.

Pregnancy and breastfeeding: This drug is either not recommended for use by women who are pregnant or breastfeeding, or the precise effects are not known and it should therefore only be used with caution and under medical advice.

Alcohol: Alcohol should not be consumed, or only consumed with caution - after medical advice has been sought - while you are taking this drug.

Driving and operating machinery: This drug may have some effect on your driving ability, so it is advisable not to drive or operate machinery while taking it.

PERGOLIDE
Brand name: Celance
Type of drug: Dopaminergic drug
Uses: To treat the symptoms of Parkinson's disease.
How it works: Reduces tremor and rigidity and improves movement in sufferers.
Possible adverse effects: Headache, sleepiness, hallucinations and confusion, fall in blood pressure.
Availability: Available only with a prescription from a doctor.
Other information: Patient should be warned of the adverse effects, mainly hallucination and confusion.
CAUTIONS
Children: This drug is either not recommended for children, or is recommended only for children above a certain age.
Pregnancy and breastfeeding: This drug is either not recommended for use by women who are pregnant or breastfeeding, or the precise effects are not known and it should therefore only be used with caution and under medical advice.
Alcohol: No known problems if taken with alcohol.
Driving and operating machinery: This drug may have some effect on your driving ability, so it is advisable not to drive or operate machinery while taking it.

PERINDOPRIL
Brand name: Coversyl
Type of drug: ACE inhibitor
Uses: Used to treat raised blood pressure and congestive heart failure.
How it works: Reduces constriction of the arteries and lowers blood volume, with the result that the blood pressure falls.
Possible adverse effects: Too much of a fall in blood pressure, leading to light-headedness and dizziness. Nausea, flushing.
Availability: Available only with a prescription from a doctor.
Other information: Supplied as tablets.

CAUTIONS

Children: There are no commonly reported problems associated with prescribing this medication for children.

Pregnancy and breastfeeding: This drug is either not recommended for use by women who are pregnant or breastfeeding, or the precise effects are not known and it should therefore only be used with caution and under medical advice.

Alcohol: No known problems if taken with alcohol.

Driving and operating machinery: There are no commonly reported problems which may impact on the ability to drive or operate machinery. However, many drugs can cause dizziness or drowsiness in a few people, so it is wise to see how the drug affects you before driving or working with dangerous machinery.

PERMETHRIN

Brand name: Lyclear

Type of drug: Insecticide

Uses: To treat head lice and scabies.

How it works: Paralyses the parasites that cause the infestation.

Possible adverse effects: Burning and stinging. Any itching, redness or swelling of the scalp should be reported.

Availability: Available with or without a prescription (over-the-counter).

Other information: Avoid contact with the eyes, do not apply to broken or infected skin. Follow the instructions carefully to maximise treatment.

CAUTIONS

Children: There are no commonly reported problems associated with prescribing this medication for children.

Pregnancy and breastfeeding: This drug is either not recommended for use by women who are pregnant or breastfeeding, or the precise effects are not known and it should therefore only be used with caution and under medical advice.

Alcohol: No known problems if taken with alcohol.

Driving and operating machinery: There are no commonly reported problems which may impact on the ability to drive or operate machinery. However, many drugs can cause dizziness or drowsiness in a few people, so it is wise to see how the drug affects you before driving or working with dangerous machinery.

PETHIDINE

Brand name: Pethidine

Type of drug: Opioid analgesic

Uses: For moderate to severe pain, such as during labour and after an operation.

How it works: Takes effect quickly, but lasts for a shorter time than alternative pain relief.

Possible adverse effects: Dizziness, sweating, dry mouth, nausea, confusion, vomiting.

Availability: Available only with a prescription from a doctor.

Other information: Potentially habit-forming, although this is unlikely to be a problem if the drug is used appropriately.

CAUTIONS

Children: There are no commonly reported problems associated with prescribing this medication for children.

Pregnancy and breastfeeding: This drug is either not recommended for use by women who are pregnant or breastfeeding, or the precise effects are not known and it should therefore only be used with caution and under medical advice.

Alcohol: Alcohol should not be consumed, or only consumed with caution - after medical advice has been sought - while you are taking this drug.

Driving and operating machinery: This drug may have some effect on your driving ability, so it is advisable not to drive or operate machinery while taking it.

PHENAZOCINE

Brand name: Narphen

Type of drug: Opioid analgesic

Uses: For the treatment of severe pain. Particularly used for gall-bladder and pancreatic pain.

How it works: Works in a similar way to morphine to relieve severe pain.

Possible adverse effects: Nausea, vomiting, drowsiness and constipation.

Availability: Available only with a prescription from a doctor.

Other information: May produce drug dependence, but is unlikely to do so if used appropriately.

CAUTIONS

Children: This drug is either not recommended for children, or is recommended only for children above a certain age.

Pregnancy and breastfeeding: This drug is either not recommended for use by women who are pregnant or breastfeeding, or the precise effects are not known and it should therefore only be used with caution and under medical advice.

Alcohol: Alcohol should not be consumed, or only consumed with caution - after medical advice has been sought - while you are taking this drug.

Driving and operating machinery: This drug may have some effect on your driving ability, so it is advisable not to drive or operate machinery while taking it.

PHENINDIONE

Brand name: Dindevan

Type of drug: Anti-coagulant

Uses: To prevent and treat deep-vein thrombosis, atrial fibrillation and pulmonary embolism.

How it works: Alters the composition of the blood, making it 'thinner'.

Possible adverse effects: Haemorrhage, rash, diarrhoea, nausea.

Availability: Available only with a prescription from a doctor.

Other information: Supplied as tablets. Urine may be discoloured.

CAUTIONS

Children: This drug is either not recommended for children, or is recommended only for children above a certain age.

Pregnancy and breastfeeding: This drug is either not recommended for use by women who are pregnant or breastfeeding, or the precise effects are not known and it should therefore only be used with caution and under medical advice.

Alcohol: Alcohol should not be consumed, or only consumed with caution - after medical advice has been sought - while you are taking this drug.

Driving and operating machinery: This drug may have some effect on your driving ability, so it is advisable not to drive or operate machinery while taking it.

PHENOBARBITONE

Brand name: Phenobarbitol Sodium, Gardenal Sodium

Type of drug: Anti-convulsant

Uses: To treat all forms of epilepsy other than sufferers who have a sense of absence (absence seizures).

How it works: Suppresses the spread of seizure activity in the brain and acts as a depressant.

Possible adverse effects: Drowsiness, lethargy, weakness, depression.

Availability: Available only with a prescription from a doctor.

Other information: Patient must not stop taking the drug suddenly, as some symptoms of withdrawal may be experienced.

CAUTIONS

Children: This drug is either not recommended for children, or is recommended only for children above a certain age.

Pregnancy and breastfeeding: This drug is either not recommended for use by women who are pregnant or breastfeeding, or the precise effects are not known and it should therefore only be used with caution and under medical advice.

Alcohol: Alcohol should not be consumed, or only consumed with caution - after medical advice has been sought - while you are taking this drug.

Driving and operating machinery: This drug may have some effect on your driving ability, so it is advisable not to drive or operate machinery while taking it.

PHENOXYMETHYLPENICILLIN

Brand name: Stabillin V-K, Tenkicin

Type of drug: Penicillin antibiotic

Uses: Used to treat a wide variety of infections. Respiratory tract, tonsillitis, pharyngitis, ear and gum infections. Also scarlet fever, rheumatic fever and sickle cell disease.

How it works: A synthetic drug which destroys the organisms that are causing the infection.

Possible adverse effects: Nausea, diarrhoea, itching, rashes, joint pain. Long-term use may increase the risk of infections with thrush.

Availability: Available only with a prescription from a doctor.

Other information: Not for patients who are allergic to penicillin.

CAUTIONS

Children: There are no commonly reported problems associated with prescribing this medication for children.

Pregnancy and breastfeeding: No specific problems documented, but any medication should be taken with utmost caution by women who are either pregnant or breastfeeding, and only after professional medical or pharmaceutical advice has been sought.

Alcohol: No known problems if taken with alcohol.

Driving and operating machinery: There are no commonly reported problems which may impact on the ability to drive or operate machinery. However, many drugs can cause dizziness or drowsiness in a few people, so it is wise to see how the drug affects you before driving or working with dangerous machinery.

PHENTERMINE

Brand name: Duromine, Ionamin

Type of drug: Appetite suppressant

Uses: For use only in severe cases of obesity.

How it works: Suppresses the appetite and boosts energy levels.

Possible adverse effects: Dizziness, drowsiness, confusion, dry mouth headache. Risk of dependence.

Availability: Available only with a prescription from a doctor.

Other information: Patients are advised to swallow the medication whole, not to chew or crush the tablet. Should also avoid caffeine-containing drinks. Patients should report if they suffer palpitations or dyspnoea.

CAUTIONS

Children: This drug is either not recommended for children, or is recommended only for children above a certain age.

Pregnancy and breastfeeding: This drug is either not recommended for use by women who are pregnant or breastfeeding, or the precise effects are not known and it should therefore only be used with caution and under medical advice.

Alcohol: Alcohol should not be consumed, or only consumed with caution - after medical advice has been sought - while you are taking this drug.

Driving and operating machinery: This drug may have some effect on

your driving ability, so it is advisable not to drive or operate machinery while taking it.

PHENYLBUTAZONE
Brand name: Butacote
Type of drug: Non-steroidal anti-inflammatory
Uses: To treat rheumatic diseases such as ankylosing spondylitis. Also can be used as a pain relief treatment and reduces high temperature.
How it works: Has a pain-killing and anti-inflammatory effect and is effective at treating continuous or regular pain.
Possible adverse effects: Salt retention, interferes with several enzyme processes. If sore throat, mouth ulcers, fevers or bruising occur, notify a doctor immediately.
Availability: Available only with a prescription from a doctor.
Other information: Do not take if allergic to aspirin.
CAUTIONS
Children: This drug is either not recommended for children, or is recommended only for children above a certain age.
Pregnancy and breastfeeding: This drug is either not recommended for use by women who are pregnant or breastfeeding, or the precise effects are not known and it should therefore only be used with caution and under medical advice.
Alcohol: No known problems if taken with alcohol.
Driving and operating machinery: There are no commonly reported problems which may impact on the ability to drive or operate machinery. However, many drugs can cause dizziness or drowsiness in a few people, so it is wise to see how the drug affects you before driving or working with dangerous machinery.

PHENYLEPHRINE
Brand name: Minims Phenylephrine
Type of drug: Decongestant
Uses: Used to treat hay fever and colds, to dilate the pupils and as a treatment for a fall in blood pressure.
How it works: Has a decongestant action. Constricts the blood vessels in the eye and dilates the pupils.

Possible adverse effects: Raised blood pressure, headache. Stinging of the eye in eye-treatment.

Availability: Available with or without a prescription (over the counter).

Other information: Prolonged use of the nasal spray may result in rebound congestion.

CAUTIONS

Children: This drug is either not recommended for children, or is recommended only for children above a certain age.

Pregnancy and breastfeeding: This drug is either not recommended for use by women who are pregnant or breastfeeding, or the precise effects are not known and it should therefore only be used with caution and under medical advice.

Alcohol: No known problems if taken with alcohol.

Driving and operating machinery: This drug may have some effect on your driving ability, so it is advisable not to drive or operate machinery while taking it.

PHENYLPROPANOLAMINE

Brand name: Dimotapp, Eskornade

Type of drug: Sympathomimetic

Uses: Used to treat sinusitis, head colds and hay fever.

How it works: Has a decongestant effect by reducing inflammation and swelling of the blood vessels within the lining of the nose.

Possible adverse effects: Raised blood pressure, palpitations, headaches.

Availability: Available with or without a prescription (over the counter).

Other information: Should not be used for long periods of time, as can raise blood pressure.

CAUTIONS

Children: This drug is either not recommended for children, or is recommended only for children above a certain age.

Pregnancy and breastfeeding: This drug is either not recommended for use by women who are pregnant or breastfeeding, or the precise effects are not known and it should therefore only be used with caution and under medical advice.

Alcohol: No known problems if taken with alcohol.

Driving and operating machinery: This drug may have some effect on your driving ability, so it is advisable not to drive or operate machinery while taking it.

PHENYTOIN
Brand name: Epanutin, Pentran
Type of drug: Anti-convulsant
Uses: Treatment of epilepsy, migraine and some abnormal heart rhythms.
How it works: Reduces the abnormal electrical discharges within the brain that lead to seizures.
Possible adverse effects: Dizziness, confusion, nausea and vomiting, difficulty in sleeping. Most adverse effects only occur with long-term use.
Availability: Available only with a prescription from a doctor.
Other information: Patient should take drug with food or milk to minimise side effects. A higher dose of contraceptive will be required.
CAUTIONS
Children: There are no commonly reported problems associated with prescribing this medication for children.
Pregnancy and breastfeeding: This drug is either not recommended for use by women who are pregnant or breastfeeding, or the precise effects are not known and it should therefore only be used with caution and under medical advice.
Alcohol: Alcohol should not be consumed, or only consumed with caution - after medical advice has been sought - while you are taking this drug.
Driving and operating machinery: This drug may have some effect on your driving ability, so it is advisable not to drive or operate machinery while taking it.

PILOCARPINE
Brand name: Minims Pilocarpine, Ocusert Pilo, Salagen, Sno Pilo
Type of drug: Glaucoma treatment
Uses: Treatment of acute and chronic glaucoma.
How it works: Narrows the pupil within the eye. Can be given as slow release Ocuserts, which are put under the eyelid once a week.
Possible adverse effects: Changes to vision, including blurring and poor sight at night. Headaches and irritation of the eye are also possible.

Availability: Available only with a prescription from a doctor.

Other information: Prescribed as eye drops and Ocuserts (slow-release inserts which are placed under the eyelid once a week).

CAUTIONS

Children: There are no commonly reported problems associated with prescribing this medication for children.

Pregnancy and breastfeeding: No specific problems documented, but any medication should be taken with utmost caution by women who are either pregnant or breastfeeding, and only after professional medical or pharmaceutical advice has been sought.

Alcohol: No known problems if taken with alcohol.

Driving and operating machinery: This drug may have some effect on your driving ability, so it is advisable not to drive or operate machinery while taking it.

PIPERAZINE

Brand name: Expelix, Pripsen

Type of drug: Anthelmintic

Uses: To treat infestations of threadworm and roundworm.

How it works: Paralyses the worms and enables the body to eliminate them.

Possible adverse effects: Very rare. Consult a doctor if there are any signs of a rash, or itching.

Availability: Available with or without a prescription (over the counter).

Other information: Roundworm treatment is usually completed in one dose, but it may need to be repeated in severe cases. Threadworm treatment may take up to seven days. Follow the instructions carefully.

CAUTIONS

Children: There are no commonly reported problems associated with prescribing this medication for children.

Pregnancy and breastfeeding: This drug is either not recommended for use by women who are pregnant or breastfeeding, or the precise effects are not known and it should therefore only be used with caution and under medical advice.

Alcohol: No known problems if taken with alcohol.

Driving and operating machinery: This drug may have some effect on

your driving ability, so it is advisable not to drive or operate machinery while taking it.

PIROXICAM

Brand name: Feldene, Flamatrol, Kentene, Larapram, Piroflam, Pirozip.

Type of drug: Non-steroidal anti-inflammatory, gout treatment

Uses: Relieves the symptoms of osteoarthritis, rheumatoid arthritis, and ankylosing spondylitis.

How it works: Reduces pain, stiffness and inflammation which occur with the above conditions. Does not cure the underlying condition.

Possible adverse effects: Stomach pain and nausea.

Availability: Available only with a prescription from a doctor.

Other information: Patient should avoid aspirin and seek medical approval with other over-the-counter preparations.

CAUTIONS

Children: There are no commonly reported problems associated with prescribing this medication for children.

Pregnancy and breastfeeding: This drug is either not recommended for use by women who are pregnant or breastfeeding, or the precise effects are not known and it should therefore only be used with caution and under medical advice.

Alcohol: Alcohol should not be consumed, or only consumed with caution - after medical advice has been sought - while you are taking this drug.

Driving and operating machinery: This drug may have some effect on your driving ability, so it is advisable not to drive or operate machinery while taking it.

PIZOTIFEN

Brand name: Sanomigran

Type of drug: Anti-migraine

Uses: Used to treat migraine, vascular and cluster headaches.

How it works: Works in a similar way to some anti-depressants. It is thought to block the effect of some of the chemicals that act on the blood vessels in the brain.

Possible adverse effects: Drowsiness, increased appetite, weight gain.

Availability: Available only with a prescription from a doctor.

Other information: Can cause weight gain during long periods of use.

CAUTIONS

Children: There are no commonly reported problems associated with prescribing this medication for children.

Pregnancy and breastfeeding: This drug is either not recommended for use by women who are pregnant or breastfeeding, or the precise effects are not known and it should therefore only be used with caution and under medical advice.

Alcohol: Alcohol should not be consumed, or only consumed with caution - after medical advice has been sought - while you are taking this drug.

Driving and operating machinery: This drug may have some effect on your driving ability, so it is advisable not to drive or operate machinery while taking it.

PODOPHYLLOTOXIN

Brand name: Condyline, Warticon

Type of drug: Wart and callus preparation

Uses: Used to treat external genital warts.

How it works: Kills the causative organism and destroys the wart.

Possible adverse effects: Can cause considerable skin irritation. Severe toxicity can occur if there is excessive use of the medication.

Availability: Available only with a prescription from a doctor.

Other information: Should be washed off the treated area after six hours. Protect skin around the affected area with a soft paraffin preparation.

CAUTIONS

Children: This drug is either not recommended for children, or is recommended only for children above a certain age.

Pregnancy and breastfeeding: This drug is either not recommended for use by women who are pregnant or breastfeeding, or the precise effects are not known and it should therefore only be used with caution and under medical advice.

Alcohol: No known problems if taken with alcohol.

Driving and operating machinery: There are no commonly reported problems which may impact on the ability to drive or operate machinery. However, many drugs can cause dizziness or drowsiness in a few people,

so it is wise to see how the drug affects you before driving or working with dangerous machinery.

PRAVASTATIN

Brand name: Lipostat

Type of drug: Lipid lowering

Uses: Used to treat people with raised blood cholesterol levels.

How it works: Prevents the formation of cholesterol which is associated with coronary artery disease.

Possible adverse effects: Nausea, constipation, flatulence, insomnia, dizziness, chest pain, fatigue.

Availability: Available only with a prescription from a doctor.

Other information: Patient should be instructed to eat a low fat, low cholesterol diet and take exercise. A doctor should be notified of any adverse aches and pains. Drug is best taken at bedtime.

CAUTIONS

Children: This drug is either not recommended for children, or is recommended only for children above a certain age.

Pregnancy and breastfeeding: This drug is either not recommended for use by women who are pregnant or breastfeeding, or the precise effects are not known and it should therefore only be used with caution and under medical advice.

Alcohol: Alcohol should not be consumed, or only consumed with caution - after medical advice has been sought - while you are taking this drug.

Driving and operating machinery: There are no commonly reported problems which may impact on the ability to drive or operate machinery. However, many drugs can cause dizziness or drowsiness in a few people, so it is wise to see how the drug affects you before driving or working with dangerous machinery.

PRAZOSIN

Brand name: Alphavase, Hypovase

Type of drug: Anti-hypertensive

Uses: Used as a treatment for high blood pressure and conditions caused by poor circulation, such as Raynaud's disease. Also given to relieve symptoms associated with an enlarged prostate gland.

How it works: Relaxes the blood vessel walls, enabling more blood to flow through.

Possible adverse effects: Dizziness and fainting on first rising. Nausea, headache, faintness and drowsiness. First dose may cause a dramatic drop in blood pressure and will be given when the patient is lying down.

Availability: Available only with a prescription from a doctor.

Other information: Patient should seek medical approval before taking any over-the-counter preparations. Must not stop taking drug suddenly.

CAUTIONS

Children: This drug is either not recommended for children, or is recommended only for children above a certain age.

Pregnancy and breastfeeding: This drug is either not recommended for use by women who are pregnant or breastfeeding, or the precise effects are not known and it should therefore only be used with caution and under medical advice.

Alcohol: Alcohol should not be consumed, or only consumed with caution - after medical advice has been sought - while you are taking this drug.

Driving and operating machinery: This drug may have some effect on your driving ability, so it is advisable not to drive or operate machinery while taking it.

PREDNISOLONE

Brand name: Deltacortril, Deltastab, Minims prednisolone, Precortisyl, Predenema, Predfoam, Pred Forte, Predsol

Type of drug: Corticosteroid

Uses: Corticosteroid used to treat a range of skin diseases, allergies, some blood disorders, inflammatory bowel disease and arthritis.

How it works: Stimulates the production of enzymes needed to reduce the inflammatory response. Suppresses the immune system by reducing activity and volume of the lymphatic system, thus reducing the inflammatory response.

Possible adverse effects: Indigestion and acne. More serious side effects are possible when taken for long periods. These include diabetes and glaucoma. Discuss with your doctor.

Availability: Available only with a prescription from a doctor.

Other information: Alcohol can increase the risk of peptic ulcers.

CAUTIONS

Children: This drug is either not recommended for children, or is recommended only for children above a certain age.

Pregnancy and breastfeeding: No specific problems documented, but any medication should be taken with utmost caution by women who are either pregnant or breastfeeding, and only after professional medical or pharmaceutical advice has been sought.

Alcohol: Alcohol should not be consumed, or only consumed with caution - after medical advice has been sought - while you are taking this drug.

Driving and operating machinery: There are no commonly reported problems which may impact on the ability to drive or operate machinery. However, many drugs can cause dizziness or drowsiness in a few people, so it is wise to see how the drug affects you before driving or working with dangerous machinery.

PRIMIDONE

Brand name: Mysoline

Type of drug: Anti-convulsant

Uses: To treat all forms of seizures except absence seizures. Also sometimes used to treat tremors.

How it works: Has a depressant effect on the central nervous system.

Possible adverse effects: Drowsiness, light-headedness, fatigue.

Availability: Available only with a prescription from a doctor.

Other information: Drug can render oral contraceptives ineffective. Supplied as tablets or a liquid which should be shaken well before use.

CAUTIONS

Children: There are no commonly reported problems associated with prescribing this medication for children.

Pregnancy and breastfeeding: This drug is either not recommended for use by women who are pregnant or breastfeeding, or the precise effects are not known and it should therefore only be used with caution and under medical advice.

Alcohol: Alcohol should not be consumed, or only consumed with caution - after medical advice has been sought - while you are taking this drug.

Driving and operating machinery: This drug may have some effect on

your driving ability, so it is advisable not to drive or operate machinery while taking it.

PROBENECID

Brand name: Benemid

Type of drug: Gout treatment

Uses: Used to treat gout.

How it works: It increases the excretion of uric acid by the kidneys, which results in the reduction of the raised blood uric acid levels which are symptomatic of the condition.

Possible adverse effects: Nausea, vomiting, sore gums and increased passing of urine.

Availability: Available only with a prescription from a doctor.

Other information: Do not use with aspirin. Patient should drink 8-10 glasses of fluid daily.

CAUTIONS

Children: There are no commonly reported problems associated with prescribing this medication for children.

Pregnancy and breastfeeding: No specific problems documented, but any medication should be taken with utmost caution by women who are either pregnant or breastfeeding, and only after professional medical or pharmaceutical advice has been sought.

Alcohol: No known problems if taken with alcohol.

Driving and operating machinery: There are no commonly reported problems which may impact on the ability to drive or operate machinery. However, many drugs can cause dizziness or drowsiness in a few people, so it is wise to see how the drug affects you before driving or working with dangerous machinery.

PROCHLORPERAZINE

Brand name: Buccastem, Proziere, Stemetil

Type of drug: Anti-emetic and anti-psychotic

Uses: Control of nausea and vomiting which occurs with some ear disorders. Can also be used as a tranquilliser for psychiatric disorders.

How it works: Acts on the central nervous system to relieve symptoms, but is not a cure.

Possible adverse effects: Drowsiness, dry mouth, dizziness and involuntary movements similar to those seen in people with Parkinson's disease.

Availability: Available only with a prescription from a doctor.

Other information: Patient should avoid excessive exposure to sun and to extreme temperatures.

CAUTIONS

Children: There are no commonly reported problems associated with prescribing this medication for children.

Pregnancy and breastfeeding: This drug is either not recommended for use by women who are pregnant or breastfeeding, or the precise effects are not known and it should therefore only be used with caution and under medical advice.

Alcohol: Alcohol should not be consumed, or only consumed with caution - after medical advice has been sought - while you are taking this drug.

Driving and operating machinery: This drug may have some effect on your driving ability, so it is advisable not to drive or operate machinery while taking it.

PROCYCLIDINE

Brand name: Arpicolin, Kemadrin

Type of drug: Anti-Parkinsonism

Uses: To treat some of the symptoms of Parkinson's disease.

How it works: Relieves muscle rigidity and excess salivation. It is particularly effective in the early stages of the disease.

Possible adverse effects: Dizziness, dry mouth, constipation, blurred vision.

Availability: Available only with a prescription from a doctor.

Other information: Prolonged use of this drug can cause glaucoma.

CAUTIONS

Children: This drug is either not recommended for children, or is recommended only for children above a certain age.

Pregnancy and breastfeeding: This drug is either not recommended for use by women who are pregnant or breastfeeding, or the precise effects are not known and it should therefore only be used with caution and under medical advice.

Alcohol: Alcohol should not be consumed, or only consumed with caution

- after medical advice has been sought - while you are taking this drug.

Driving and operating machinery: This drug may have some effect on your driving ability, so it is advisable not to drive or operate machinery while taking it.

PROGESTERONE

Brand name: Cyclogest, Gestone

Type of drug: Female sex hormone

Uses: Used for the treatment of amenorrhoea and as an contraceptive.

How it works: As a contraceptive it suppresses ovulation.

Possible adverse effects: Acne, rashes, fluid retention, weight changes, gastrointestinal disturbances.

Availability: Available only with a prescription from a doctor.

Other information: A doctor should be consulted if there is any excessive bleeding.

CAUTIONS

Children: Unlikely to be prescribed.

Pregnancy and breastfeeding: This drug is either not recommended for use by women who are pregnant or breastfeeding, or the precise effects are not known and it should therefore only be used with caution and under medical advice.

Alcohol: No known problems if taken with alcohol.

Driving and operating machinery: There are no commonly reported problems which may impact on the ability to drive or operate machinery. However, many drugs can cause dizziness or drowsiness in a few people, so it is wise to see how the drug affects you before driving or working with dangerous machinery.

PROGUANIL

Brand name: Paludrine

Type of drug: Anti-malarial

Uses: As protection against malaria in infected areas.

How it works: Prevents development of the disease, but may need to be taken in conjunction with other drugs in order to be effective.

Possible adverse effects: These are rare, but may include stomach irritation, which usually settles with continued treatment.

Availability: Available with or without a prescription (over-the-counter).

Other information: The drug should be taken one week before travelling and for four weeks after returning. Care should be taken to avoid getting bitten.

CAUTIONS

Children: There are no commonly reported problems associated with prescribing this medication for children.

Pregnancy and breastfeeding: This drug is either not recommended for use by women who are pregnant or breastfeeding, or the precise effects are not known and it should therefore only be used with caution and under medical advice.

Alcohol: No known problems if taken with alcohol.

Driving and operating machinery: There are no commonly reported problems which may impact on the ability to drive or operate machinery. However, many drugs can cause dizziness or drowsiness in a few people, so it is wise to see how the drug affects you before driving or working with dangerous machinery.

PROMETHAZINE

Brand name: Avomine, Phenergan, Sominex

Type of drug: Antihistamine, anti-emetic

Uses: Used to treat nausea, various skin allergies and motion sickness.

How it works: Has an effect similar to that of antihistamines. Relieves itching and can also relieve nausea and vomiting caused by inner ear problems such as Meniere's disease and travel sickness. Its sedative effect means it is also given as a premedication before surgery.

Possible adverse effects: Drowsiness, dry mouth and blurred vision.

Availability: Available with or without a prescription (over-the-counter).

Other information: For motion sickness the patient should take the drug 30-60 minutes before travelling.

CAUTIONS

Children: There are no commonly reported problems associated with prescribing this medication for children.

Pregnancy and breastfeeding: This drug is either not recommended for use by women who are pregnant or breastfeeding, or the precise effects are not known and it should therefore only be used with caution and under medical advice.

Alcohol: Alcohol should not be consumed, or only consumed with caution - after medical advice has been sought - while you are taking this drug.

Driving and operating machinery: This drug may have some effect on your driving ability, so it is advisable not to drive or operate machinery while taking it.

PROPAFENONE

Brand name: Arythmol

Type of drug: Anti-arrhythmic

Uses: Is used to treat disorders of heart rhythm.

How it works: Changes the chemicals which determine the heart rhythm to slow and steady the heartbeat.

Possible adverse effects: Constipation, blurred vision, dizziness, dry mouth, nausea, vomiting and fatigue.

Availability: Available only with a prescription from a doctor.

Other information: Patient should report any signs of infection.

CAUTIONS

Children: There are no commonly reported problems associated with prescribing this medication for children.

Pregnancy and breastfeeding: This drug is either not recommended for use by women who are pregnant or breastfeeding, or the precise effects are not known and it should therefore only be used with caution and under medical advice.

Alcohol: No known problems if taken with alcohol.

Driving and operating machinery: There are no commonly reported problems which may impact on the ability to drive or operate machinery. However, many drugs can cause dizziness or drowsiness in a few people, so it is wise to see how the drug affects you before driving or working with dangerous machinery.

PROPRANOLOL

Brand name: Angilol, Apsolol, Berkolol, Beta-Prograne, Cardinol, Inderal, Inderal-LA, Propanix

Type of drug: Beta-blocker and anti-anxiety

Uses: Used to treat high blood pressure, and heart disorders, such as angina and arrhythmia. The drug can also be used to control the symptoms associated with an overactive thyroid and severe anxiety. Also used to prevent migraines.

How it works: Reduces the amount of action needed by the heart, reduces the heart rate, dilates the blood vessels, with the result that the heart rate is slowed and steadied.

Possible adverse effects: Tiredness and nausea usually only last for a short time.

Availability: Available only with a prescription from a doctor.

Other information: Patient to check with doctor before taking any other over-the-counter preparations.

CAUTIONS

Children: This drug is either not recommended for children, or is recommended only for children above a certain age.

Pregnancy and breastfeeding: This drug is either not recommended for use by women who are pregnant or breastfeeding, or the precise effects are not known and it should therefore only be used with caution and under medical advice.

Alcohol: No known problems if taken with alcohol.

Driving and operating machinery: There are no commonly reported problems which may impact on the ability to drive or operate machinery. However, many drugs can cause dizziness or drowsiness in a few people, so it is wise to see how the drug affects you before driving or working with dangerous machinery.

PROPYLTHIOURACIL

Brand name: Propylthiouracil

Type of drug: Anti-thyroid

Uses: The management of an overactive thyroid.

How it works: Helps to restore normal function to the thyroid gland.

Possible adverse effects: Skin rashes and itches. Sometimes the ability to fight infection may be reduced, so any sign of a sore throat or mouth ulceration should be reported to a doctor.

Availability: Available only with a prescription from a doctor.

Other information: Regular blood tests will monitor effect on thyroid function.

CAUTIONS

Children: There are no commonly reported problems associated with prescribing this medication for children.

Pregnancy and breastfeeding: This drug is either not recommended for use by women who are pregnant or breastfeeding, or the precise effects are not known and it should therefore only be used with caution and under medical advice.

Alcohol: No known problems if taken with alcohol.

Driving and operating machinery: There are no commonly reported problems which may impact on the ability to drive or operate machinery. However, many drugs can cause dizziness or drowsiness in a few people, so it is wise to see how the drug affects you before driving or working with dangerous machinery.

PYRAZINAMIDE

Brand name: Rifater, Zinamide

Type of drug: Anti-tuberculous

Uses: Used in conjunction with other drugs to treat tuberculosis.

How it works: Acts on the bacteria which are causing the infection.

Possible adverse effects: Liver damage with fever, nausea and vomiting.

Availability: Available only with a prescription from a doctor.

Other information: Patient should be made fully aware of all side effects and report any immediately. Treatment may be continued for up to 18 months.

CAUTIONS

Children: This drug is either not recommended for children, or is recommended only for children above a certain age.

Pregnancy and breastfeeding: This drug is either not recommended for use by women who are pregnant or breastfeeding, or the precise effects are not known and it should therefore only be used with caution and under medical advice.

Alcohol: No known problems if taken with alcohol.

Driving and operating machinery: There are no commonly reported problems which may impact on the ability to drive or operate machinery. However, many drugs can cause dizziness or drowsiness in a few people, so it is wise to see how the drug affects you before driving or working with dangerous machinery.

PYRIDOSTIGMINE
Brand name: Mestinon
Type of drug: Anti-cholinesterases
Uses: To treat myasthenia gravis, a rare autoimmune condition.
How it works: Acts as a muscle stimulant to improve the muscle tone by strengthening the signals sent down the nerves which are faulty in this condition.
Possible adverse effects: Nausea, vomiting, diarrhoea and abdominal cramps, sweating and increased saliva.
Availability: Available only with a prescription from a doctor.
Other information: Tablets should be swallowed whole, not chewed or crushed. Patient should be taught to how to evaluate any changes in muscle strength.
CAUTIONS
Children: This drug is either not recommended for children, or is recommended only for children above a certain age.
Pregnancy and breastfeeding: This drug is either not recommended for use by women who are pregnant or breastfeeding, or the precise effects are not known and it should therefore only be used with caution and under medical advice.
Alcohol: No known problems if taken with alcohol.
Driving and operating machinery: This drug may have some effect on your driving ability, so it is advisable not to drive or operate machinery while taking it.

PYRIMETHAMINE
Brand name: Daraprim
Type of drug: Anti-malarial
Uses: To treat infections with malaria. Not used in the prevention of malaria.
How it works: Treats infections which are resistant to other antimalarial drugs. Usually given in conjunction with other drugs to increase the power.
Possible adverse effects: Skin rashes and insomnia. Long-term use may lead to folic acid deficiency.
Availability: Available only with a prescription from a doctor.

Other information: Blood will be tested regularly and vitamin supplements may be given during treatment.

CAUTIONS

Children: This drug is either not recommended for children, or is recommended only for children above a certain age.

Pregnancy and breastfeeding: This drug is either not recommended for use by women who are pregnant or breastfeeding, or the precise effects are not known and it should therefore only be used with caution and under medical advice.

Alcohol: No known problems if taken with alcohol.

Driving and operating machinery: There are no commonly reported problems which may impact on the ability to drive or operate machinery. However, many drugs can cause dizziness or drowsiness in a few people, so it is wise to see how the drug affects you before driving or working with dangerous machinery.

QUINAPRIL

Brand name: Accupro, Accuretic

Type of drug: ACE inhibitor

Uses: To treat raised blood pressure and congestive heart failure.

How it works: Dilates the blood vessels, reduces sodium and water retention, with the result that the blood pressure is lowered.

Possible adverse effects: Chest pain, nausea, indigestion, abdominal pains, headache, insomnia, blurred vision.

Availability: Available only with a prescription from a doctor.

Other information: Drug should be taken on an empty stomach. Patient should avoid salt substitutes. Patient should take care in hot weather, or if taking exercise, to avoid over-heating and dehydration.

CAUTIONS

Children: This drug is either not recommended for children, or is recommended only for children above a certain age.

Pregnancy and breastfeeding: This drug is either not recommended for use by women who are pregnant or breastfeeding, or the precise effects are not known and it should therefore only be used with caution and under medical advice.

Alcohol: No known problems if taken with alcohol.

Driving and operating machinery: There are no commonly reported problems which may impact on the ability to drive or operate machinery. However, many drugs can cause dizziness or drowsiness in a few people, so it is wise to see how the drug affects you before driving or working with dangerous machinery.

QUINIDINE
Brand name: Kinidin Durules
Type of drug: Anti-arrhythmic
Uses: To treat disorders of heart rhythm such as atrial fibrillation, paroxysmal supraventricular tachycardia and premature atrial contractions.
How it works: Acts on the electrical impulses in the heart to enable it to beat more steadily and effectively.
Possible adverse effects: Vertigo, headache, nausea, diarrhoea, fever.
Availability: Available only with a prescription from a doctor.
Other information: Patient must report rash, fever, ringing in the ears or visual disturbances.
CAUTIONS
Children: There are no commonly reported problems associated with prescribing this medication for children.
Pregnancy and breastfeeding: This drug is either not recommended for use by women who are pregnant or breastfeeding, or the precise effects are not known and it should therefore only be used with caution and under medical advice.
Alcohol: No known problems if taken with alcohol.
Driving and operating machinery: There are no commonly reported problems which may impact on the ability to drive or operate machinery. However, many drugs can cause dizziness or drowsiness in a few people, so it is wise to see how the drug affects you before driving or working with dangerous machinery.

QUININE
Brand name: Quinine
Type of drug: Anti-malarial and muscle relaxant
Uses: For the treatment of malaria and it is also used to treat nocturnal leg cramps.

How it works: Is often an effective treatment for malaria when other treatments have failed. Also has a muscle relaxant effect.

Possible adverse effects: Tinnitus, headache, nausea, hot and flushed skin.

Availability: Available only with a prescription from a doctor.

Other information: If the patient suffers from hearing impairment it should be reported it immediately.

CAUTIONS

Children: There are no commonly reported problems associated with prescribing this medication for children.

Pregnancy and breastfeeding: No specific problems documented, but any medication should be taken with utmost caution by women who are either pregnant or breastfeeding, and only after professional medical or pharmaceutical advice has been sought.

Alcohol: No known problems if taken with alcohol.

Driving and operating machinery: This drug may have some effect on your driving ability, so it is advisable not to drive or operate machinery while taking it.

RALTITREXED

Brand name: Tomudex

Type of drug: Anti-cancer

Uses: To treat cancer of the colon.

How it works: Prevents the cancer cells from dividing and therefore from multiplying.

Possible adverse effects: Blood disorders and stomach and bowel upsets. Anaemia and impaired liver function can occur but they do not produce symptoms and are reversible.

Availability: Available only with a prescription from a doctor.

Other information: Given by intravenous infusions. Regular blood counts will be carried out.

CAUTIONS

Children: There are no commonly reported problems associated with prescribing this medication for children.

Pregnancy and breastfeeding: This drug is either not recommended for use by women who are pregnant or breastfeeding, or the precise effects are

not known and it should therefore only be used with caution and under medical advice.

Alcohol: No known problems if taken with alcohol.

Driving and operating machinery: There are no commonly reported problems which may impact on the ability to drive or operate machinery. However, many drugs can cause dizziness or drowsiness in a few people, so it is wise to see how the drug affects you before driving or working with dangerous machinery.

RAMIPRIL

Brand name: Tritace

Type of drug: ACE inhibitor and anti-hypertensive

Uses: To treat high blood pressure and heart failure after a heart attack.

How it works: Dilates the blood vessels so that blood can flow around the body more freely.

Possible adverse effects: Nausea, dizziness, cough, headache.

Availability: Available only with a prescription from a doctor.

Other information: Blood pressure and heart function will be regularly checked.

CAUTIONS

Children: This drug is either not recommended for children, or is recommended only for children above a certain age.

Pregnancy and breastfeeding: This drug is either not recommended for use by women who are pregnant or breastfeeding, or the precise effects are not known and it should therefore only be used with caution and under medical advice.

Alcohol: Alcohol should not be consumed, or only consumed with caution - after medical advice has been sought - while you are taking this drug.

Driving and operating machinery: This drug may have some effect on your driving ability, so it is advisable not to drive or operate machinery while taking it.

RANITIDINE

Brand name: Zantac

Type of drug: Anti-ulcer

Uses: Treatment of stomach and duodenal ulcers. Used in conjunction with other drugs to treat the Helicobacter pylori infection. Also used to treat reflux oesophagitis.

How it works: Reduces the amount of acid produced and thus enables the ulcers to heal.

Possible adverse effects: Rare, but occasional headaches.

Availability: Available only with a prescription from a doctor.

Other information: Patient must swallow medication whole with water.

CAUTIONS

Children: There are no commonly reported problems associated with prescribing this medication for children.

Pregnancy and breastfeeding: No specific problems documented, but any medication should be taken with utmost caution by women who are either pregnant or breastfeeding, and only after professional medical or pharmaceutical advice has been sought.

Alcohol: Alcohol should not be consumed, or only consumed with caution - after medical advice has been sought - while you are taking this drug.

Driving and operating machinery: There are no commonly reported problems which may impact on the ability to drive or operate machinery. However, many drugs can cause dizziness or drowsiness in a few people, so it is wise to see how the drug affects you before driving or working with dangerous machinery.

RIFABUTIN

Brand name: Mycobutin

Type of drug: Anti-tuberculous

Uses: To treat tuberculosis, often in patients who are suffering from HIV or AIDS.

How it works: The drug has an antibiotic action and will often be used in conjunction with other drugs for maximum effect.

Possible adverse effects: Nausea and vomiting, abdominal pain, diarrhoea.

Availability: Available only with a prescription from a doctor.

Other information: Can interact with oral contraceptives.

CAUTIONS

Children: This drug is either not recommended for children, or is recommended only for children above a certain age.

Pregnancy and breastfeeding: This drug is either not recommended for use by women who are pregnant or breastfeeding, or the precise effects are not known and it should therefore only be used with caution and under medical advice.

Alcohol: No known problems if taken with alcohol.

Driving and operating machinery: There are no commonly reported problems which may impact on the ability to drive or operate machinery. However, many drugs can cause dizziness or drowsiness in a few people, so it is wise to see how the drug affects you before driving or working with dangerous machinery.

RIFAMPICIN

Brand name: Rifadin, Rimactane

Type of drug: Anti-tuberculous

Uses: To treat tuberculosis (TB) and leprosy.

How it works: Has an antibiotic action and is used in conjunction with other anti-TB drugs to maximise effect.

Possible adverse effects: Headache, fatigue, and orange-red coloured urine.

Availability: Available only with a prescription from a doctor.

Other information: May render oral contraceptives ineffective and disrupt menstrual cycle.

CAUTIONS

Children: This drug is either not recommended for children, or is recommended only for children above a certain age.

Pregnancy and breastfeeding: This drug is either not recommended for use by women who are pregnant or breastfeeding, or the precise effects are not known and it should therefore only be used with caution and under medical advice.

Alcohol: Alcohol should not be consumed, or only consumed with caution - after medical advice has been sought - while you are taking this drug.

Driving and operating machinery: There are no commonly reported problems which may impact on the ability to drive or operate machinery. However, many drugs can cause dizziness or drowsiness in a few people, so it is wise to see how the drug affects you before driving or working with dangerous machinery.

RISPERIDONE

Brand name: Risperdal

Type of drug: Anti-emetic and anti-psychotic

Uses: Treatment of long-term psychiatric disorders such as schizophrenia.

How it works: Affects the chemicals in the brain, with the result that symptoms such as hallucinations, though disturbances and aggression are reduced. Reduces the tendency to become emotionally and socially withdrawn; also helps with other symptoms such as anxiety and depression.

Possible adverse effects: Insomnia, anxiety, headache, poor concentration.

Availability: Available only with a prescription from a doctor.

Other information: If used for a long time, some movement disorders may occur.

CAUTIONS

Children: There are no commonly reported problems associated with prescribing this medication for children.

Pregnancy and breastfeeding: This drug is either not recommended for use by women who are pregnant or breastfeeding, or the precise effects are not known and it should therefore only be used with caution and under medical advice.

Alcohol: Alcohol should not be consumed, or only consumed with caution - after medical advice has been sought - while you are taking this drug.

Driving and operating machinery: This drug may have some effect on your driving ability, so it is advisable not to drive or operate machinery while taking it.

RITONAVIR

Brand name: Norvir

Type of drug: Anti-viral

Uses: To treat HIV infection.

How it works: Inhibits the activity of an enzyme which is vital for the survival of the HIV virus.

Possible adverse effects: Nausea, vomiting, diarrhoea, flushing, weakness, headache.

Availability: Available only with a prescription from a doctor.

Other information: Patient to report use of any other over-the-counter preparations in case of drug interactions.

CAUTIONS

Children: This drug is either not recommended for children, or is recommended only for children above a certain age.

Pregnancy and breastfeeding: This drug is either not recommended for use by women who are pregnant or breastfeeding, or the precise effects are not known and it should therefore only be used with caution and under medical advice.

Alcohol: No known problems if taken with alcohol.

Driving and operating machinery: There are no commonly reported problems which may impact on the ability to drive or operate machinery. However, many drugs can cause dizziness or drowsiness in a few people, so it is wise to see how the drug affects you before driving or working with dangerous machinery.

ROPINIROLE

Brand name: Requip

Type of drug: Anti-Parkinsonism

Uses: To treat some of the signs and symptoms of Parkinson's disease.

How it works: Thought to stimulate the part of the brain that is not working effectively in patients with Parkinson's disease.

Possible adverse effects: Nausea, vomiting, abdominal pains, sleepiness and oedema. Occasionally hallucinations may occur.

Availability: Available only with a prescription from a doctor.

Other information: The patient should be warned to rise slowly immediately after sitting or lying down to avoid becoming dizzy. Nausea will be minimised if this drug is taken with food.

CAUTIONS

Children: This drug is either not recommended for children, or is recommended only for children above a certain age.

Pregnancy and breastfeeding: This drug is either not recommended for use by women who are pregnant or breastfeeding, or the precise effects are not known and it should therefore only be used with caution and under medical advice.

Alcohol: Alcohol should not be consumed, or only consumed with caution - after medical advice has been sought - while you are taking this drug.

Driving and operating machinery: This drug may have some effect on your driving ability, so it is advisable not to drive or operate machinery while taking it.

SALBUTAMOL

Brand name: Aerolin, Airomir, Asmaven, Maxivent, Salamol, Salbulin, Ventodisks, Ventolin, Volmax

Type of drug: Bronchodilator

Uses: To treat lung disorders (eg, asthma, chronic bronchitis emphysema).

How it works: Improves air flow through the lungs, enabling the sufferer to breathe more easily.

Possible adverse effects: Muscle tremor, anxiety and restlessness.

Availability: Available only with a prescription from a doctor.

Other information: If requiring more than eight puffs in 24 hours, consult your doctor.

CAUTIONS

Children: There are no commonly reported problems associated with prescribing this medication for children.

Pregnancy and breastfeeding: This drug is either not recommended for use by women who are pregnant or breastfeeding, or the precise effects are not known and it should therefore only be used with caution and under medical advice.

Alcohol: No known problems if taken with alcohol.

Driving and operating machinery: This drug may have some effect on your driving ability, so it is advisable not to drive or operate machinery while taking it.

SALMETEROL

Brand name: Serevent

Type of drug: Bronchodilator

Uses: Long-term maintenance treatment of people with asthma.

How it works: Dilates the airways to enable the sufferer to breathe more easily.

Possible adverse effects: Tremor, headaches, palpitations.

Availability: Available only with a prescription from a doctor.

Other information: This medication is not to appropriate for the relief of acute attacks of asthma; another type of medication should be used in those cases. Salmeterol should not be used more than twice daily; if the drug does not meet your requirements, consult your doctor.

CAUTIONS

Children: There are no commonly reported problems associated with prescribing this medication for children.

Pregnancy and breastfeeding: This drug is either not recommended for use by women who are pregnant or breastfeeding, or the precise effects are not known and it should therefore only be used with caution and under medical advice.

Alcohol: No known problems if taken with alcohol.

Driving and operating machinery: There are no commonly reported problems which may impact on the ability to drive or operate machinery. However, many drugs can cause dizziness or drowsiness in a few people, so it is wise to see how the drug affects you before driving or working with dangerous machinery.

SAQUINAVIR

Brand name: Invirase

Type of drug: Anti-viral

Uses: To treat HIV infection.

How it works: Prevents the HIV virus from reaching maturity.

Possible adverse effects: Nausea, vomiting, headache, diarrhoea, abdominal discomfort.

Availability: Available only with a prescription from a doctor.

Other information: The drug is best taken two hours after a full meal. This drug will usually be given in conjunction with other medication.

CAUTIONS

Children: This drug is either not recommended for children, or is recommended only for children above a certain age.

Pregnancy and breastfeeding: This drug is either not recommended for use by women who are pregnant or breastfeeding, or the precise effects are not known and it should therefore only be used with caution and under medical advice.

Alcohol: No known problems if taken with alcohol.

Driving and operating machinery: There are no commonly reported

problems which may impact on the ability to drive or operate machinery. However, many drugs can cause dizziness or drowsiness in a few people, so it is wise to see how the drug affects you before driving or working with dangerous machinery.

SERTINDOLE

Brand name: Serdolect

Type of drug: Anti-psychotic

Uses: Used to treat schizophrenia.

How it works: Reduces the symptoms of the disorder.

Possible adverse effects: Insomnia, anxiety, headache, drowsiness, blurred vision, nausea.

Availability: Available only with a prescription from a doctor.

Other information: Not prescribed for new patients, although people already treated with this drug will continue with it.

CAUTIONS

Children: There are no commonly reported problems associated with prescribing this medication for children.

Pregnancy and breastfeeding: This drug is either not recommended for use by women who are pregnant or breastfeeding, or the precise effects are not known and it should only be used with caution, after medical advice.

Alcohol: No known problems if taken with alcohol.

Driving and operating machinery: There are no commonly reported problems which may impact on the ability to drive or operate machinery. However, many drugs can cause dizziness or drowsiness in a few people, so it is wise to see how the drug affects you before driving or working with dangerous machinery.

SERTRALINE

Brand name: Lustral

Type of drug: Anti-depressant

Uses: Treatment of depression.

How it works: Improves the mood, increases energy and stimulates an interest in day-to-day living without the sedative effects of similar drugs.

Possible adverse effects: Nausea and diarrhoea.

Availability: Available only with a prescription from a doctor.

Other information: Patient should check with the doctor before using other over-the-counter preparations.

CAUTIONS

Children: This drug is either not recommended for children, or is recommended only for children above a certain age.

Pregnancy and breastfeeding: This drug is either not recommended for use by women who are pregnant or breastfeeding, or the precise effects are not known and it should only be used with caution, after medical advice.

Alcohol: Alcohol should not be consumed, or only consumed with caution - after medical advice has been sought - while you are taking this drug.

Driving and operating machinery: This drug may have some effect on your driving ability, so it is advisable not to drive or operate machinery while taking it.

SILDENAFIL

Brand name: Viagra

Type of drug: Impotence treatment

Uses: Treatment of erectile dysfunction.

How it works: Enables impotent men to attain and maintain an erection.

Possible adverse effects: Indigestion, headache, flushing, dizziness, visual disturbances, nasal congestion.

Availability: Available only with a prescription from a doctor.

Other information: Should not be used at the same time as other impotence treatments or for people with heart problems. This drug will not be prescribed on the NHS unless the problem is caused by a medical disorder.

CAUTIONS

Alcohol: Alcohol should not be consumed, or only consumed with caution - after medical advice has been sought - while you are taking this drug.

Driving and operating machinery: This drug may have some effect on your driving ability, so it is advisable not to drive or operate machinery while taking it.

SIMVASTATIN

Brand name: Zocor

Type of drug: Lipid lowering

Uses: Treatment of people who have high levels of fat in their blood and who are at risk of developing heart disease.

How it works: Lowers level of cholesterol in the blood, particularly in people who have not responded to other forms of treatment and who are at risk of developing heart disease.

Possible adverse effects: Nausea and diarrhoea are rare and will usually resolve, but prolonged treatment can damage the liver.

Availability: Available only with a prescription from a doctor.

Other information: Regular tests to assess liver function will be carried out.

CAUTIONS

Children: This drug is either not recommended for children, or is recommended only for children above a certain age.

Pregnancy and breastfeeding: This drug is either not recommended for use by women who are pregnant or breastfeeding, or the precise effects are not known and it should therefore only be used with caution and under medical advice.

Alcohol: Alcohol should not be consumed, or only consumed with caution - after medical advice has been sought - while you are taking this drug.

Driving and operating machinery: There are no commonly reported problems which may impact on the ability to drive or operate machinery. However, many drugs can cause dizziness or drowsiness in a few people, so it is wise to see how the drug affects you before driving or working with dangerous machinery.

SODIUM AUROTHIOMALATE

Brand name: Myocrisin

Type of drug: Anti-rheumatic

Uses: To treat progressive rheumatoid arthritis.

How it works: Slows and halts progression of the disease, but does not repair damage that has already occurred.

Possible adverse effects: Side effects can be serious, such as blood disorders, rashes and impaired kidney function and mouth ulcers.

Availability: Available only with a prescription from a doctor.

Other information: Patient should report a sore throat, mouth ulcers, fever, infection, rashes, immediately. The drug can take several months to reach full effectiveness.

CAUTIONS

Children: There are no commonly reported problems associated with prescribing this medication for children.

Pregnancy and breastfeeding: No specific problems documented, but any medication should be taken with utmost caution by women who are either pregnant or breastfeeding, and only after professional medical or pharmaceutical advice has been sought.

Alcohol: No known problems if taken with alcohol.

Driving and operating machinery: There are no commonly reported problems which may impact on the ability to drive or operate machinery. However, many drugs can cause dizziness or drowsiness in a few people, so it is wise to see how the drug affects you before driving or working with dangerous machinery.

SODIUM CROMOGLYCATE

Brand name: Cromogem, Intal, Nalcrom, Opticrom, Rynacrom

Type of drug: Anti-allergy

Uses: Used to treat allergies and asthma.

How it works: Reduces the frequency and severity of asthma attacks which are brought on by cold air or exercise. Also effective as a preventive treatment for hay fever and conjunctivitis.

Possible adverse effects: Coughing, wheezing and throat irritation.

Availability: Available with or without a prescription (over-the-counter).

Other information: This medication is not effective for the relief of an asthmatic attack. May take up to six weeks for benefits to be felt.

CAUTIONS

Children: There are no commonly reported problems associated with prescribing this medication for children.

Pregnancy and breastfeeding: No specific problems documented, but any medication should be taken with utmost caution by women who are either pregnant or breastfeeding, and only after professional medical or pharmaceutical advice has been sought.

Alcohol: No known problems if taken with alcohol.

Driving and operating machinery: There are no commonly reported problems which may impact on the ability to drive or operate machinery. However, many drugs can cause dizziness or drowsiness in a few people,

so it is wise to see how the drug affects you before driving or working with dangerous machinery.

SODIUM VALPROATE

Brand name: Convulex (valproic acid), Epilim, Orlept

Type of drug: Anti-convulsant

Uses: Treatment of several different types of epilepsy.

How it works: Reduces electrical activity in the brain to prevent epileptic seizures.

Possible adverse effects: Side effects are very uncommon.

Availability: Available only with a prescription from a doctor.

Other information: Blood will be tested to monitor levels in the blood.

CAUTIONS

Children: There are no commonly reported problems associated with prescribing this medication for children.

Pregnancy and breastfeeding: This drug is either not recommended for use by women who are pregnant or breastfeeding, or the precise effects are not known and it should therefore only be used with caution and under medical advice.

Alcohol: Alcohol should not be consumed, or only consumed with caution - after medical advice has been sought - while you are taking this drug.

Driving and operating machinery: This drug may have some effect on your driving ability, so it is advisable not to drive or operate machinery while taking it.

SOMATROPIN

Brand name: Genotropin, Humatrope, Norditropin, Saizen, Zomacton

Type of drug: Pituitary hormone

Uses: To treat growth problems caused by a deficiency in growth hormone produced by the pituitary gland.

How it works: A synthetic form of growth hormone, it performs the same function - promoting normal growth and development. It stimulates skeletal, linear bone, muscle and organ growth.

Possible adverse effects: These are rare but include headache and nausea.

Availability: Available only with a prescription from a doctor.

Other information: Treatment will continue throughout childhood until an acceptable height is reached. Treatment may be stopped for a few months and then restarted depending on rate of growth.

CAUTIONS

Children: There are no commonly reported problems associated with prescribing this medication for children.

Pregnancy and breastfeeding: This drug is either not recommended for use by women who are pregnant or breastfeeding, or the precise effects are not known and it should therefore only be used with caution and under medical advice.

Alcohol: No known problems if taken with alcohol.

Driving and operating machinery: There are no commonly reported problems which may impact on the ability to drive or operate machinery. However, many drugs can cause dizziness or drowsiness in a few people, so it is wise to see how the drug affects you before driving or working with dangerous machinery.

SPECTINOMYCIN

Brand name: Trobicin

Type of drug: Antibiotic

Uses: Used to treat gonorrhoea in patients who cannot tolerate penicillin or other antibiotics.

How it works: Binds to the infective organism and prevents it from replicating.

Possible adverse effects: Nausea, dizziness, fever.

Availability: Available only with a prescription from a doctor.

Other information: Sexual partners must also be treated.

CAUTIONS

Children: This drug is either not recommended for children, or is recommended only for children above a certain age.

Pregnancy and breastfeeding: This drug is either not recommended for use by women who are pregnant or breastfeeding, or the precise effects are not known and it should only be used with caution, after medical advice.

Alcohol: No known problems if taken with alcohol.

Driving and operating machinery: There are no commonly reported

problems which may impact on the ability to drive or operate machinery. However, many drugs can cause dizziness or drowsiness in a few people, so it is wise to see how the drug affects you before driving or working with dangerous machinery.

SPIRONOLACTONE

Brand name: Aldactone, Laractone, Spiroctan, Spirolone, Spirospare

Type of drug: Potassium-sparing diuretic

Uses: Treatment of fluid build-up (oedema) caused by heart failure. Also used to treat oedema caused by liver and kidney problems and some kinds of pre-menstrual syndrome.

How it works: Acts on the kidneys to encourage the expulsion of excess fluid from the body.

Possible adverse effects: Nausea.

Availability: Available only with a prescription from a doctor.

Other information: Blood tests will be taken regularly to check kidneys are working.

CAUTIONS

Children: There are no commonly reported problems associated with prescribing this medication for children.

Pregnancy and breastfeeding: This drug is either not recommended for use by women who are pregnant or breastfeeding, or the precise effects are not known and it should therefore only be used with caution and under medical advice.

Alcohol: No known problems if taken with alcohol.

Driving and operating machinery: This drug may have some effect on your driving ability, so it is advisable not to drive or operate machinery while taking it.

STAVUDINE

Brand name: Zerit

Type of drug: Anti-viral

Uses: To treat HIV infections.

How it works: Acts on the DNA of the virus to inhibit its replication.

Possible adverse effects: Headache, fever, dizziness, nausea, abdominal upsets.

Availability: Available only with a prescription from a doctor.

Other information: Patient should report any tingling or numbness in limbs.

CAUTIONS

Children: This drug is either not recommended for children, or is recommended only for children above a certain age.

Pregnancy and breastfeeding: This drug is either not recommended for use by women who are pregnant or breastfeeding, or the precise effects are not known and it should therefore only be used with caution and under medical advice.

Alcohol: No known problems if taken with alcohol.

Driving and operating machinery: There are no commonly reported problems which may impact on the ability to drive or operate machinery. However, many drugs can cause dizziness or drowsiness in a few people, so it is wise to see how the drug affects you before driving or working with dangerous machinery.

STILBOESTROL

Brand name: Apstil

Type of drug: Female sex hormone and anti-cancer

Uses: To treat cancer of the breast in women after the menopause. Also occasionally used to treat prostate cancer in men.

How it works: A synthetic hormone, it suppresses the effects of male sex hormones.

Possible adverse effects: In women it can cause nausea, vomiting, sore breasts, swollen ankles and withdrawal bleeding. In men it can lead to impotence.

Availability: Available only with a prescription from a doctor.

Other information: There is a risk of gallstones with long-term use of this drug.

CAUTIONS

Children: This drug is either not recommended for children, or is recommended only for children above a certain age.

Pregnancy and breastfeeding: This drug is either not recommended for use by women who are pregnant or breastfeeding, or the precise effects are not known and it should therefore only be used with caution and under medical advice.

Alcohol: No known problems if taken with alcohol.

Driving and operating machinery: There are no commonly reported problems which may impact on the ability to drive or operate machinery. However, many drugs can cause dizziness or drowsiness in a few people, so it is wise to see how the drug affects you before driving or working with dangerous machinery.

STREPTOKINASE

Brand name: Kabikinase, Streptase

Type of drug: Thrombolytic

Uses: Used to treat life-threatening deep-vein thrombosis and pulmonary embolisms.

How it works: An enzyme which dissolves the blood clots and is particularly effective at dissolving recently formed ones. It is also used in conjunction with other drugs to treat wounds and ulcers.

Possible adverse effects: Nausea, vomiting, bleeding. It can cause allergic reactions, so any sign of this should be reported to a doctor.

Availability: Available only with a prescription from a doctor.

Other information: Usually given as an injection but is supplied in powder form for the treatment of wounds.

CAUTIONS

Children: This drug is either not recommended for children, or is recommended only for children above a certain age.

Pregnancy and breastfeeding: This drug is either not recommended for use by women who are pregnant or breastfeeding, or the precise effects are not known and it should therefore only be used with caution and under medical advice.

Alcohol: Alcohol should not be consumed, or only consumed with caution - after medical advice has been sought - while you are taking this drug.

Driving and operating machinery: This drug may have some effect on your driving ability, so it is advisable not to drive or operate machinery while taking it.

SUCRALFATE

Brand name: Antepsin

Type of drug: Ulcer-healing

Uses: To promote the healing of gastric and duodenal ulcers.

How it works: Forms a barrier over the ulcer which protects it from further attack by stomach acid and gives it the opportunity to heal.

Possible adverse effects: Constipation, diarrhoea, nausea, indigestion and gastric discomfort.

Availability: Available only with a prescription from a doctor.

Other information: This medication should be taken on an empty stomach at least one hour before meals.

CAUTIONS

Children: This drug is either not recommended for children, or is recommended only for children above a certain age.

Pregnancy and breastfeeding: This drug is either not recommended for use by women who are pregnant or breastfeeding, or the precise effects are not known and it should therefore only be used with caution and under medical advice.

Alcohol: Alcohol should not be consumed, or only consumed with caution - after medical advice has been sought - while you are taking this drug.

Driving and operating machinery: There are no commonly reported problems which may impact on the ability to drive or operate machinery. However, many drugs can cause dizziness or drowsiness in a few people, so it is wise to see how the drug affects you before driving or working with dangerous machinery.

SULCONAZOLE NITRATE

Brand name: Exelderm

Type of drug: Anti-fungal

Uses: To treat fungal skin infections such as those which cause athlete's foot.

How it works: Inhibits the growth of fungi and yeast.

Possible adverse effects: Skin irritation.

Availability: Available only with a prescription from a doctor.

Other information: Avoid contact with the eyes. Relief should be apparent within a few days, but the full course of treatment should be completed to prevent re-occurrence.

CAUTIONS

Children: There are no commonly reported problems associated with prescribing this medication for children.

Pregnancy and breastfeeding: No specific problems documented, but any medication should be taken with utmost caution by women who are either pregnant or breastfeeding, and only after professional medical or pharmaceutical advice has been sought.

Alcohol: No known problems if taken with alcohol.

Driving and operating machinery: There are no commonly reported problems which may impact on the ability to drive or operate machinery. However, many drugs can cause dizziness or drowsiness in a few people, so it is wise to see how the drug affects you before driving or working with dangerous machinery.

SULPHASALAZINE

Brand name: Salazopyrin

Type of drug: Inflammatory bowel disease and anti-rheumatic drug

Uses: Treatment of conditions which cause inflammation of the bowel, such as ulcerative colitis and Crohn's disease. Can also be beneficial in the treatment of rheumatoid arthritis.

How it works: Has an anti-inflammatory effect.

Possible adverse effects: Adverse effects are more likely with high doses. Nausea, appetite loss, headache and joint pain. May cause orange or yellow urine.

Availability: Available only with a prescription from a doctor.

Other information: It is important to drink a lot of fluid when taking this medication. Treatment will often be long-term.

CAUTIONS

Children: There are no commonly reported problems associated with prescribing this medication for children.

Pregnancy and breastfeeding: This drug is either not recommended for use by women who are pregnant or breastfeeding, or the precise effects are not known and it should therefore only be used with caution and under medical advice.

Alcohol: No known problems if taken with alcohol.

Driving and operating machinery: There are no commonly reported problems which may impact on the ability to drive or operate machinery. However, many drugs can cause dizziness or drowsiness in a few people,

so it is wise to see how the drug affects you before driving or working with dangerous machinery.

SUMATRIPTAN
Brand name: Imigran
Type of drug: Anti-migraine
Uses: Relieves acute migraine attacks without the need to identify an aura.
How it works: Stops the blood vessels in the brain from dilating - the cause of migraine attacks.
Possible adverse effects: Most disappear within an hour. Include tingling, flushing and a heavy feeling.
Availability: Available only with a prescription from a doctor.
Other information: Should only be used to treat attacks, not as a preventive measure.
CAUTIONS
Children: This drug is either not recommended for children, or is recommended only for children above a certain age.
Pregnancy and breastfeeding: This drug is either not recommended for use by women who are pregnant or breastfeeding, or the precise effects are not known and it should only be used with caution, after medical advice.
Alcohol: No known problems if taken with alcohol.
Driving and operating machinery: This drug may have some effect on your driving ability, so it is advisable not to drive or operate machinery while taking it.

TACALCITOL
Brand name: Curatoderm
Type of drug: Anti-psoriasis
Uses: To treat psoriasis.
How it works: Slows down the division of keratin-making cells in the skin and thus prevents the formation of the plaques which are characteristic of psoriasis.
Possible adverse effects: Local skin irritation.
Availability: Available only with a prescription from a doctor.
Other information: Wash hands immediately after use and avoid contact with the eyes. Can affect hormonal contraception.

CAUTIONS

Children: This drug is either not recommended for children, or is recommended only for children above a certain age.

Pregnancy and breastfeeding: This drug is either not recommended for use by women who are pregnant or breastfeeding, or the precise effects are not known and it should therefore only be used with caution and under medical advice.

Alcohol: No known problems if taken with alcohol.

Driving and operating machinery: There are no commonly reported problems which may impact on the ability to drive or operate machinery. However, many drugs can cause dizziness or drowsiness in a few people, so it is wise to see how the drug affects you before driving or working with dangerous machinery.

TAMOXIFEN

Brand name: Emblon, Fentamox, Noltam, Nolvadex, Oestrifen, Tamofen

Type of drug: Anti-cancer

Uses: Used to treat breast cancer.

How it works: The exact mechanism of this medication is unknown, but it is thought to block some of the hormonal action that the cancer cells require for survival.

Possible adverse effects: Nausea, vomiting, diarrhoea.

Availability: Available only with a prescription from a doctor.

Other information: A barrier contraceptive is recommended during treatment.

CAUTIONS

Children: This drug is either not recommended for children, or is recommended only for children above a certain age.

Pregnancy and breastfeeding: This drug is either not recommended for use by women who are pregnant or breastfeeding, or the precise effects are not known and it should therefore only be used with caution and under medical advice.

Alcohol: No known problems if taken with alcohol.

Driving and operating machinery: This drug may have some effect on your driving ability, so it is advisable not to drive or operate machinery while taking it.

TAMSULOSIN

Brand name: Flomax MR

Type of drug: Urinary retention treatment

Uses: Used to relieve the symptoms of urinary retention.

How it works: It relaxes the muscles in the bladder neck, with the result that urine flow is improved.

Possible adverse effects: Dizziness, headache, decrease in blood pressure.

Availability: Available only with a prescription from a doctor.

Other information: Patient should not chew or crush the tablets. Patient should get up slowly from bed or chair at the beginning of therapy.

CAUTIONS

Children: There are no commonly reported problems associated with prescribing this medication for children.

Pregnancy and breastfeeding: This drug is either not recommended for use by women who are pregnant or breastfeeding, or the precise effects are not known and it should therefore only be used with caution and under medical advice.

Alcohol: No known problems if taken with alcohol.

Driving and operating machinery: This drug may have some effect on your driving ability, so it is advisable not to drive or operate machinery while taking it.

TEMAZEPAM

Brand name: Normison

Type of drug: Sleeping aid

Uses: Treatment of insomnia.

How it works: Depresses the action of part of the brain. Acts within 30 minutes and has a short-term effect to help induce sleep.

Possible adverse effects: Occasional daytime drowsiness.

Availability: Available only with a prescription from a doctor.

Other information: Should only be taken for short periods as can be habit-forming.

CAUTIONS

Children: There are no commonly reported problems associated with prescribing this medication for children.

Pregnancy and breastfeeding: This drug is either not recommended for

use by women who are pregnant or breastfeeding, or the precise effects are not known and it should therefore only be used with caution and under medical advice.

Alcohol: Alcohol should not be consumed, or only consumed with caution - after medical advice has been sought - while you are taking this drug.

Driving and operating machinery: This drug may have some effect on your driving ability, so it is advisable not to drive or operate machinery while taking it.

TENOXICAM

Brand name: Mobiflex

Type of drug: Non-steroidal anti-inflammatory

Uses: To treat pain in rheumatic disease and similar disorders.

How it works: Has an anti-inflammatory effect which alleviates the symptoms but does not treat the underlying condition.

Possible adverse effects: Irritates the stomach, so can cause nausea, diarrhoea and occasionally bleeding. Any sign of these should be reported to a doctor.

Availability: Available only with a prescription from a doctor.

Other information: Supplied either as an injection or as tablets.

CAUTIONS

Children: This drug is either not recommended for children, or is recommended only for children above a certain age.

Pregnancy and breastfeeding: No specific problems documented, but any medication should be taken with utmost caution by women who are either pregnant or breastfeeding, and only after professional medical or pharmaceutical advice has been sought.

Alcohol: No known problems if taken with alcohol.

Driving and operating machinery: There are no commonly reported problems which may impact on the ability to drive or operate machinery. However, many drugs can cause dizziness or drowsiness in a few people, so it is wise to see how the drug affects you before driving or working with dangerous machinery.

TERAZOSIN

Brand name: Hytrin

Type of drug: Anti-hypertensive

Uses: To treat mild to moderate raised blood pressure. Also used to treat urinary tract blockages.

How it works: Relaxes the smooth muscle of blood vessels to enable the blood to flow more freely through them.

Possible adverse effects: Dizziness, light-headedness, low blood pressure, headache, fatigue, oedema.

Availability: Available only with a prescription from a doctor.

Other information: Dizziness may occur with the first dose.

CAUTIONS

Children: There are no commonly reported problems associated with prescribing this medication for children.

Pregnancy and breastfeeding: No specific problems documented, but any medication should be taken with utmost caution by women who are either pregnant or breastfeeding, and only after professional medical or pharmaceutical advice has been sought.

Alcohol: No known problems if taken with alcohol.

Driving and operating machinery: This drug may have some effect on your driving ability, so it is advisable not to drive or operate machinery while taking it.

TERBINAFINE

Brand name: Lamisil

Type of drug: Anti-fungal

Uses: To treat fungal skin infections such as athlete's foot, jock itch or ringworm.

How it works: Causes the fungal cells to die.

Possible adverse effects: Abdominal discomfort.

Availability: Available only with a prescription from a doctor.

Other information: Avoid contact with eyes, nose and mouth. Use only as directed.

CAUTIONS

Children: There are no commonly reported problems associated with prescribing this medication for children.

Pregnancy and breastfeeding: This drug is either not recommended for use by women who are pregnant or breastfeeding, or the precise effects are

not known and it should therefore only be used with caution and under medical advice.

Alcohol: No known problems if taken with alcohol.

Driving and operating machinery: There are no commonly reported problems which may impact on the ability to drive or operate machinery. However, many drugs can cause dizziness or drowsiness in a few people, so it is wise to see how the drug affects you before driving or working with dangerous machinery.

TERBUTALINE

Brand name: Bricanyl, Monovent

Type of drug: Bronchodilator

Uses: Treatment of lung spasms associated with asthma, bronchitis and emphysema.

How it works: Acts on the muscles within the lungs, with the result that the small airways of the lungs are expanded.

Possible adverse effects: Nausea, anxiety, tremor and nervousness.

Availability: Available only with a prescription from a doctor.

Other information: If drug produces no relief the patient should report immediately. Must also check use of over-the-counter preparations.

CAUTIONS

Children: This drug is either not recommended for children, or is recommended only for children above a certain age.

Pregnancy and breastfeeding: This drug is either not recommended for use by women who are pregnant or breastfeeding, or the precise effects are not known and it should therefore only be used with caution and under medical advice.

Alcohol: No known problems if taken with alcohol.

Driving and operating machinery: This drug may have some effect on your driving ability, so it is advisable not to drive or operate machinery while taking it.

TERFENADINE

Brand name: Aller-eze, Boots Antihistamine Tablets, Histafen, Seldane, Terfenor, Terfex, Terfinax, Triludan.

Type of drug: Antihistamine

Uses: For the relief of rhinitis and hayfever and other similar allergies. Also for skin allergies such as hives.

How it works: Acts in the same way as other antihistamines, but without the accompanying sedative effect. Reduces sneezing and irritation of the eyes and nose.

Possible adverse effects: Rare, although indigestion and abdominal pain can occur in some cases.

Availability: Most of this drug type are available with or without a prescription (over-the-counter). Triludan, however, is available only with a prescription from a doctor.

Other information: Patient should avoid grapefruit juice. Patients who have arrhythmias should avoid this medication.

CAUTIONS

Children: There are no commonly reported problems associated with prescribing this medication for children.

Pregnancy and breastfeeding: This drug is either not recommended for use by women who are pregnant or breastfeeding, or the precise effects are not known and it should therefore only be used with caution and under medical advice.

Alcohol: Alcohol should not be consumed, or only consumed with caution - after medical advice has been sought - while you are taking this drug.

Driving and operating machinery: This drug may have some effect on your driving ability, so it is advisable not to drive or operate machinery while taking it.

TESTOSTERONE

Brand name: Primoteston Depot, Restandol, Sustanon, Virormone

Type of drug: Male sex hormone

Uses: It is used to treat under-development of the testes in males. It is also used to treat cancer of the breast in women.

How it works: Compensates for deficiency in hormone.

Possible adverse effects: Increase in weight, prostate abnormalities, headache, nausea, depression.

Availability: Available only with a prescription from a doctor.

Other information: Regular checks will be made to monitor the effect of treatment.

CAUTIONS

Children: This drug is either not recommended for children, or is recommended only for children above a certain age.

Pregnancy and breastfeeding: This drug is either not recommended for use by women who are pregnant or breastfeeding, or the precise effects are not known and it should therefore only be used with caution and under medical advice.

Alcohol: No known problems if taken with alcohol.

Driving and operating machinery: There are no commonly reported problems which may impact on the ability to drive or operate machinery. However, many drugs can cause dizziness or drowsiness in a few people, so it is wise to see how the drug affects you before driving or working with dangerous machinery.

TETRACYCLINE

Brand name: Achromycin, Sustamycin, Tetrabid, Tetrachel, Topicycline

Type of drug: Tetracycline antibiotic

Uses: To treat chest infections such as bronchitis, and other types of infection such as acne.

How it works: Prevents the bacteria from multiplying.

Possible adverse effects: Nausea, vomiting, diarrhoea, headache and dizziness.

Availability: Available only with a prescription from a doctor.

Other information: Discontinue use of the drug if the condition stays the same.

CAUTIONS

Children: This drug is either not recommended for children, or is recommended only for children above a certain age.

Pregnancy and breastfeeding: This drug is either not recommended for use by women who are pregnant or breastfeeding, or the precise effects are not known and it should therefore only be used with caution and under medical advice.

Alcohol: No known problems if taken with alcohol.

Driving and operating machinery: There are no commonly reported problems which may impact on the ability to drive or operate machinery. However, many drugs can cause dizziness or drowsiness in a few people,

so it is wise to see how the drug affects you before driving or working with dangerous machinery.

THEOPHYLLINE

Brand name: Lasma Nuelin, Theo-Dur, Uniphyllin Continus; [aminophylline] Pecram, Phyllocontin Continus

Type of drug: Bronchodilator

Uses: Treatment and prevention of acute lung spasms in people with asthma, bronchitis and emphysema.

How it works: Allows the air passages to expand and stimulates the heart and the nervous system to recover.

Possible adverse effects: Headache, nausea, vomiting and anxiety - usually related to dosage.

Availability: Available without a prescription (over-the-counter).

Other information: Often given as a slow-release preparation. Overdose should be treated as a medical emergency.

CAUTIONS

Children: There are no commonly reported problems associated with prescribing this medication for children.

Pregnancy and breastfeeding: This drug is either not recommended for use by women who are pregnant or breastfeeding, or the precise effects are not known and it should only be used with caution, after medical advice.

Alcohol: Alcohol should not be consumed, or only consumed with caution - after medical advice has been sought - while you are taking this drug.

Driving and operating machinery: There are no commonly reported problems which may impact on the ability to drive or operate machinery. However, many drugs can cause dizziness or drowsiness in a few people, so it is wise to see how the drug affects you before driving or working with dangerous machinery.

THIABENDAZOLE

Brand name: Mintezol

Type of drug: Anthelmintic

Uses: To treat infections with, among others, roundworm, threadworm, pinworm and whipworm.

How it works: Kills the infective organisms.

Possible adverse effects: Anorexia, nausea and vomiting, diarrhoea, headache and drowsiness.

Availability: Available only with a prescription from a doctor.

Other information: Good hygiene is vital to prevent re-infection.

CAUTIONS

Children: There are no commonly reported problems associated with prescribing this medication for children.

Pregnancy and breastfeeding: This drug is either not recommended for use by women who are pregnant or breastfeeding, or the precise effects are not known and it should only be used with caution, after medical advice.

Alcohol: No known problems if taken with alcohol.

Driving and operating machinery: This drug may have some effect on your driving ability, so it is advisable not to drive or operate machinery while taking it.

THIORIDAZINE

Brand name: Melleril, Rideril

Type of drug: Anti-psychotic

Uses: Treatment of a range of psychiatric problems, including schizophrenia, mania, dementia.

How it works: Has a tranquillising effect which reduces aggression and abnormal behaviour.

Possible adverse effects: Drowsiness, dry mouth, blocked nose. Can cause eye problems if taken in large doses.

Availability: Available only with a prescription from a doctor.

Other information: If sore throat, dizziness or difficulty in urinating, develops your doctor should be informed immediately.

CAUTIONS

Children: There are no commonly reported problems associated with prescribing this medication for children.

Pregnancy and breastfeeding: This drug is either not recommended for use by women who are pregnant or breastfeeding, or the precise effects are not known and it should therefore only be used with caution and under medical advice.

Alcohol: Alcohol should not be consumed or only consumed with caution - after medical advice has been sought - while you are taking this drug.

Driving and operating machinery: This drug may have some effect on your driving ability, so it is advisable not to drive or operate machinery while taking it.

THYROXINE
Brand name: Eltroxin
Type of drug: Thyroid hormone
Uses: Treatment of an under-active thyroid gland.
How it works: Replaces vital hormones which are not being produced by the thyroid gland. Also prescribed for some people with thyroid cancer.
Possible adverse effects: Rare, and usually related to dosage.
Availability: Available only with a prescription from a doctor.
Other information: Regular blood tests will be taken.
CAUTIONS
Children: There are no commonly reported problems associated with prescribing this medication for children.
Pregnancy and breastfeeding: No specific problems documented, but any medication should be taken with utmost caution by women who are either pregnant or breastfeeding, and only after professional medical or pharmaceutical advice has been sought.
Alcohol: No known problems if taken with alcohol.
Driving and operating machinery: There are no commonly reported problems which may impact on the ability to drive or operate machinery. However, many drugs can cause dizziness or drowsiness in a few people, so it is wise to see how the drug affects you before driving or working with dangerous machinery.

TIBOLONE
Brand name: Livial
Type of drug: Hormone replacement therapy
Uses: To treat the symptoms of the menopause, including sweating, depression, decreased sex drive and hot flushes.
How it works: Replaces hormones which are depleted after either a naturally occurring menopause or one brought on by surgical treatment.
Possible adverse effects: Rare. Vaginal bleeding is possible if prescribed within one year of the menopause.

Availability: Available only with a prescription from a doctor.

Other information: Not used as a way of preventing osteoporosis. Not usually prescribed within 10 months of the last period. Unlike other HRT it does not need to be taken in conjunction with progestogen.

CAUTIONS

Children: This drug is either not recommended for children, or is recommended only for children above a certain age.

Pregnancy and breastfeeding: This drug is either not recommended for use by women who are pregnant or breastfeeding, or the precise effects are not known and it should therefore only be used with caution and under medical advice.

Alcohol: No known problems if taken with alcohol.

Driving and operating machinery: There are no commonly reported problems which may impact on the ability to drive or operate machinery. However, many drugs can cause dizziness or drowsiness in a few people, so it is wise to see how the drug affects you before driving or working with dangerous machinery.

TILUDRONIC ACID

Brand name: Skelid

Type of drug: Bisphosphonate

Uses: To treat Paget's disease.

How it works: Promotes normal bone formation.

Possible adverse effects: Stomach pain, nausea, diarrhoea, dizziness and headache.

Availability: Available only with a prescription from a doctor.

Other information: The patient must avoid food for two hours before and after taking this medication. Also, calcium products and antacids should be avoided.

CAUTIONS

Children: This drug is either not recommended for children, or is recommended only for children above a certain age.

Pregnancy and breastfeeding: This drug is either not recommended for use by women who are pregnant or breastfeeding, or the precise effects are not known and it should therefore only be used with caution and under medical advice.

Alcohol: No known problems if taken with alcohol.

Driving and operating machinery: There are no commonly reported problems which may impact on the ability to drive or operate machinery. However, many drugs can cause dizziness or drowsiness in a few people, so it is wise to see how the drug affects you before driving or working with dangerous machinery.

TIMOLOL

Brand name: Betim, Blocadren, Glaucol, Timoptol

Type of drug: Anti-hypertensive

Uses: Treatment of high blood pressure (hypertension), heart attack, glaucoma and to prevent migraine.

How it works: Slows and steadies the heartbeat, prevents heart muscle damage and reduces blood pressure.

Possible adverse effects: Tiredness, blurred vision, headache.

Availability: Available only with a prescription from a doctor.

Other information: Administered as tablets, or eye drops if given for glaucoma.

CAUTIONS

Children: This drug is either not recommended for children, or is recommended only for children above a certain age.

Pregnancy and breastfeeding: This drug is either not recommended for use by women who are pregnant or breastfeeding, or the precise effects are not known and it should therefore only be used with caution and under medical advice.

Alcohol: Alcohol should not be consumed or only consumed with caution - after medical advice has been sought - while you are taking this drug.

Driving and operating machinery: This drug may have some effect on your driving ability, so it is advisable not to drive or operate machinery while taking it.

TIOCONAZOLE

Brand name: Trosyl

Type of drug: Anti-fungal

Uses: Used to treat fungal infections of the skin and vagina.

How it works: Alters the cell wall of the fungus and disables it.

Possible adverse effects: Skin irritations, burning discharge.

Availability: Available only with a prescription from a doctor.

Other information: Pessaries should be inserted high into the vagina. Sexual intercourse should be avoided during treatment to minimise the risk of re-infection.

CAUTIONS

Children: There are no commonly reported problems associated with prescribing this medication for children.

Pregnancy and breastfeeding: This drug is either not recommended for use by women who are pregnant or breastfeeding, or the precise effects are not known and it should therefore only be used with caution and under medical advice.

Alcohol: No known problems if taken with alcohol.

Driving and operating machinery: There are no commonly reported problems which may impact on the ability to drive or operate machinery. However, many drugs can cause dizziness or drowsiness in a few people, so it is wise to see how the drug affects you before driving or working with dangerous machinery.

TOLBUTAMIDE

Brand name: Rastinon

Type of drug: Anti-diabetic

Uses: Treatment of diabetes in adults who are still producing small amounts of insulin.

How it works: Stimulates the pancreas to produce more insulin.

Possible adverse effects: Dizziness, clamminess, which may indicate that the blood sugar is too low.

Availability: Available only with a prescription from a doctor.

Other information: Should be taken in conjunction with a diabetic diet. Urine will be tested regularly for sugar. An overdose should be treated as a medical emergency.

CAUTIONS

Children: This drug is either not recommended for children, or is recommended only for children above a certain age.

Pregnancy and breastfeeding: This drug is either not recommended for use by women who are pregnant or breastfeeding, or the precise effects are not known and it should therefore only be used with caution and under medical advice.

Alcohol: Alcohol should not be consumed, or only consumed with caution - after medical advice has been sought - while you are taking this drug.

Driving and operating machinery: There are no commonly reported problems which may impact on the ability to drive or operate machinery. However, many drugs can cause dizziness or drowsiness in a few people, so it is wise to see how the drug affects you before driving or working with dangerous machinery.

TRANDOLAPRIL

Brand name: Gopten, Odrik

Type of drug: ACE inhibitor

Uses: To treat mild to moderate raised blood pressure.

How it works: Acts as a vasodilator which enables the blood to flow more freely and the pressure to be lowered.

Possible adverse effects: Low blood pressure, light-headedness, dizziness, headache, fatigue.

Availability: Available only with a prescription from a doctor.

Other information: Patient should report immediately any signs of infection, sore throat, swelling, difficulty in breathing. Also best to avoid sodium substitutes. Caution must be exercised in hot weather.

CAUTIONS

Children: This drug is either not recommended for children, or is recommended only for children above a certain age.

Pregnancy and breastfeeding: This drug is either not recommended for use by women who are pregnant or breastfeeding, or the precise effects are not known and it should therefore only be used with caution and under medical advice.

Alcohol: No known problems if taken with alcohol.

Driving and operating machinery: There are no commonly reported problems which may impact on the ability to drive or operate machinery. However, many drugs can cause dizziness or drowsiness in a few people, so it is wise to see how the drug affects you before driving or working with dangerous machinery.

TRANEXAMIC ACID

Brand name: Cykolkapron

Type of drug: Anti-fibrinolytic

Uses: To treat bleeding in various situations, menorrhagia, dental extractions, nose bleeds.

How it works: Affects the clotting mechanism of the blood to prevent unwanted bleeding.

Possible adverse effects: Nausea, vomiting, diarrhoea, and drop in blood pressure. Report any visual disturbances immediately to your medical practitioner.

Availability: Available only with a prescription from a doctor.

Other information: Regular eye tests will be performed on people undergoing long-term treatment.

CAUTIONS

Children: There are no commonly reported problems associated with prescribing this medication for children.

Pregnancy and breastfeeding: No specific problems documented, but any medication should be taken with utmost caution by women who are either pregnant or breastfeeding, and only after professional medical or pharmaceutical advice has been sought.

Alcohol: No known problems if taken with alcohol.

Driving and operating machinery: There are no commonly reported problems which may impact on the ability to drive or operate machinery. However, many drugs can cause dizziness or drowsiness in a few people, so it is wise to see how the drug affects you before driving or working with dangerous machinery.

TRAZODONE

Brand name: Molipaxin

Type of drug: Anti-depressant

Uses: Treatment of depression, particularly for people who have difficulty in sleeping.

How it works: Lifts the mood and restores interest in day-to-day living.

Possible adverse effects: Less likely than with many anti-depressants, but some people experience drowsiness.

Availability: Available only with a prescription from a doctor.

Other information: It is advisable to lie down for 30 minutes after taking medication.

CAUTIONS

Children: This drug is either not recommended for children, or is recommended only for children above a certain age.

Pregnancy and breastfeeding: This drug is either not recommended for use by women who are pregnant or breastfeeding, or the precise effects are not known and it should therefore only be used with caution and under medical advice.

Alcohol: Alcohol should not be consumed, or only consumed with caution - after medical advice has been sought - while taking this drug.

Driving and operating machinery: This drug may have some effect on your driving ability, so it is advisable not to drive or operate machinery while taking it.

TRETINOIN

Brand name: Retin-A, Retinova

Type of drug: Vitamin A derivative

Uses: Topical treatment for acne and, in some cases, wrinkles.

How it works: Promotes the growth of healthy skin cells.

Possible adverse effects: Skin irritation and sensitivity, including peeling and redness.

Availability: Available only with a prescription from a doctor.

Other information: Avoid excessive exposure to the sun and wear a sunscreen during treatment. Follow the instructions carefully.

CAUTIONS

Children: There are no commonly reported problems associated with prescribing this medication for children.

Pregnancy and breastfeeding: This drug is either not recommended for use by women who are pregnant or breastfeeding, or the precise effects are not known and it should therefore only be used with caution and under medical advice.

Alcohol: No known problems if taken with alcohol.

Driving and operating machinery: There are no commonly reported problems which may impact on the ability to drive or operate machinery. However, many drugs can cause dizziness or drowsiness in a few people, so it is wise to see how the drug affects you before driving or working with dangerous machinery.

TRIAMCINOLONE ACETONIDE

Brand name: Adcortyl

Type of drug: Corticosteroid

Uses: Topical treatment of severe inflammatory skin conditions for which other treatments have failed to work.

How it works: Suppresses the body's inflammatory response which causes the condition and thus alleviates the symptoms of eczema without providing a cure.

Possible adverse effects: Worsening of any skin infection present, skin irritation.

Availability: Available only with a prescription from a doctor.

Other information: Supplied as a cream, ointment or paste. Follow the instructions carefully.

CAUTIONS

Children: This drug is either not recommended for children, or is recommended only for children above a certain age.

Pregnancy and breastfeeding: This drug is either not recommended for use by women who are pregnant or breastfeeding, or the precise effects are not known and it should therefore only be used with caution and under medical advice.

Alcohol: No known problems if taken with alcohol.

Driving and operating machinery: There are no commonly reported problems which may impact on the ability to drive or operate machinery. However, many drugs can cause dizziness or drowsiness in a few people, so it is wise to see how the drug affects you before driving or working with dangerous machinery.

TRIAMTERENE

Brand name: Dytac, Dytide, Frusene, Kalspare, Triamax Co, Triam-Co

Type of drug: Diuretic

Uses: Treatment of high blood pressure (hypertension) and oedema.

How it works: Acts on the kidneys to encourage the body to eliminate excess fluid.

Possible adverse effects: Rare. Can stain urine blue, but this is harmless.

Availability: Available only with a prescription from a doctor.

Other information: Supplied as capsules.

CAUTIONS

Children: There are no commonly reported problems associated with prescribing this medication for children.

Pregnancy and breastfeeding: This drug is either not recommended for use by women who are pregnant or breastfeeding, or the precise effects are not known and it should therefore only be used with caution and under medical advice.

Alcohol: No known problems if taken with alcohol.

Driving and operating machinery: There are no commonly reported problems which may impact on the ability to drive or operate machinery. However, many drugs can cause dizziness or drowsiness in a few people, so it is wise to see how the drug affects you before driving or working with dangerous machinery.

TRIMEPRAZINE

Brand name: Vallergan

Type of drug: Antihistamine

Uses: To help relieve itching.

How it works: Suppresses the allergic symptoms, one of which is the itching sensation.

Possible adverse effects: Drowsiness, dizziness, headache.

Availability: Available only with a prescription from a doctor.

Other information: A sunscreen should be worn during treatment because of the photosensitising effect of this medication.

CAUTIONS

Children: There are no commonly reported problems associated with prescribing this medication for children.

Pregnancy and breastfeeding: This drug is either not recommended for use by women who are pregnant or breastfeeding, or the precise effects are not known and it should therefore only be used with caution and under medical advice.

Alcohol: Alcohol should not be consumed, or only consumed with caution - after medical advice has been sought - while you are taking this drug.

Driving and operating machinery: This drug may have some effect on your driving ability, so it is advisable not to drive or operate machinery while taking it.

TRIMETHOPRIM

Brand name: Ipral, Monotrim, Trimogal, Trimopan, Triprimix, Bactrim, Chemotrim, Comixco

Type of drug: Anti-bacterial

Uses: Treatment of infections, particularly of the urinary tract and respiratory tract.

How it works: Has an anti-bacterial effect: destroys the infective organism.

Possible adverse effects: Rare when taken on its own, but rash, nausea and a sore throat are possible.

Availability: Available only with a prescription from a doctor.

Other information: Often taken together with another antibacterial drug, sulphamethoxazole.

CAUTIONS

Children: There are no commonly reported problems associated with prescribing this medication for children.

Pregnancy and breastfeeding: This drug is either not recommended for use by women who are pregnant or breastfeeding, or the precise effects are not known and it should only be used with caution, after medical advice.

Alcohol: No known problems if taken with alcohol.

Driving and operating machinery: There are no commonly reported problems which may impact on the ability to drive or operate machinery. However, many drugs can cause dizziness or drowsiness in a few people, so it is wise to see how the drug affects you before driving or working with dangerous machinery.

TRIMETREXATE

Brand name: Neutrexin

Type of drug: Anti-microbial

Uses: To treat Pneumocystis Carinii Pneumonia in AIDS patients who have not responded to other treatments.

How it works: Acts to disable the infective organism.

Possible adverse effects: Vomiting, diarrhoea, rashes, blood disorders.

Availability: Available only with a prescription from a doctor.

Other information: This medication is usually given as an injection in hospital.

CAUTIONS

Children: There are no commonly reported problems associated with prescribing this medication for children.

Pregnancy and breastfeeding: This drug is either not recommended for use by women who are pregnant or breastfeeding, or the precise effects are not known and it should therefore only be used with caution and under medical advice.

Alcohol: No known problems if taken with alcohol.

Driving and operating machinery: There are no commonly reported problems which may impact on the ability to drive or operate machinery. However, many drugs can cause dizziness or drowsiness in a few people, so it is wise to see how the drug affects you before driving or working with dangerous machinery.

TRIPTORELIN

Brand name: De-capeptyl SR

Type of drug: Hormone antagonist

Uses: Used to treat advanced prostate cancer and endometriosis.

How it works: In cancer it neutralises the male sex hormones which the tumour needs to survive. In endometriosis it reduces the production of female hormones.

Possible adverse effects: Nausea, vomiting, diarrhoea, dry mouth.

Availability: Available only with a prescription from a doctor.

Other information: Should not be used by women at high risk of developing osteoporosis.

CAUTIONS

Children: There are no commonly reported problems associated with prescribing this medication for children.

Pregnancy and breastfeeding: No specific problems documented, but any medication should be taken with utmost caution by women who are either pregnant or breastfeeding, and only after professional medical or pharmaceutical advice has been sought.

Alcohol: No known problems if taken with alcohol.

Driving and operating machinery: There are no commonly reported problems which may impact on the ability to drive or operate machinery. However, many drugs can cause dizziness or drowsiness in a few people,

so it is wise to see how the drug affects you before driving or working with dangerous machinery.

TULOBUTEROL

Brand name: Respacal
Type of drug: Adrenoceptor stimulant
Uses: To treat asthma and other reversible airways disease.
How it works: Relaxes the muscles in the lung, enabling air to flow more freely through them.
Possible adverse effects: Tremor and palpitations.
Availability: Available only with a prescription from a doctor.
Other information: Could cause a potentially serious fall in the blood potassium level.
CAUTIONS
Children: There are no commonly reported problems associated with prescribing this medication for children.
Pregnancy and breastfeeding: This drug is either not recommended for use by women who are pregnant or breastfeeding, or the precise effects are not known and it should therefore only be used with caution and under medical advice.
Alcohol: No known problems if taken with alcohol.
Driving and operating machinery: There are no commonly reported problems which may impact on the ability to drive or operate machinery. However, many drugs can cause dizziness or drowsiness in a few people, so it is wise to see how the drug affects you before driving or working with dangerous machinery.

UROKINASE

Brand name: Ukidan
Type of drug: Fibrinolytic
Uses: To treat deep-vein thrombosis and other blood clots.
How it works: Affects the clotting mechanism of the blood, with the result that it is 'thinned' and clots can more easily dissolve.
Possible adverse effects: Nausea, vomiting, fever and bleeding.
Availability: Available only with a prescription from a doctor.
Other information: Will usually be administered as an injection.

CAUTIONS

Children: There are no commonly reported problems associated with prescribing this medication for children.

Pregnancy and breastfeeding: This drug is either not recommended for use by women who are pregnant or breastfeeding, or the precise effects are not known and it should therefore only be used with caution and under medical advice.

Alcohol: No known problems if taken with alcohol.

Driving and operating machinery: There are no commonly reported problems which may impact on the ability to drive or operate machinery. However, many drugs can cause dizziness or drowsiness in a few people, so it is wise to see how the drug affects you before driving or working with dangerous machinery.

URSODEOXYCHOLIC ACID

Brand name: Destolit, Ursofalk

Type of drug: Bile acid preparation

Uses: Treatment of gallstones.

How it works: A naturally occurring chemical, it affects cholesterol levels, with the effect that the gallstones dissolve within three to 18 months.

Possible adverse effects: Rare, but can include diarrhoea, indigestion and a rash.

Availability: Available only with a prescription from a doctor.

Other information: Oral contraceptives may not be so effective. Ultrasound examinations may be carried out to check progress of treatment.

CAUTIONS

Children: This drug is either not recommended for children, or is recommended only for children above a certain age.

Pregnancy and breastfeeding: This drug is either not recommended for use by women who are pregnant or breastfeeding, or the precise effects are not known and it should therefore only be used with caution and under medical advice.

Alcohol: No known problems if taken with alcohol.

Driving and operating machinery: There are no commonly reported problems which may impact on the ability to drive or operate machinery.

However, many drugs can cause dizziness or drowsiness in a few people, so it is wise to see how the drug affects you before driving or working with dangerous machinery.

VALPROIC ACID

Brand name: Convulex

Type of drug: Anti-convulsant

Uses: For treating all forms of epileptic seizure.

How it works: Alters the chemicals in the brain.

Possible adverse effects: Gastric irritation, nausea, tremor, oedema, hair loss.

Availability: Available only with a prescription from a doctor.

Other information: Patient should swallow tablets whole. May take a week for treatment to be effective.

CAUTIONS

Children: There are no commonly reported problems associated with prescribing this medication for children.

Pregnancy and breastfeeding: This drug is either not recommended for use by women who are pregnant or breastfeeding, or the precise effects are not known and it should therefore only be used with caution and under medical advice.

Alcohol: Alcohol should not be consumed, or only consumed with caution - after medical advice has been sought - while you are taking this drug.

Driving and operating machinery: This drug may have some effect on your driving ability, so it is advisable not to drive or operate machinery while taking it.

VENLAFAXINE

Brand name: Efexor

Type of drug: Anti-depressant

Uses: To treat depression.

How it works: Improves mood, energy levels and interest in daily life.

Possible adverse effects: Nausea, dizziness, lethargy, blurred vision, weight loss. Blood pressure can increase.

Availability: Available only with a prescription from a doctor.

Other information: Patient to check before buying any over-the-counter preparations. Patient to report any rashes or other allergic reactions.

CAUTIONS

Children: This drug is either not recommended for children, or is recommended only for children above a certain age.

Pregnancy and breastfeeding: This drug is either not recommended for use by women who are pregnant or breastfeeding, or the precise effects are not known and it should therefore only be used with caution and under medical advice.

Alcohol: Alcohol should not be consumed, or only consumed with caution - after medical advice has been sought - while you are taking this drug.

Driving and operating machinery: This drug may have some effect on your driving ability, so it is advisable not to drive or operate machinery while taking it.

VERAPAMIL

Brand name: Berkatens, Cordilox, Securon-SR, Univer

Type of drug: Anti-angina, anti-arrhythmic, anti-hypertensive

Uses: Treatment of heart problems such as high blood pressure, rhythm disorders and angina.

How it works: Interferes with the electrical signals in the heart and the blood vessels. Reduces the frequency of angina attacks.

Possible adverse effects: Headache, constipation, nausea, swollen ankles.

Availability: Available only with a prescription from a doctor.

Other information: Patient must report any shortness of breath or swelling of hands and feet.

CAUTIONS

Children: There are no commonly reported problems associated with prescribing this medication for children.

Pregnancy and breastfeeding: This drug is either not recommended for use by women who are pregnant or breastfeeding, or the precise effects are not known and it should therefore only be used with caution and under medical advice.

Alcohol: Alcohol should not be consumed, or only consumed with caution - after medical advice has been sought - while you are taking this drug.

Driving and operating machinery: This drug may have some effect on your driving ability, so it is advisable not to drive or operate machinery while taking it.

VIGABATRIN

Brand name: Sabril

Type of drug: Anti-convulsant

Uses: For the treatment of epilepsy.

How it works: Affects the chemicals in the brain so that epileptic seizures are minimised.

Possible adverse effects: Drowsiness, dizziness and fatigue.

Availability: Available only with a prescription from a doctor.

Other information: Patients should report any visual disturbances.

CAUTIONS

Children: There are no commonly reported problems associated with prescribing this medication for children.

Pregnancy and breastfeeding: This drug is either not recommended for use by women who are pregnant or breastfeeding, or the precise effects are not known and it should therefore only be used with caution and under medical advice.

Alcohol: No known problems if taken with alcohol.

Driving and operating machinery: This drug may have some effect on your driving ability, so it is advisable not to drive or operate machinery while taking it.

VILOXAZINE

Brand name: Vivalan

Type of drug: Anti-depressant

Uses: To treat depression.

How it works: Treats the symptoms of depressive illness without undue sedation, thus enabling sufferers to lead a more normal day-to-day life.

Possible adverse effects: Nausea, vomiting, headache, dry mouth, rapid heart beat, drowsiness.

Availability: Available only with a prescription from a doctor.

Other information: It is advisable to avoid stopping taking this drug abruptly.

CAUTIONS

Children: This drug is either not recommended for children, or is recommended only for children above a certain age.

Pregnancy and breastfeeding: This drug is either not recommended for use by women who are pregnant or breastfeeding, or the precise effects are not known and it should therefore only be used with caution and under medical advice.

Alcohol: No known problems if taken with alcohol.

Driving and operating machinery: There are no commonly reported problems which may impact on the ability to drive or operate machinery. However, many drugs can cause dizziness or drowsiness in a few people, so it is wise to see how the drug affects you before driving or working with dangerous machinery.

WARFARIN

Brand name: Marevan

Type of drug: Anti-coagulant

Uses: To prevent blood clots.

How it works: 'Thins' the blood to stop the formation of clots which can settle in the lung, heart, brain and legs.

Possible adverse effects: Bleeding. Any signs of blood in the vomit or faeces or unexplained bruising should be reported to your doctor as soon as possible.

Availability: Available only with a prescription from a doctor.

Other information: Caution must be taken to avoid any injuries, as these could cause excessive bleeding.

CAUTIONS

Children: There are no commonly reported problems associated with prescribing this medication to children.

Pregnancy and breastfeeding: This drug is either not recommended for use by women who are pregnant or breastfeeding, or the precise effects are not known and it should therefore only be used with caution and under medical advice.

Alcohol: Alcohol should not be consumed, or only consumed with caution - after medical advice has been sought - while you are taking this drug.

Driving and operating machinery: This drug may have some effect on

your driving ability, so it is advisable not to drive or operate machinery while taking it.

ZALCITABINE (ddC)

Brand name: Hivid

Type of drug: AIDS and immune deficiency drug

Uses: Treatment of AIDS and other disorders of the immune system.

How it works: Interferes with the genetic material of the virus to stop it replicating.

Possible adverse effects: Bowel problems, nausea, loss of appetite, stomach pain and fatigue. The drug can adversely affect the nerves, pancreas or liver.

Availability: Available only with a prescription from a doctor.

Other information: Blood tests are taken regularly to assess the treatment's effect on the liver and pancreas. The drug is usually taken in conjunction with two other drugs (zidovudine and didanosine). A barrier contraceptive is recommended.

CAUTIONS

Children: This drug is either not recommended for children, or is recommended only for children above a certain age.

Pregnancy and breastfeeding: This drug is either not recommended for use by women who are pregnant or breastfeeding, or the precise effects are not known and it should therefore only be used with caution and under medical advice.

Alcohol: Alcohol should not be consumed, or only consumed with caution - after medical advice has been sought - while you are taking this drug.

Driving and operating machinery: There are no commonly reported problems which may impact on the ability to drive or operate machinery. However, many drugs can cause dizziness or drowsiness in a few people, so it is wise to see how the drug affects you before driving or working with dangerous machinery.

ZIDOVUDINE

Brand name: Retrovir

Type of drug: AIDS and immune deficiency treatment

Uses: Treatment of AIDS.

How it works: Reduces the frequency and severity of infections associated with AIDS. Used as treatment for and prevention of infections.

Possible adverse effects: Anaemia (characterized by paleness, shortness of breath and fatigue). Also, nausea, headache, tiredness, and loss of appetite.

Availability: Available only with a prescription from a doctor.

Other information: A blood transfusion may be necessary.

CAUTIONS

Children: There are no commonly reported problems associated with prescribing this medication for children.

Pregnancy and breastfeeding: This drug is either not recommended for use by women who are pregnant or breastfeeding, or the precise effects are not known and it should therefore only be used with caution and under medical advice.

Alcohol: No known problems if taken with alcohol.

Driving and operating machinery: There are no commonly reported problems which may impact on the ability to drive or operate machinery. However, many drugs can cause dizziness or drowsiness in a few people, so it is wise to see how the drug affects you before driving or working with dangerous machinery.

ZOLPIDEM

Brand name: Stilnoct

Type of drug: Sleeping aid

Uses: To treat insomnia in the short term.

How it works: Has a hypnotic effect in order to induce sleep without having the muscle relaxant properties of other sleeping aids.

Possible adverse effects: Diarrhoea, nausea and vomiting. Vertigo and dizziness.

Availability: Available only with a prescription from a doctor.

Other information: Drug should not be taken with or after a meal. Patient should report when drug no longer effective.

CAUTIONS

Children: This drug is either not recommended for children, or is recommended only for children above a certain age.

Pregnancy and breastfeeding: This drug is either not recommended for

use by women who are pregnant or breastfeeding, or the precise effects are not known and it should therefore only be used with caution and under medical advice.

Alcohol: Alcohol should not be consumed, or only consumed with caution - after medical advice has been sought - while you are taking this drug.

Driving and operating machinery: This drug may have some effect on your driving ability, so it is advisable not to drive or operate machinery while taking it.

ZOPICLONE

Brand name: Zimovane

Type of drug: Sleeping aid

Uses: Treatment of insomnia (difficulty in sleeping). It is particularly suitable for sleeplessness which is due to international travel or shift work and not accompanied by anxiety.

How it works: Has a hypnotic effect which helps to induce sleep.

Possible adverse effects: Bitter taste in the mouth, daytime sleepiness.

Availability: Available only with a prescription from a doctor.

Other information: For infrequent use only, as can be habit-forming after even one week.

CAUTIONS

Children: This drug is either not recommended for children, or is recommended only for children above a certain age.

Pregnancy and breastfeeding: This drug is either not recommended for use by women who are pregnant or breastfeeding, or the precise effects are not known and it should therefore only be used with caution and under medical advice.

Alcohol: Alcohol should not be consumed, or only consumed with caution - after medical advice has been sought - while you are taking this drug.

Driving and operating machinery: This drug may have some effect on your driving ability, so it is advisable not to drive or operate machinery while taking it.

OVER-THE-COUNTER MEDICINES

Over-the-counter (OTC) medicines are those which can be bought from either a pharmacist or other retail outlet, without the need for a prescription from a doctor.

Medicines which are available OTC are relatively mild and designed to help with the treatment of minor ailments at home. Many of the available products are not 'cures' but aim to relieve the symptoms of the problem so that the illness can run its course. For example, the many cold remedies available OTC do not attack the virus that causes colds, but relieve the sufferer of the discomfort of symptoms, such as sore throat or headache.

The minor conditions which are generally suitable for treatment with OTC medicines include: aches and pains, constipation and diarrhoea, coughs and colds, travel sickness, tummy upsets, skin conditions and low-grade infections such as thrush and cystitis.

However, as with all types of medicines, OTC products can be harmful or simply ineffective if they are not used, stored and disposed of properly. For this reason they should be treated with the same care as prescription medicines or any other dangerous chemicals you may keep in the house.

When buying OTC preparations it is worth making use of the expertise of a pharmacist. Pharmacists are trained, independent professionals who are willing to answer questions or give advice about the suitability of the medicines they sell. When you are discussing the suitability of a particular treatment with a pharmacist, ensure that you tell them about any prescription drugs you are taking or any other illnesses or allergies you, or the patient, may have.

When you are preparing to take the medicine, or to give it to someone else, always ensure that you read the packet carefully, taking note of how much you should take, when, and any other specific instructions such as whether it should be taken with food. Do not take any medication when you are pregnant or breastfeeding without first taking advice. Take extra care when giving medicines to children - they are not mini adults and their doses need to be carefully calculated by experts. Follow the advice on the packet or, if in doubt, ask your pharmacist.

Finally, but most importantly, remember to dispose of any unused medicines carefully and safely.

HOW TO USE THIS SECTION

The aim of this section is to give some basic information about the range of over-the-counter preparations available. The information is intended as guidance only and does not provide all you need to know about a product before deciding whether or not to use it. Most importantly, it should not be used as a substitute for talking to a qualified professional, and any queries you may have about a particular medicine should be addressed either to your GP or a pharmacist. Be aware, too, that OTC medicines should not be used by certain groups of people - for example, children of a certain age or people with long-standing conditions such as asthma or diabetes.

The most commonly used OTC products are listed below in alphabetical order, with the information arranged as follows:

Name: The branded name under which the product is sold.
Use: A brief description of the disorder the product treats and how it works.
Dose: The frequency and amount of each dose or, in the case of creams and lotions, each application.

AAA SPRAY

Use: An aerosol spray for soothing sore throats. It contains benzocaine, a local anaesthetic.

Dose: Adults should apply two sprays every 2-3 hours. The maximum dose is 16 sprays over 24 hours. For children over six years, half the adult dose should be given, with a maximum of 8 sprays over 24 hours. This treatment is not recommended for children under six years.

ACNE-AID

Use: This is a cleansing bar for the treatment of acne and greasy skin.

Dose: The cleansing bar should be used in the same way as an ordinary soap. This treatment is not recommended for children under 15 years.

ACNIDAZIL

Use: A cream for the treatment of acne, containing benzoyl peroxide and micanazole, an anti-microbial.

Dose: The cream should be applied to clean, dry skin once a day for the first week. In the second week it should be applied twice a day, and then for 4-8 weeks. This treatment is not recommended for children under 15 years.

ACRIFLEX CREAM

Use: This is a cream for the treatment of minor burns, cuts and grazes, containing chlorhexidine, an antiseptic.

Dose: The cream should be smoothed onto the affected area and then applied again after 15 minutes if required.

ACTAL

Use: Available in tablet form for relieving indigestion and settle digestive discomfort. The tablets contain an antacid.

Dose: 1-2 tablets should be taken as required. The maximum dose is 16 tablets over 24 hours. This treatment is not recommended for children under 12 years.

ACTIFED

Use: These are tablets for hayfever that contain triprolidine, an antihistamine, and pseudoephedrine, a decongestant.

Dose: One tablet should be taken up to four times a day. This treatment is not recommended for children under 12 years.

ACTIFED COMPOUND LINCTUS

Use: This is a liquid remedy for the treatment of coughs, containing dextromethorphan, a cough suppressant, pseudoephedrine, a decongestant and triprolidine, an antihistamine.

Dose: Adults should take 10 ml every four to six hours. Children (6-12 years) should be given 5 ml every 4-6 hours. Children (2-5 years) should be given 2.5 ml every four to six hours. Take a maximum of four doses in 24 hours. This treatment is not recommended for children under two years.

ACTIFED EXPECTORANT

Use: A liquid remedy for the treatment of coughs. It contains guaiphenesin, an expectorant, pseudoephedrine, a decongestant and an antihistamine.

Dose: Adults should take 10 ml every four to six hours. Children (6-12 years) should be given 5 ml every 4-6 hours. Children (2-5 years) should be given 2.5 ml every 4-6 hours. This treatment is not recommended for children under two years.

ACTIFED SYRUP

Use: A liquid remedy for relieving cold, flu and hayfever symptoms. It contains triprolidine, an antihistamine and pseudoephedrine, a decongestant.

Dose: Adults should take 10 ml every 4-6 hours, with a maximum of 4 doses over 24 hours. Children (2-12 years) should be given 2.5-10 ml, according to age. Always read the label. This treatment is not recommended for children under two years. This product is also available in tablet form.

ADCORTYL IN ORABASE

Use: Available in the form of a paste for the treatment of mouth ulcers, containing triamcinolone, a corticosteroid.

Dose: The paste should be applied to the affected area up to three times a day after meals, and then once at night. The treatment can be used for up to five days.

ADULT MELTUS DRY COUGH ELIXIR

Use: A liquid remedy for the treatment of coughs, containing dextromethorphan, a suppressant, and pseudoephedrine, a decongestant.

Dose: Adults should take 5-10 ml four times a day. This treatment is not recommended for children under 12 years.

ADULT MELTUS EXPECTORANT

Use: A liquid remedy for the treatment of coughs, containing guaiphenesin, an expectorant, cetylp yearidium, an antiseptic, purified honey and sucrose.

Dose: Adults should take 5-10 ml every 3-4 hours. This treatment is not recommended for children under 12 years.

ADULT MELTUS EXPECTORANT WITH DECONGESTANT

Use: A liquid remedy for the treatment of coughs, containing guaiphenesin, an expectorant, and pseudoephedrine, a decongestant.

Dose: 10 ml should be taken four times a day. This treatment is not recommended for children under 12 years.

ADVIL COLD AND SINUS TABLETS

Use: These are tablets for relieving cold and flu symptoms, containing ibuprofen and pseudoephedrine, a decongestant.

Dose: 1-2 tablets should be taken every 4-6 hours. Take a maximum of six tablets over 24 hours. This treatment is not recommended for children under 12 years.

ADVIL EXTRA STRENGTH IBUPROFEN

Use: Analgesic tablets which can be used for general pain relief, containing 400 mg ibuprofen.

Dose: One tablet, which can be taken up to three times a day. A maximum of three tablets can be taken over 24 hours. This treatment is not recommended for children under 12 years.

ADVIL IBUPROFEN

Use: These are analgesic tablets for general pain relief containing 200 mg ibuprofen.

Dose: 1-2 tablets should be taken with or just after a meal every 4-6 hours.

Take a maximum of six tablets over 24 hours. This treatment is not recommended for children under 12 years.

AFRAZINE NASAL SPRAY

Use: This is a spray for clearing nasal congestion caused by a cold, sinusitis or hayfever. It contains oxymetazoline, a decongestant.

Dose: Adults and children over 5 years should apply 2-3 sprays into each nostril morning and night. The spray should not be used continuously for more than one week. This treatment is not recommended for children under 5 years.

AFTER BITE

Use: A pen that dispenses ammonia for soothing bites, stings and irritated or itchy skin.

Dose: The pen should be applied as often as required. This treatment is not recommended for children under 2 years.

ALGESAL

Use: This is a cream rub which can be applied to the skin to alleviate muscular aches and pains. It contains a rubefacient and salicylate, an aspirin derivative.

Dose: The cream should be massaged into the affected part of the body up to three times a day. This treatment is not recommended for children under six years.

ALGICON

Use: Available in tablet form for easing the symptoms of acidic stomach, heartburn and indigestion. The tablets contain antacids and an alginate. They have a high sugar content, so diabetics should check with a doctor prior to use.

Dose: 1-2 tablets should be taken four times a day after meals and on retiring. This treatment is not recommended for children under 12 years. The product is also available in liquid form.

ALGIPAN RUB

Use: A cream rub for the treatment of muscular aches and pains, containing rubefacients and a salicylate, an aspirin derivative.

Dose: The cream should be rubbed into the affected area 2-3 times a day. This treatment is not recommended for children under six years.

ALKA-SELTZER

Use: Effervescent tablets which contain an antacid and an analgesic for the relief of headache and upset stomach caused by excess alcohol or over-eating. The tablets contain 324 mg of aspirin, sodium bicarbonate and citric acid.

Dose: Two tablets should be dissolved in water every four hours. The maximum dose is eight tablets over 24 hours. This treatment is not recommended for children under 12 years.

ALKA-SELTZER XS

Use: Effervescent tablets containing an antacid and an analgesic for the relief of headache, upset stomach and general pain caused by excess alcohol or over-eating. The tablets contain 267 mg of aspirin, 133 mg of paracetamol, sodium bicarbonate, citric acid and caffeine.

Dose: 1-2 tablets should be dissolved in water. The maximum dosage is eight tablets over 24 hours. This treatment is not recommended for children under 12 years.

ALLER-EZE CREAM

Use: A cream for relieving itching and irritation caused by bites, stings and rashes. It contains clemastine, an antihistamine.

Dose: This treatment should be applied as and when required.

ALLER-EZE ORIGINAL FORMULA

Use: Available in tablet form for relieving the symptoms of hayfever. The tablets contain clemastine, an antihistamine.

Dose: Adults should take one tablet in the morning and one at night. For children (3-12 years), read the label for variations in dosage. This treatment is not recommended for children under three years.

ALLER-EZE PLUS

Use: These are tablets for relieving the symptoms of hayfever. They contain clemastine, an antihistamine and phenylpropanolamine, a decongestant.

Dose: One tablet should be taken every six hours. There is a maximum dose of four tablets over 24 hours. This treatment is not recommended for children under 12 years.

ALPHOSYL SHAMPOO 2-IN-1

Use: This is a medicated shampoo for the treatment of dandruff. It contains coal tar and a hair conditioner.

Dose: Apply as an ordinary shampoo every 2-3 days.

ALPKA KERI BATH OIL

Use: This is an emollient bath additive containing various oils, including lanolin, for the relief and treatment of eczema and dermatitis.

Dose: Should be added to bath water.

ALTACITE

Use: Available in tablet form for the relief of indigestion and heartburn.

Dose: Adults should take two tablets between meals and on retiring. Children (6-12 years) should take half the adult dose. This treatment is not recommended for children under six years.

ALTACITE PLUS

Use: These are antacid tablets for the relief of indigestion and heartburn. They contain dimethicone to aid the release of trapped wind.

Dose: Adults should take two tablets between meals and on retiring. Children (8-12 years) should take one tablet between meals and one at bedtime. This treatment is not recommended for children under eight years.

ALUDROX

Use: These are antacid tablets for the relief of indigestion and heartburn.

Dose: Adults should take 1-2 tablets four times a day and on retiring. Children (6-12 years) should take one tablet 2-3 times a day. This treatment is not recommended for children under six years. The product is also available in liquid form.

ANACAL RECTAL OINTMENT

Use: An ointment for the treatment and relief of piles. It contains mucopolysaccharide, which is thought to strengthen tissue in the anus.

Dose: The ointment should be applied to the affected area 1-4 times a day. This treatment is not recommended for children under 12 years.

ANACAL SUPPOSITORIES

Use: A treatment for piles available in the form of a suppository tablet. It contains mucopolysaccharide, which is thought to strengthen the tissue in the anus.

Dose: Insert one suppository once or twice a day. This treatment is not recommended for children under 12 years.

ANADIN

Use: Analgesic tablets which can be used for general pain relief, containing 325mg of aspirin, and caffeine.

Dose: Adults should take 1-2 tablets every four hours. The maximum dose is 12 tablets over 24 hours. This treatment is not recommended for children under 12 years.

ANADIN MAXIMUM STRENGTH

Use: Analgesic capsules which can be used for general pain relief, containing 500mg of aspirin, and caffeine.

Dose: Adults should take 1-2 capsules every four hours. There is a maximum dose of eight capsules over 24 hours. This treatment is not recommended for children under 12 years.

ANADIN EXTRA

Use: Analgesic tablets which can be used for general pain relief, containing 300mg of aspirin and 200 mg of paracetamol.

Dose: Adults should take two tablets every four hours. There is a maximum dose of eight tablets over 24 hours. This treatment is not recommended for children under 12 years. The product is also available in the form of soluble tablets with caffeine.

ANADIN IBUPROFEN

Use: Analgesic tablets which can be used for general pain relief, containing 200mg of ibuprofen.

Dose: Adults should take 1-2 tablets 2-3 times a day. There is a maximum dose of six tablets over 24 hours. This treatment is not recommended for children under 12 years.

ANADIN PARACETAMOL

Use: Analgesic tablets which can be used for general pain relief and contains 500mg of paracetamol.

Dose: Adults should take two tablets every four hours. There is a maximum dose of eight tablets over 24 hours. Children (6-12 years) should take half to one tablet every four hours. This treatment is not recommended for children under six years.

ANBESOL

Use: This treatment is available in liquid form for the relief and treatment of mouth ulcers. It contains lidocaine, an anaesthetic, and chlorocresol and cetylp yearidium, which are antiseptics.

Dose: Two applications to the affected area, allowing at least 30 minutes between applications. Use a maximum of eight applications over 24 hours.

ANBESOL ADULT STRENGTH GEL

Use: This is a gel for the relief and treatment of mouth ulcers. It contains lidocaine, an anaesthetic, and chlorocresol and cetylp yearidium, which are antiseptics.

Dose: Adults should apply the gel up to four times a day for one week. This treatment is not recommended for young children.

ANBESOL TEETHING GEL

Use: A gel for the relief of teething pain in babies, containing lidocaine, an anaesthetic, and various antiseptics.

Dose: The gel should be applied onto the affected area no more than four times a day.

ANDREWS ANTACID

Use: Available in tablet form for relieving the symptoms of upset stomach, indigestion and heartburn. The tablets contain various antacids.

Dose: Adults should take 1-2 tablets as needed. The maximum dose is 12 tablets over 24 hours. This treatment is not recommended for children under 12 years. The product is available in various flavours.

ANDREWS ORIGINAL SALTS

Use: Available in powder form for relieving an upset stomach. It contains antacids and sodium.

Dose: Adults should take one teaspoon or one sachet dissolved in water. Take a maximum of four doses over 24 hours. Children over three years should be given half the adult dose. This treatment is not recommended for children under three years.

ANETHAINE

Use: Available in the form of a cream for the treatment and relief of itching and irritation caused by bites and stings, containing a mild anaesthetic.

Dose: The cream should be applied to the affected area 2-3 times a day for up to three days. This treatment is not recommended for children under three years.

ANODESYN OINTMENT

Use: This is an ointment for the treatment of piles, containing benzocaine, a mild local anaesthetic, and allantoin, an astringent.

Dose: Adults should use the ointment twice a day and after each bowel movement. This treatment is not recommended for children under 12 years. The cream should not be used for more than one week unless advised otherwise by a doctor.

ANODESYN SUPPOSITORIES

Use: A suppository for the treatment and relief of piles, containing lignocaine, a mild local anaesthetic, and allantoin, an astringent.

Dose: Insert one suppository in the morning and one in the evening, and after each bowel movement. This treatment is not recommended for children under 12 years. The suppositories should not be used for more than two weeks unless advised otherwise by a doctor.

ANTHISAN CREAM

Use: A cream for the treatment and relief of itching and irritation caused by bites and stings, containing an antihistamine.

Dose: The cream should be applied to the affected area 2-3 times a day for up to three days. This treatment is not recommended for children under three years.

ANTHISAN PLUS STING RELIEF SPRAY

Use: A spray with a metered dose for the treatment and relief of itching and irritation caused by stings, rashes and bites. It contains an antihistamine and a mild anaesthetic.

Dose: To deliver a single dose, the nozzle head should be pressed once. Do this two or three times to the affected part. The spray can be used up to three times a day. This treatment is not recommended for children under three years.

ANUSOL OINTMENT AND CREAM

Use: Available in cream and ointment form for the treatment and relief of piles, containing bismuth, balsam of Peru and zinc oxide, all of which are astringents.

Dose: Should be applied at night and in the morning, and after each bowel movement. This treatment is not recommended for children under 12 years.

ANUSOL SUPPOSITORIES

Use: A suppository for the treatment and relief of piles, containing bismuth, balsam of Peru and zinc oxide.

Dose: One suppository should be inserted into the anus at night and one in the morning, and after each bowel movement. This treatment is not recommended for children under 12 years.

ANUSOL PLUS HC OINTMENT

Use: This is an ointment for the treatment and relief of piles, containing similar ingredients to those in the suppositories with the added ingredient of hydrocortisone, a steroid.

Dose: The ointment should be applied sparingly to the affected area at night and in the morning and after each bowel movement. This treatment is not recommended for children under 18 years. The ointment should not be used for more than seven days. The product is also available in suppository form.

AQUA-BAN

Use: Available in tablet form to relieve pre-menstrual water retention. It is a mild diuretic and contains caffeine.

Dose: Two tablets should be taken three times a day for the 4-5 days before a period is due. The tablets should not be taken for more than five days in one month.

ARRET

Use: Available in capsule form to stop diarrhoea. It contains loperamide.

Dose: Take two capsules initially and then one capsule after every loose bowel movement. Take a maximum of eight capsules over 24 hours. This treatment is not recommended for children under 12 years.

ASILONE ANTACID LIQUID

Use: A liquid remedy for the relief of indigestion, heartburn and upset stomach. It contains antacids, and dimethicone, an anti-flatulent.

Dose: 5-10 ml should be taken after meals and on retiring or as required. Take a maximum of 40 ml over 24 hours. This treatment is not recommended for children under 12 years.

ASILONE ANTACID TABLETS

Use: These tablets are for the relief of indigestion, heartburn, excess gas and an upset stomach, containing antacids.

Dose: 1-2 tablets should be taken before meals and at bedtime. This treatment is not recommended for children under 12 years.

ASKIT POWDERS

Use: An analgesic dissolvable powder which can be used for general pain relief. The powder contains 530mg of aspirin, aloxiprin and caffeine.

Dose: One sachet of powder should be mixed with water and taken every four hours. Take a maximum of six powders over 24 hours. This treatment is not recommended for children under 12 years.

ASPRO CLEAR

Use: These are effervescent analgesic tablets for the relief of general pain, containing 300 mg of aspirin.

Dose: 2-3 tablets should be dissolved in water every three hours. Take a maximum of 13 tablets over 24 hours. This treatment is not recommended for children under 12 years.

ATKINSON AND BARKER'S INFANT GRIPE MIXTURE

Use: A liquid remedy for the relief of colic and wind in infants, containing sodium bicarbonate, an antacid, dill and caraway oils.

Dose: 2.5-10 ml should be given every four hours depending on age. Always read the label. This treatment is not recommended for babies under one month.

AUDAX EAR DROPS

Use: These are drops for softening earwax. The drops contain a mild analgesic and an ingredient to soften the wax.

Dose: The ear should be filled with the liquid and plugged with cotton wool. Repeat this treatment twice a day for four days. This treatment is not recommended for children under one year.

AVOCA WART & VERRUCA SET

Use: This treatment is available as a kit for the removal of warts and verrucae. The kit contains a caustic pencil, an emery file, dressings and protector pads.

Dose: The pencil should be applied to the wart or verruca for one to two minutes and re-applied after 24 hours if required. Protect with the dressings provided. Use a maximum of three treatments for warts and six for verrucae.

AVOMINE

Use: Available in tablet form for the relief of travel sickness, containing promethazine, an antihistamine.

Dose: To prevent travel sickness, adults and children over 10 years should take one tablet on the night before a long journey or two hours before starting a shorter journey.

BABY MELTUS COUGH LINCTUS

Use: This is a liquid remedy for the treatment of coughs. It contains acetic acid, a soothing ingredient.

Dose: Babies (3-12 months) should be given 2.5 ml every two to three hours. Babies (13-30 months) should be given 5 ml every 2-3 hours. Babies over 30 months should be given 10 ml every 2-3 hours. This treatment is not recommended for babies under three months.

BALMOSA CREAM

Use: This is a cream rub for the relief of muscular aches and pains, containing rubefacients and a salicylate, an aspirin derivative.

Dose: The cream should be massaged into the affected area as required. This treatment is not recommended for children under six years.

BANSOR

Use: This treatment is available in liquid form for the treatment of bad breath and infections of the mouth and gums. It contains cetrimide, an anti-microbial.

Dose: To relieve sore gums apply a few drops to the affected area.

BAYER ASPIRIN

Use: Analgesic tablets which can be used for general pain relief, containing 300mg of aspirin.

Dose: 1-3 tablets should be taken every four hours. Take a maximum of 12 tablets over 24 hours. This treatment is not recommended for children under 12 years.

BAZUKA GEL

Use: A gel for the treatment of corns, calluses, warts and verrucae that comes an applicator and an emery board containing salicylic acid. The gel dries to form a water-resistant barrier over the affected area.

Dose: 1-2 drops should be applied to the corn or callus each night, then the area should be rubbed down once a week with the emery board. This treatment is not recommended for children under six years. The product is also available in Extra Strength form.

BECONASE ALLERGY

Use: Available in the form of a nasal spray for easing the congestion caused by hayfever. It contains beclomethasone, a steroid.

Dose: Two sprays should be applied into each nostril morning and evening. This treatment is not recommended for children under 12 years.

BEECHAMS ALL-IN-ONE

Use: This treatment is available in liquid form to alleviate the symptoms of colds and flu. It contains paracetamol, phenylephrine, a decongestant and guaiphenesin, an expectorant.

Dose: 20 ml should be taken up to twice a day. This treatment is not recommended for children under 12 years.

BEECHAMS FLU-PLUS CAPLETS

Use: These are tablets for treatment of the symptoms of colds and flu, containing paracetamol, phenylephrine, a decongestant and caffeine.

Dose: Two capsules should be taken every 4-6 hours if required. Take a maximum of eight capsules over 24 hours. This treatment is not recommended for children under 12 years.

BEECHAMS FLU-PLUS HOT LEMON

Use: Available in the form of sachets of powder for relieving the symptoms of colds and flu. Each sachet contains paracetamol, phenylephrine, a decongestant and vitamin C.

Dose: One sachet should be dissolved in a mug of hot water every 4-6 hours. Take a maximum of four sachets over 24 hours. Treatment is not recommended for children under 12 years. Also available in other flavours.

BEECHAMS LEMON TABLETS

Use: Lemon flavoured tablets for the treatment of cold and flu symptoms, containing aspirin.

Dose: 1-2 tablets should be taken every 3-4 hours. Take a maximum of 12 tablets over 24 hours. This treatment is not recommended for children under 12 years.

BEECHAMS POWDERS

Use: These are sachets of powder that contain aspirin and caffeine for relieving the symptoms of colds and flu.

Dose: One sachet should be dissolved in hot water and taken every 3-4 hours. Take a maximum of six sachets over 24 hours. This treatment is not recommended for children under 12 years.

BEECHAMS POWDERS CAPSULES

Use: These are capsules for relieving the symptoms of colds and flu. They contain paracetamol, phenylephrine, a decongestant and caffeine.

Dose: Adults should take two capsules every 3-4 hours if required. Take a maximum of 12 capsules over 24 hours. Children (6-12 years) should take one capsule every three to four hours, with a maximum dose of six capsules in 24 hours. This treatment is not recommended for children under six years.

BEECHAMS WARMERS BLACKCURRANT

Use: Available in the form of sachets of powder for relieving the symptoms of colds and flu. Each sachet contains paracetamol, phenylephrine, a decongestant and vitamin C.

Dose: One sachet should be dissolved in hot water and taken every four hours. Take a maximum of six sachets over 24 hours. This treatment is not recommended for children under 12 years. The product is also available in other flavours.

BENADRYL ALLERGY RELIEF

Use: Available in capsule form for easing the symptoms of hayfever. Each capsule contains acrivastine, an antihistamine.

Dose: One capsule should be taken up to three times a day. This treatment is not recommended for children under 12 years, or for the elderly.

BENYLIN CHESTY COUGHS

Use: This is a liquid remedy for the treatment of coughs, containing diphenhydramine, an antihistamine and menthol.

Dose: Adults should take 10 ml four times a day. Children (6-12 years) should take 5 ml four times a day. This treatment is not recommended for children under six years. A non-drowsy version is also available.

BENYLIN CHILDREN'S CHESTY COUGHS

Use: A liquid remedy for the treatment of chesty coughs, containing guaiphenesin, an expectorant.

Dose: Children (6-12 years) should be given 10 ml four times a day, with a maximum of four doses a day. Children (1-5 years) should be given 5 ml four times a day, with a maximum of four doses a day. This treatment is not recommended for babies under one year.

BENYLIN CHILDREN'S COUGHS AND COLDS

Use: This is a sugar- and colour-free liquid remedy for treatment of the symptoms of coughs and colds. It contains dextromethorphan, a cough suppressant and triprolidine, an antihistamine.

Dose: Children (6-12 years) should take 10 ml 3-4 times a day. Children (2-5 years) should be given 5 ml 3-4 times a day. Children (1-2 years) should be given 2.5 ml 3-4 times a day. This treatment is not recommended for children under one year.

BENYLIN CHILDREN'S DRY COUGHS

Use: A liquid remedy for the treatment of dry coughs, containing pholcodine, a cough suppressant.

Dose: Children (6-12 years) should be given 10-15 ml three times a day. Children (1-5 years) should be given 5 ml three times a day. This treatment is not recommended for children under one year.

BENYLIN CHILDREN'S NIGHT COUGHS

Use: A liquid remedy for the treatment of coughs. It contains diphenhydramine, an antihistamine, and menthol.

Dose: Children (6 years and over) should take 10 ml no more than four times a day. Children (1-5 years) should take 5 ml no more than four times a day. This treatment is not recommended for children under one year.

BENYLIN COUGH AND CONGESTION

Use: This is a liquid remedy for the treatment of coughs, containing diphenhydramine, an antihistamine, dextromethorphan, a cough suppressant, pseudoephedrine, a decongestant and menthol.

Dose: Adults should take 10 ml no more than four times a day. Children (6-12 years) should take 5 ml no more than four times a day. This treatment is not recommended for children under six years.

BENYLIN DAY AND NIGHT COLD TREATMENT

Use: These are tablets for the treatment of colds and flu. The yellow tablets should be taken in the day and contain paracetamol and phenylpropanolamine, a decongestant. The blue night time tablets contain paracetamol and diphenhydramine, an antihistamine.

Dose: One yellow tablet should be taken three times a day and one blue tablet should be taken at night. This treatment is not recommended for children under six years.

BENYLIN DRY COUGHS

Use: A liquid remedy for the treatment of dry coughs, containing dextromethorphan, a cough suppressant, diphenhydramine, an antihistamine and menthol.

Dose: Adults should take 10 ml four times a day. Children (6-12 years) should take 5 ml four times a day. This treatment is not recommended for children under six years. A non-drowsy version is also available.

BENYLIN FOUR FLU LIQUID

Use: A liquid remedy for relieving the symptoms of colds and flu. The liquid contains pseudoephedrine, a decongestant, diphenhydramine, an antihistamine and paracetamol.

Dose: Adults should take 20 ml four times a day. Children (6-12 years) should take 10 ml four times a day. This treatment is not recommended for children under six years. Hot drink and tablet forms are also available.

BENYLIN WITH CODEINE

Use: This is a liquid remedy for the treatment of coughs, containing codeine, a cough suppressant and diphenhydramine, an antihistamine.

Dose: Adults should take 10 ml four times a day. Children (6-12 years) should be given 5 ml four times a day. This treatment is not recommended for children under six years.

BETACEPT ACNE WASH

Use: A liquid facial wash for the treatment of acne and spots, containing povidone iodine, an anti-microbial.

Dose: The wash should be used twice a day until the symptoms have disappeared. This treatment is not recommended for children under 15 years. Check the label for warnings about povidone iodine.

BETADINE SHAMPOO

Use: This is a medicated shampoo for the treatment of dandruff, containing povidone iodine, an anti-microbial.

Dose: Should be applied twice a week as an ordinary shampoo. Adults should use two to three capfuls. Children (2-12 years) should use 1-2 capfuls. This treatment is not recommended for children under two years.

BETADINE SKIN CLEANSER

Use: This is a liquid facial wash for the treatment of acne and spots. It contains povidone iodine, an anti-microbial.

Dose: The liquid should be applied with a damp sponge, lathered and left on for three to five minutes; then the skin should be rinsed with warm water and dried. Repeat this twice a day. This treatment is not recommended for children under two years. Read the label for warnings about povidone iodine.

BETADINE SPRAY

Use: A dry powder spray for the treatment of minor burns, scalds, cuts and grazes. It contains povidone iodine, an anti-microbial.

Dose: The spray should be applied onto the affected area once or twice a day as required, and covered with a clean dressing. This treatment is not recommended for children under two years.

BIORAL

Use: Available in the form of a gel for the treatment of mouth ulcers, containing carbenoxolone, which promotes healing of the ulcers.

Dose: The gel should be rubbed into the affected area after meals and at bedtime. The gel should be allowed to remain in contact with the ulcer for as long as possible. This treatment is not recommended for children.

BIRLEY'S ANTACID POWDER
Use: An antacid powder remedy for relieving the symptoms of indigestion and heartburn.
Dose: Adults should take 5 ml in water after each meal, or twice a day. Check the label for the correct dosage for children.

BISMAG
Use: These are antacid tablets for relieving the symptoms of indigestion, heartburn and gastritis.
Dose: 2-4 tablets should be taken after meals. Repeat this dose after 15 minutes if required. Can also be taken on retiring. This treatment is not recommended for children under 12 years.

BISODOL ANTACID POWDER
Use: A remedy for indigestion and heartburn available in powder form, containing antacids and sodium.
Dose: 5 ml of the powder should be dissolved in water after meals. This treatment is not recommended for children. The product is also available in tablet form.

BISODOL HEARTBURN
Use: These are tablets for relieving the symptoms of indigestion and heartburn, containing antacids and sodium.
Dose: Adults should chew 1-2 tablets as required. Children (6-12 years) should chew one tablet after meals and at bedtime. This treatment is not recommended for children under six years.

BLISTEZE
Use: This is a cream for the treatment of cold sores. It contains ammonia, a soothing ingredient.
Dose: The cream should be applied to the affected area every two hours or as required.

BN LINIMENT

Use: A liniment for muscular aches and pains, containing rubefacients and a salicylate, an aspirin derivative.

Dose: The cream should be massaged into the affected part 2-3 times a day. For children over six years the liniment should be diluted with equal parts of olive oil before applying it to the affected part. This treatment is not recommended for children under six years.

BOCASAN

Use: This is a mouthwash available in powder form, for the treatment of bad breath and general mouth and gum infections. The powders contain sodium perborate - an anti-microbial, and a cleanser.

Dose: One sachet should be dissolved in water and used as a mouthwash three times a day after meals. Repeat this treatment for seven days. This treatment is not recommended for children under five years.

BONJELA

Use: This is a gel for the treatment of cold sores and mouth ulcers, containing choline salicylate, an aspirin derivative, and cetalkonium, an antiseptic.

Dose: A small quantity of the gel should be applied to the affected area every three hours. Use a maximum of six applications in 24 hours.

BONJELA ORAL PAIN-RELIEVING GEL

Use: A gel for easing teething pain in babies, containing choline salicylate - an analgesic, and an antiseptic.

Dose: The gel should be applied to the gums every three hours. Use a maximum of six applications over 24 hours. This treatment is not recommended for babies under four months.

BRADOSOL

Use: Lozenges for relieving sore throats, containing benzalkonium chloride, an antibacterial.

Dose: One lozenge should be sucked as required. This treatment is not recommended for children under five years. Available in various flavours.

BRADOSOL PLUS
Use: Lozenges for relieving sore throats, containing domiphen bromide, an antibacterial, and lignocaine, an anaesthetic.
Dose: One lozenge should be sucked every 2-3 hours. Take a maximum of eight lozenges every 24 hours. This treatment is not recommended for children under 12 years.

BRASIVOL
Use: This is an abrasive paste used for the treatment of acne. It is available in two grades.
Dose: The affected area should be moistened, and the paste then rubbed in vigorously. Repeat this one to three times a day. The finer grade should be used first, and then the stronger grade progressed to if needed. This treatment is not recommended for children under 15 years.

BROLENE EYE DROPS
Use: Eye drops for the treatment of infections of the eye, containing propamidine, an anti-microbial.
Dose: 1-2 drops should be applied into the affected eye up to four times a day.

BROLENE EYE OINTMENT
Use: An ointment for the treatment of eye infections, including conjunctivitis and styes, containing dibromopropamidine, an anti-microbial.
Dose: The ointment should be applied to the infected eye/s twice a day.

BRONALIN DECONGESTANT
Use: A liquid remedy for the treatment of colds and flu, containing pseudoephedrine, a decongestant.
Dose: Adults should take 10 ml three times a day. Children (6-12 years) should be given 5 ml three times a day. Children (2-5 years) should be given 2.5 ml three times a day. This treatment is not recommended for children under two years.

BRONALIN DRY COUGH ELIXIR
Use: A liquid remedy for the treatment of coughs, containing

dextromethorphan, a suppressant, and pseudoephedrine, a decongestant.

Dose: Adults should take 5-10 ml four times a day. Children (6-12 years) should be given 2.5 ml four times a day. This treatment is not recommended for children under six years.

BRONALIN EXPECTORANT LINCTUS

Use: A liquid remedy for the treatment of coughs, containing diphenhydramine, an antihistamine and sodium citrate and ammonium bicarbonate, both expectorants.

Dose: Adults should take 5-10 ml four times a day if required. Children (6-12 years) should take 5 ml four times a day if required. This treatment is not recommended for children under six years.

BRONALIN JUNIOR LINCTUS

Use: A liquid remedy for the treatment of coughs, containing diphenhydramine, an antihistamine and sodium citrate, an expectorant.

Dose: 5-10 ml, according to age, should be taken three times a day. Read the label for the correct dosage. This treatment is not recommended for children under one year.

BRUSH OFF COLD SORE LOTION

Use: This is a lotion treatment for cold sores, containing povidone iodine, an antiseptic.

Dose: The lotion should be applied twice a day.

BURNEZE

Use: A spray for the treatment of minor burns and scalds. It contains benzocaine, an anaesthetic.

Dose: The spray should be applied onto the affected area and then again after 15 minutes if required.

BUSCOPAN TABLETS

Use: These are tablets containing an antispasmodic, for relieving period pains.

Dose: Two tablets should be taken up to four times a day when necessary.

BUTTERCUP SYRUP (ORIGINAL)

Use: A liquid remedy for relieving coughs, containing capsicum and squill, both expectorants.

Dose: Adults should take 10 ml three times a day. Children over two years should be given 5 ml. This treatment is not recommended for children under two years. The product is also available in honey and lemon flavour.

BUTTERCUP INFANT COUGH SYRUP

Use: A liquid remedy for relieving coughs, containing ipecacuanha, an expectorant, menthol and liquid glucose.

Dose: Children (1-5 years) should be given 5 ml 3-4 times a day. This treatment is not recommended for children under one year.

CABDRIVER'S COUGH LINCTUS

Use: A liquid remedy for the treatment of coughs, containing dextromethorphan - a cough suppressant - terpin, menthol, pumilio pine oil and eucalyptus oil.

Dose: 5 ml should be taken every four hours. This treatment is not recommended for children under 12 years.

CALADRYL CREAM

Use: A cream containing an antihistamine for relieving bites, stings, rashes and sunburn.

Dose: The cream should be applied to the affected part 2-3 times a day as required. The product is also available as a lotion.

CALGEL TEETHING GEL

Use: A gel for relieving teething pains in babies, containing lignocaine - an anaesthetic - and an antiseptic.

Dose: The cream should be applied up to six times a day, leaving a minimum of 20 minutes between applications. This treatment is not recommended for babies under three months.

CALIFIG CALIFORNIA SYRUP OF FIGS

Use: A liquid remedy for the treatment of constipation, containing senna, a stimulant laxative.

Dose: 7.5-30 ml (depending on age) should be taken on retiring. Read the label for the correct dosage. This treatment is not recommended for children under one year.

CALIMAL ANTIHISTAMINE TABLETS

Use: Tablets for relieving the symptoms of hayfever, containing chlorpheniramine, an antihistamine.

Dose: Adults should take one tablet 3-4 times a day. Children (6-12 years) should take half to one tablet 3-4 times a day. This treatment is not recommended for children under six years.

CALPOL INFANT SUSPENSION

Use: A strawberry flavoured analgesic liquid for general pain relief, containing 120 mg of paracetamol in every 5 ml.

Dose: A maximum of four doses can be taken over 24 hours. Babies (3-12 months) should be given 2.5 ml every four hours if required, with no more than 20 ml in 24 hours. Children (1-5 years) should be given 5-10 ml every four hours. This treatment is not recommended for babies under three months.

CALPOL SIX PLUS SUSPENSION

Use: A strawberry flavoured analgesic for general pain relief that is sugar- and colour-free, containing 250 mg of paracetamol in every 5 ml.

Dose: A maximum of four doses can be taken in 24 hours. Children (6-12 years) should be given 5-10 ml every four hours if required. For children under six years use Calpol Infant Suspension.

CANESTEN 1% CREAM

Use: A cream treatment for the treatment of nappy rash, containing clotrimazole, an antifungal.

Dose: The cream should be massaged gently into clean, dry skin 2-3 times a day.

CANESTEN AF CREAM

Use: An antifungal cream containing clotrimazole for the treatment of athlete's foot.

Dose: The cream should be rubbed gently into the affected area 2-3 times a day, and should be used for four weeks.

CANESTEN AF POWDER

Use: A powder treatment for athlete's foot, containing clotrimazole.

Dose: The powder should be sprinkled onto the affected area 2-3 times a day. It is also advisable to dust the inside of socks and footwear each day. This treatment may be continued for four weeks.

CANESTEN AF SPRAY

Use: A spray treatment for athlete's foot, containing clotrimazole, an antifungal ingredient.

Dose: The feet should be washed and dried, particularly between the toes. The product should then be sprayed thinly all over the affected area 2-3 times a day. The treatment should be continued for one month.

CANESTEN COMBI

Use: A combination treatment for thrush comprising of a cream containing 1 per cent clotrimazole - an antifungal drug - and one pessary containing 500 mg of clotrimazole. An applicator is included in the pack.

Dose: One pessary should be inserted into the vagina at night. The cream should be applied twice daily to the external area around the vagina and also applied to the partner's penis.

CANESTEN HYDROCORTISONE

Use: A cream for the treatment of athlete's foot, containing clotrimazole - an antifungal - and a steroid.

Dose: The cream should be applied thinly to the affected area and rubbed in gently. The product should not be used for more than seven days.

CANESTEN 1% CREAM

Use: A cream treatment for the treatment of nappy rash, containing clotrimazole, an antifungal.

Dose: The cream should be massaged gently into clean, dry skin 2-3 times a day.

CANESTEN 1 PESSARY

Use: A pessary for the treatment of thrush, containing 500 mg of clotrimazole, an antifungal drug. An applicator is included in the pack.

Dose: The pessary should be inserted into the vagina at night. This is a single-dose treatment.

CANESTEN 10% VAGINAL CREAM

Use: A cream for the treatment of thrush, containing 10 per cent clotrimazole, an antifungal drug. An applicator is included in the pack.

Dose: The cream should be applied once into the vagina.

CAPASAL SHAMPOO

Use: A shampoo remedy for the treatment of cradle cap in children, containing coal tar, coconut oil and salicylic acid.

Dose: Shampoo the baby's head, rinse and repeat. The treatment can be applied once daily if necessary.

CAPASAL THERAPEUTIC SHAMPOO

Use: A medicated shampoo for the treatment of dandruff, containing coal tar, salicylic acid and coconut oil.

Dose: Should be used as a shampoo when required.

CAPRIN

Use: Analgesic tablets which can be used for general pain relief, containing 300 mg of aspirin.

Dose: 1-3 tablets should be taken 3-4 times a day. Take a maximum of 12 tablets over 24 hours. This treatment is not recommended for children under 12 years.

CARBELLON

Use: Antacid tablets for relieving indigestion, heartburn and gastritis.

Dose: Adults should take 2-4 tablets three times a day. Children over six years should be given two tablets three times a day. This treatment is not recommended for children under six years.

CARNATION CALLUS CAPS

Use: A medicated plaster containing salicylic acid for the treatment of corns and calluses.

Dose: The plaster should be applied to the affected area and changed after three days. The callus can be removed after six days. This treatment is not recommended for children under 16 years.

CARNATION CORN CAPS

Use: Medicated plasters for the treatment of corns, containing salicylic acid.

Dose: The plaster should be applied and changed every two days. The corn can be removed after six days. This treatment is not recommended for children under 15 years unless advised otherwise by a doctor. Do not use for more than 10 days, and do not use more than five caps in that time.

CARNATION VERRUCA CARE

Use: Medicated pads used for the removal of verrucae, containing salicylic acid.

Dose: The pad should be applied and changed every two days, for up to 10 days. The treatment can be repeated after a month. This treatment is not recommended for children under six years, unless advised otherwise by a doctor.

CATARRH-EX

Use: Capsules for relieving catarrh, containing phenylephrine, a decongestant, paracetamol and caffeine.

Dose: 1-2 capsules should be taken every 4-6 hours. Take a maximum of eight capsules in 24 hours.

CEANEL CONCENTRATE

Use: A medicated shampoo for the treatment of dandruff, containing various anti-microbials.

Dose: Should be used as a shampoo three times a week for one week, then twice a week as required.

CEPTON

Use: A wash for the treatment of acne, containing chlorhexidine, an antimicrobial.

Dose: The wash should be applied to clean skin and left for one minute before rinsing off thoroughly. This treatment is not recommended for children under 15 years. The product is also available in the form of a lotion.

CERUMOL EAR DROPS

Use: Ear drops for removing earwax, containing a mild analgesic and an ingredient for softening the wax.

Dose: Five drops should be applied into the affected ear and left for 20 minutes. This should be repeated two to three times a day for three days.

CETAVLEX

Use: A cream for the treatment of minor burns, scalds, cuts and grazes, containing cetrimide, an antiseptic.

Dose: The cream should be applied to the affected area as required.

CETRIMIDE CREAM

Use: An antiseptic cream for the treatment of minor wounds or irritations of the skin, containing cetrimide.

Dose: The cream should be applied to the affected area or smeared on a dressing to cover the wound.

CLARITEYES

Use: Eye drops for relieving irritated eyes caused by hayfever. They contain sodium cromoglycate, an anti-inflammatory.

Dose: 1-2 drops should be applied to each affected eye up to four times a day. This treatment is not recommended for children under five years.

CLARITYN ALLERGY

Use: Tablets for relieving the symptoms of hayfever, containing loratadine, an antihistamine.

Dose: One tablet should be taken daily. This treatment is not recommended for children under 12 years.

CLARITYN ALLERGY SYRUP

Use: A liquid remedy for relieving the symptoms of hayfever. It contains loratadine, an antihistamine.

Dose: Adults should take 10 ml once a day. Children (2-5 years) should be given half the adult dose. This treatment is not recommended for children under two years.

CLEARASIL

Use: A cream for the treatment of acne and spots, containing benzoyl peroxide.

Dose: The cream should be applied once a day for one week. Increase applications to twice a day after one week if there are no adverse effects. This treatment is not recommended for children under 12 years.

CLEARASIL TREATMENT CREAM (REGULAR)

Use: A cream treatment for acne and spots, containing triclosan, an antimicrobial, and sulphur.

Dose: The cream should be applied twice daily to clean skin. This treatment is not recommended for children under 15 years.

CLINITAR CREAM

Use: A cream for the treatment of dermatitis and eczema, containing coal tar.

Dose: The cream should be applied once or twice a day as required.

CLINITAR SHAMPOO

Use: A medicated shampoo for the treatment of dandruff, containing coal tar.

Dose: The shampoo should be used up to three times a week

COCOIS SCALP OINTMENT

Use: An ointment for the treatment of dandruff, containing coal tar.

Dose: The ointment should be applied to the scalp once a week as necessary. For severe conditions apply daily for three to seven days.

Shampoo the hair one hour after using the ointment. This treatment is not recommended for children under six years.

CODIS 500

Use: A soluble analgesic tablet that can be used for general pain relief. Each tablet contains 500 mg of aspirin and 8 mg of codeine phosphate.
Dose: 1-2 tablets should be dissolved in water and taken every four hours as required. Take a maximum of eight tablets over 24 hours. This treatment is not recommended for children under 12 years.

COJENE

Use: Analgesic tablets which can be used for general pain relief, containing 300 mg of aspirin, 8 mg of codeine phosphate and caffeine.
Dose: 1-2 tablets should be taken every four hours. Take a maximum of six tablets in 24 hours. This treatment is not recommended for children under 12 years.

COLOFAC IBS

Use: A tablet remedy for easing the symptoms of irritable bowel syndrome. The tablets contain mebeverine, an ingredient that helps to calm intestinal spasms.
Dose: One tablet should be taken three times a day, preferably 20 minutes before meals. This treatment is not recommended for children under 10 years.

COLPERMIN

Use: Capsules for irritable bowel syndrome, containing peppermint oil for calming intestinal spasms.
Dose: 1-2 capsules should be taken three times a day for up to two weeks. The capsules should be swallowed whole to prevent the peppermint oil irritating the throat. This treatment is not recommended for children under 15 years.

COLSOR

Use: A cream treatment for cold sores, containing tannic acid and phenol, astringents, and menthol, a soothing ingredient.

Dose: The cream should be applied as required. The product is also available in the form of a lotion.

COMPOUND W

Use: A liquid treatment for warts and verrucae, containing salicylic acid.
Dose: The liquid should be applied to the wart or verruca daily for up to 12 weeks. This treatment is not recommended for children under six years.

CONOTRANE CREAM

Use: A cream for the treatment of nappy rash, containing benzalkonium chloride - an antiseptic - and dimethicone, a soothing agent.
Dose: The cream should be applied after every nappy change.

CONTAC 400

Use: Capsules for relieving the symptoms of colds and flu, containing chlorpheniramine, an antihistamine, and phenylpropanolamine, a decongestant.
Dose: One capsule should be taken in the morning and another before retiring. This treatment is not recommended for children under 12 years.

COPHOLCO

Use: A liquid remedy for the treatment of coughs, containing pholcodine, a cough suppressant, terpin, menthol and cineole.
Dose: Adults should take 10 ml four to five times a day. Children over eight years should be given 5 ml per day. This treatment is not recommended for children under eight years.

CORLAN

Use: A tablet for the treatment of mouth ulcers, containing hydrocortisone, a corticosteroid.
Dose: One tablet should be dissolved near the site of the ulcer four times a day. This treatment is not recommended for children under 12 years, unless advised otherwise by a doctor.

CORSODYL

Use: This is a mouthwash for the treatment of mouth infections, sore gums and bad breath. It contains chlorhexidine, an anti-microbial.

Dose: The mouth should be rinsed with 10 ml of the mouthwash for one minute. This should be carried out daily for one month.

CORSODYL DENTAL GEL

Use: A gel for the treatment of mouth infections such as thrush and mouth ulcers, containing chlorhexidine, an antiseptic.
Dose: The gel should be applied directly onto the affected area once or twice a day and left for one minute.

COVONIA BRONCHIAL BALSAM

Use: A liquid remedy for the treatment of coughs, containing dextromethorphan - a cough suppressant - and menthol.
Dose: Adults should take 10 ml every four hours. Children (6-12 years) should be given 5 ml every four hours. This treatment is not recommended for children under six years. The elderly should check with their doctor or pharmacist prior to use.

COVONIA FOR CHILDREN

Use: A liquid remedy for the treatment of coughs, containing dextromethorphan - a cough suppressant - and benzoic acid.
Dose: Children should be given 5-10 ml according to age, every four to six hours as required. Read the label for the correct dosage. This treatment is not recommended for children under two years.

COVONIA MENTHOLATED COUGH MIXTURE

Use: A liquid remedy for the treatment of coughs, containing squill and liquorice - both expectorants - and menthol.
Dose: Adults should take 5-10 ml every four hours. Children (5-12 years) should be given 5 ml every four hours. This treatment is not recommended for children under five years.

COVONIA NIGHT TIME FORMULA

Use: A liquid remedy for the treatment of coughs, containing dextromethorphan, a cough suppressant, and diphenhydramine, an antihistamine.

Dose: 15 ml should be taken before retiring. This treatment is not recommended for children under five years.

CRAMPEX

Use: This is a tablet remedy for dispelling cramps, containing nicotinic acid, which improves the circulation.

Dose: 1-2 tablets should be taken before bedtime. This treatment is not recommended for children.

CREMALGIN

Use: A cream rub for relieving muscular aches and pains, containing rubefacients and a salicylate, an aspirin derivative.

Dose: The cream should be massaged into the affected area twice or three times a day. This treatment is not recommended for children under six years.

CUPAL BABY CHEST RUB

Use: This is an aromatic ointment for relieving catarrh and congestion in young children and babies over three months. The ointment contains eucalyptus and menthol oils.

Dose: The ointment should be rubbed gently into the chest, throat and back twice a day.

CUPLEX

Use: A gel containing salicylic acid for the treatment of calluses, corns, warts and verrucae.

Dose: This gel should be applied at night to the affected part. When it is dry, Cuplex produces a protective film, which should be removed in the mornings. This treatment may take between six and twelve weeks before it shows a result. The product is not recommended for young children.

CUPROFEN

Use: Analgesic tablets which can be used for general pain relief, containing 200 mg of ibuprofen.

Dose: Two tablets should be taken after food. 1-2 tablets can be taken every four hours if required. Take a maximum of six tablets in 24 hours. This treatment is not recommended for children under 12 years.

CUPROFEN IBUTOP GEL

Use: A gel containing ibuprofen for relieving muscular aches and pains, which is non-steroidal anti-inflammatory (NSAID).

Dose: The gel should be applied to the affected area, allowing at least four hours between applications. Do not use more than four times in 24 hours. This treatment is not recommended for children under 12 years.

CUPROFEN MAXIMUM STRENGTH

Use: Analgesic tablets which can be used for general pain relief, containing 400 mg of ibuprofen.

Dose: One tablet should be taken with food every eight hours. Take a maximum of three tablets in 24 hours. This treatment is not recommended for children under 12 years.

CURASH

Use: This is a powder treatment for nappy rash, containing zinc oxide, an antiseptic and an astringent.

Dose: The powder should be applied after every nappy change. Try to avoid inhalation by baby and do not apply to broken skin.

CYMALON

Use: Granules containing sodium citrate and sodium bicarbonate for relieving the symptoms of cystitis.

Dose: One sachet of the granules should be dissolved in water, and taken three times a day for two days.

CYMEX

Use: A cream treatment for cold sores, which contains cetrimide, an antiseptic, and urea, a soothing ingredient.

Dose: The cream should be applied sparingly every hour if necessary.

CYSTOLEVE

Use: Sachets of granules for the treatment of cystitis, containing sodium nitrate.

Dose: One sachet of granules should be dissolved in water three times a day for two days.

CYSTOPURIN

Use: Sachets of granules for the treatment of cystitis, containing potassium citrate.

Dose: One sachet of granules should be dissolved in water three times a day for two days.

DAKTARIN DUAL ACTION CREAM

Use: This is a cream for the treatment of athlete's foot, containing the antifungal ingredient, miconazole.

Dose: The cream should be applied twice a day to the affected area. Continue this treatment for a further 10 days after the infection has cleared up.

DAKTARIN DUAL ACTION POWDER

Use: This is a spray-on treatment for athlete's foot. The powder contains miconazole, an antifungal ingredient.

Dose: The powder should be applied to the affected area twice a day. Continue with this treatment for a further 10 days after the infection has cleared up.

DAKTARIN ORAL GEL

Use: This is a gel treatment for oral thrush, containing miconazole, an antifungal.

Dose: A small amount of the gel should be applied and held in the mouth for as long as possible and then spat out. Repeat this four times a day. The dosage for children varies according to age. Always read the label. Continue treatment for a further two days after the infection has cleared up.

DAYLEVE

Use: A cream for the treatment of stings, bites, hives, eczema and dermatitis. It contains hydrocortisone, a steroid.

Dose: The cream should be applied thinly to the affected area twice a day. This treatment is not recommended for children under 10 years.

DAY NURSE

Use: A liquid remedy for relieving the symptoms of colds and flu, containing paracetamol, phenylpropanolamine, a decongestant and dextromethorphan, a cough suppressant.

Dose: Adults should take 20 ml every four hours. Take a maximum of 80 ml over 24 hours. Children (6-12 years) should be given 10 ml every four hours. This treatment is not recommended for children under six years. The product is also available in capsule form and as a hot drink.

DDD MEDICATED CREAM

Use: A medicated antiseptic cream that is used for the treatment of minor wounds and skin irritations. It contains thymol, menthol, salicylic acid, chlorbutol and titanium dioxide.

Dose: The cream should be applied morning and evening until the problem has cleared up.

DDD MEDICATED LOTION

Use: A medicated antiseptic lotion that can be used for the treatment of minor wounds and skin irritations, containing thymol, menthol, salicylic acid, chlorobutol, methyl salicylate, glycerin and ethanol.

Dose: The cream should be applied to the affected area as needed.

DEEP FREEZE

Use: This is a cooling, spray treatment for relieving muscular aches.

Dose: The treatment should be sprayed onto the affected area as required but no more than three times in 24 hours. This treatment is not recommended for children under six years.

DEEP FREEZE COOLING GEL

Use: A gel for soothing muscular aches which contains cooling ingredients.

Dose: The gel should be rubbed into the affected area 3-4 times a day. This treatment is not recommended for children under five years.

DEEP HEAT MASSAGE LINIMENT

Use: A liniment for the treatment of muscular aches and pains, containing rubefacients and a salicylate, an aspirin derivative.

Dose: The cream should be rubbed into the affected area 3-4 times a day. This treatment is not recommended for children under five years.

DEEP HEAT MAXIMUM STRENGTH

Use: A cream for relieving muscular aches and pains, containing a rubefacient and a salicylate, an aspirin derivative.

Dose: The product should be massaged into the affected area 2-3 times a day. This treatment is not recommended for children under five years.

DEEP HEAT RUB

Use: A cream rub treatment for relieving muscular aches and pains, containing rubefacients, and a salicylate, an aspirin derivative.

Dose: The product should be massaged into the affected area 2-3 times a day. This treatment is not recommended for children under six years.

DEEP HEAT SPRAY

Use: A spray for easing muscular aches and pains, containing rubefacients and a salicylate, an aspirin derivative.

Dose: The affected area should be sprayed with 2-3 short bursts as required. This treatment is not recommended for children under six years.

DEEP RELIEF

Use: A gel treatment for relieving muscular aches and pains, containing ibuprofen, a non-steroidal anti-inflammatory (NSAID).

Dose: The gel should be massaged into the affected area up to three times a day. This treatment is not recommended for children under 12 years.

DENOREX ANTI-DANDRUFF SHAMPOO

Use: A medicated shampoo for the treatment of dandruff, containing coal tar.

Dose: Should be used as a shampoo on alternate days. Continue this treatment for 10 days, then use 2-3 times a week if required. The product is also available as a shampoo with conditioner.

DENTINOX CRADLE CAP TREATMENT SHAMPOO

Use: A shampoo for the treatment of cradle cap.

Dose: The treatment should be used as a normal shampoo at every bath time until the condition clears up.

DENTINOX INFANT COLIC DROPS

Use: A liquid remedy for relieving colic in infants, containing dimethicone, an anti-wind ingredient.

Dose: 2.5 ml should be given with or after each feed. A maximum of six doses can be given in one day. The product can be used from birth onwards.

DENTINOX TEETHING GEL

Use: A gel for soothing teething pain in babies, containing an antiseptic and lignocaine, an anaesthetic.

Dose: The gel should be applied every 20 minutes as required and is suitable for use from birth onwards.

DENTOGEN

Use: A gel for relieving toothache, containing clove oil.

Dose: The gel should be rubbed onto the affected tooth.

DEQUACAINE LOZENGES

Use: Lozenges for relieving sore throats, containing dequalinium, an antibacterial, and benzocaine, an anaesthetic.

Dose: One lozenge should be dissolved in the mouth every two hours or as required. Take a maximum of eight lozenges in 24 hours. This treatment is not recommended for children under 12 years.

DERBAC M LIQUID

Use: A liquid treatment for head lice and other similar infestations, containing malathion.

Dose: For head lice, the liquid should be applied to the affected area, combed through the hair while wet, left to dry and finally washed out after 12 hours. For pubic lice, it should be left on for 1-12 hours, or longer if possible. For scabies, it should be applied to the whole body and left for

24 hours before washing off. This treatment is not recommended for babies under six months.

DERMACORT CREAM

Use: A cream for the treatment of bites, stings, hives, eczema and dermatitis, containing hydrocortisone, a steroid.
Dose: The product should be applied to the affected area once or twice a day. This treatment is not recommended for children under 10 years.

DERMAMIST

Use: An emollient spray for the treatment of eczema and dermatitis, containing a mixture of oils.
Dose: The product should be sprayed onto the affected areas after a bath or shower.

DERMIDEX CREAM

Use: This is a cream for the treatment of bites, stings, eczema, dermatitis and hives, containing an anaesthetic and antiseptic.
Dose: The product should be applied to the affected part every three hours if necessary. Treatment is not recommended for children under four years.

DETTOL ANTISEPTIC PAIN RELIEF SPRAY

Use: A liquid antiseptic spray with a mild anaesthetic for the treatment of minor wounds and skin irritations, containing benzalkonium chloride and lidocaine hydrochloride.
Dose: The liquid should be sprayed onto the affected area as required.

DETTOL CREAM

Use: An antiseptic cream for the treatment of minor wounds or irritations of the skin, containing triclosan, chloro-xylenol and edetic acid.
Dose: The cream should be applied thinly onto the affected area.

DETTOL FRESH

Use: A liquid antiseptic and disinfectant for the treatment of minor wounds and irritations of the skin, containing benzalkonium chloride.

Dose: 50 ml should be diluted in 1 litre of water and applied to the affected area.

DETTOL LIQUID

Use: A liquid antiseptic and disinfectant for the treatment of minor wounds and irritations of the skin, containing chloroxyenol.
Dose: The liquid should be diluted with water as appropriate for its intended use.

DE WITT'S ANTACID POWDER

Use: An antacid powder for relieving indigestion and heartburn, containing sodium.
Dose: 1 teaspoon of the powder should be dissolved in water and taken after meals. This treatment is not recommended for children under 12 years. The product is also available in tablet form.

DE WITT'S THROAT LOZENGES

Use: Lozenges for relieving sore throats, containing cetylp yearidium chloride, an antibacterial.
Dose: Adults should take one lozenge every three hours. Take a maximum of eight in 24 hours. Children over six years should be given half the adult dose with a maximum of four in 24 hours. This treatment is not recommended for children under six years.

DE WITT'S WORM SYRUP

Use: A liquid remedy for removing intestinal worms. The liquid contains piperazine citrate, an anti-worm ingredient.
Dose: For threadworms, adults should take 15 ml daily for seven days. Children should be given 5-10 ml, according to age. For roundworms, adults should take one dose of 3 ml. Children should be given one dose of 10-25 ml, according to age. This treatment is not recommended for children under two years.

DIASORB

Use: Capsules for the treatment of diarrhoea, containing loperamide.
Dose: Two capsules should be taken initially, then one capsule after each

loose bowel movement. Take a maximum of eight capsules in 24 hours. This treatment is not recommended for children under 12 years.

DIFFLAM
Use: A cream for relieving muscular aches and pains, containing benzydamine, a non-steroidal anti-inflammatory (NSAID).
Dose: The cream should be massaged into the affected area three times a day. This treatment is not recommended for children under six years.

DIFLUCAN
Use: An oral capsule for the treatment of thrush, containing 150 mg of fluconazole.
Dose: One capsule should be taken orally. This is a single-dose treatment.

DIJEX
Use: A liquid remedy for relieving indigestion, heartburn and general digestive discomfort, containing an antacid.
Dose: Adults should take 5-10 ml four times a day and on retiring. Children over six years should be given 5 ml three times a day. This treatment is not recommended for children under six years.

DIMOTANE CO
Use: A liquid remedy for the treatment of coughs, containing brompheniramine, an antihistamine, pseudoephedrine, a decongestant, codeine, a cough suppressant and ethanol (alcohol).
Dose: Adults should take 5-10 ml up to four times a day. Children (4-12 years) should be given 5-7.5 ml three times a day, depending on age. Read the label for the correct dosage. This treatment is not recommended for children under four years. The product is also available in a children's formula.

DIMOTAPP ELIXIR
Use: A liquid remedy for the treatment of colds and flu, containing brompheniramine, an antihistamine and phenylephrine, a decongestant.
Dose: Adults should take 5-10 ml three times a day. Children (6-12 years) should be given 5 ml three times a day. Children (2-6 years) should be given 2.5 ml three times a day. This treatment is not recommended for

children under two years. Tablet and children's versions are also available.

DINNEFORDS TEEJEL GEL
Use: A gel for relieving teething pains in babies, containing choline salicylate, an analgesic and an antiseptic.
Dose: 2 cm of the gel should be applied to the gums every 3-4 hours as required. This treatment is not recommended for babies under four months.

DIOCALM DUAL ACTION
Use: A tablet remedy for stopping diarrhoea, containing morphine and attapulgite.
Dose: Two tablets should be taken every two to four hours as required. Take a maximum of 12 tablets in 24 hours. Children (6-12 years) should be given one tablet every 2-4 hours, with a maximum of six tablets in 24 hours. This treatment is not recommended for children under six years.

DIOCALM REPLENISH
Use: A powder remedy to stop diarrhoea. It also aids recovery after diarrhoea by replacing the water and salts lost from the body.
Dose: Adults should take 1-2 sachets dissolved in a measured amount of water, as stated on the packet, after every loose bowel movement. Children (6-12 years) should be given one sachet dissolved in water at the start of diarrhoea, with a repeat dose after every bowel movement. Take a maximum of nine sachets in 24 hours. For bottle-fed babies, use the equivalent volume as a substitute for a bottle-feed. Milk should be gradually re-introduced after 24 hours. Discuss with a doctor before giving medication to babies under 12 months.

DIOCALM ULTRA
Use: Capsules for stopping diarrhoea, containing loperamide.
Dose: Two capsules should be taken at the start of the diarrhoea, followed by one capsule after every loose bowel movement. Take a maximum of eight capsules in 24 hours. This treatment is not recommended for children under 12 years.

DIOCTYL

Use: Capsules for easing constipation, containing docusate, a stimulant laxative with a stool-softening action.

Dose: Adults can take up to five capsules through the day. The dosage should be reduced as the condition improves. This treatment is not recommended for children under 12 years. The product is also available as a solution and in a lower dose form for children.

DIORALYTE NATURAL

Use: A powder remedy to help replace the salts and water lost during an attack of diarrhoea.

Dose: Adults should take 1-2 sachets of the powder in a measured amount of water after each loose bowel movement. Children should be given one sachet. Bottle-fed infants should be given a diluted solution instead of their feed - read the instructions on the packet for the correct dosage. Always consult a doctor before giving this treatment to babies under one year. This product is also available in other flavours.

DIORALYTE RELIEF

Use: A powder formula to replace salts and water lost from the body during an attack of diarrhoea.

Dose: One sachet should be dissolved in a measured quantity of water. Read the instructions on the packet. Take a maximum of five sachets in 24 hours. The product can be taken up to 3-4 days after loose bowel movements. Consult a doctor before giving the solution to babies under one year.

DIPROBASE

Use: An emollient cream for relieving the discomfort of eczema and dermatitis, containing a mixture of oils.

Dose: The cream should be applied when necessary.

DIPROBATH

Use: An emollient bath additive for relieving the discomfort of eczema and dermatitis, containing oil.

Dose: The liquid should be added to bathwater.

DISPRIN

Use: A soluble analgesic tablet which can be used for general pain relief, containing 300 mg of aspirin.

Dose: 2-3 tablets should be taken every four hours. Take a maximum of 13 tablets in 24 hours. The treatment is not recommended for children under 12 years.

DISPRIN DIRECT

Use: Analgesic tablets which can be used for general pain relief and can be dissolved in the mouth without water. Each tablet contains 300mg of aspirin.

Dose: 1-3 tablets should be taken every four hours as required. Take a maximum of 13 tablets in 24 hours. This treatment is not recommended for children under 12 years.

DISPRIN EXTRA

Use: A soluble analgesic tablet which can be used for general pain relief, containing 300 mg of aspirin and 200 mg of paracetamol.

Dose: 1-2 tablets should be dissolved in water every four hours as required. Take a maximum of six tablets in 24 hours. This treatment is not recommended for children under 12 years.

DISPROL PARACETAMOL SUSPENSION

Use: A banana-flavoured, sugar-free analgesic liquid which can be used for general pain relief, containing 120mg of paracetamol in every 5 ml.

Dose: Babies (3-12 months) should be given 2.5-5 ml every four hours if required, with a maximum of four doses in 24 hours. Children (1-6 years) should be given 5-10 ml every four hours if required, with a maximum of four doses in 24 hours. The treatment is not recommended for babies under three months.

DO-DO CHESTEZE

Use: Tablets for the treatment of coughs, containing ephedrine, a decongestant, theophylline, a bronchodilator, and caffeine.

Dose: Adults should take no more than one tablet in four hours. Take a maximum of four tablets in 24 hours. Children over 12 years should be given a maximum of three tablets in 24 hours. This treatment is not recommended for children under 12 years.

DO-DO CHESTEZE EXPECTORANT SYRUP
Use: A liquid remedy for the treatment of coughs, containing guaiphenesin, an expectorant.
Dose: 5-10 ml should be taken every two to four hours. This treatment is not recommended for children under 12 years.

DOLVAN TABLETS
Use: Tablets for the treatment of colds and flu, containing paracetamol, diphenhydramine, an antihistamine, ephedrine, a decongestant and caffeine.
Dose: Adults should take 1-2 tablets three times a day. The elderly should take one tablet three times a day. This treatment is not recommended for children under 12 years.

DRAMAMINE
Use: Tablets for relieving travel sickness that contain an antihistamine.
Dose: Adults should take 1-2 tablets 2-3 times a day. The first dose should be taken half an hour before starting on a journey. Children, depending on age, should be given a quarter to one tablet. This treatment is not recommended for babies under one year.

DRAPOLENE CREAM
Use: A cream which can help soothe sunburn and nappy rash, containing the antiseptics, benzalkonium chloride and cetrimide.
Dose: The cream should be applied as required.

DRISTAN DECONGESTANT TABLETS
Use: Tablets for relieving the symptoms of colds and flu. Each tablet contains aspirin, chlorpheniramine, an antihistamine, phenylephrine, a decongestant and caffeine.
Dose: Two tablets should be taken four times a day. Take a maximum of eight tablets in 24 hours. This treatment is not recommended for children under 12 years.

DRISTAN NASAL SPRAY

Use: A nasal spray for clearing nasal congestion caused by sinusitis or hayfever, containing oxymetazoline, a decongestant.

Dose: Adults should take 1-2 sprays in each nostril every 8-12 hours. This treatment is not recommended for children under six years. Do not use for longer than seven days.

DUBAM SPRAY

Use: A spray treatment for easing muscular aches and pains, containing rubefacients and a salicylate, an aspirin derivative.

Dose: The product should be sprayed onto the affected area for two seconds, up to four times a day. This treatment is not recommended for children under six years. Use with caution if asthmatic or allergic to aspirin.

DULCO-LAX SUPPOSITORIES

Use: A suppository for alleviating constipation, containing the stimulant laxative, bisacodyl.

Dose: One suppository should be applied in the morning. This treatment is not recommended for children under 10 years. A lower strength version is also available for children.

DULCO-LAX TABLETS

Use: Tablets for relieving constipation. They contain bisacodyl, a stimulant laxative.

Dose: 1-2 tablets should be taken on retiring. This treatment is not recommended for children under 10 years. The product is also available in liquid form and as a children's lower strength version.

DUOFILM

Use: A liquid remedy for the treatment of warts and verrucae, containing salicylic acid and lactic acid.

Dose: The liquid should be applied once or twice a day. Allow 6-12 weeks for it to take effect. Discuss with a doctor before using the product on children. This treatment is not recommended for children under six years.

DUPHALAC SOLUTION

Use: A liquid remedy for relieving constipation, containing lactulose, an osmotic laxative.

Dose: Adults should take 15 ml twice a day. Children (5-10 years) should be given 10 ml twice a day. Children (1-5 years) should be given 5 ml twice a day. Babies under one year should be given 2.5 ml - check with a pharmacist or doctor prior to use.

E45 CREAM

Use: An emollient cream for the treatment of eczema and dermatitis, which contains a mixture of oils including hypoallergenic lanolin.

Dose: The cream should be applied to the affected area 2-3 times a day as required.

EAREX EAR DROPS

Use: Ear drops for softening and removing earwax, which contain various oils including peanut oil.

Dose: Four drops of the liquid should be applied into the affected ear and a cotton wool plug applied. Repeat morning and evening for four days until the wax clears.

EAREX PLUS DROPS

Use: Ear drops for the removal of earwax, containing a mild analgesic and an ingredient for softening wax.

Dose: The ear should be filled with the liquid and plugged with cotton wool. Use twice a day for four days. This treatment is not recommended for babies under one year.

ECDYLIN SYRUP

Use: A liquid remedy for the treatment of coughs, containing diphenhydramine, an antihistamine and ammonium chloride, an expectorant.

Dose: Adults should take 5-10 ml every 2-3 hours. Children (1-12 years) should be given 2.5-5 ml according to age. Read the label for the correct dosage. This treatment is not recommended for children under one year.

ECOSTATIN

Use: This is a cream for the treatment of athlete's foot, containing econazole, an antifungal ingredient.

Dose: Apply this product twice a day to the affected part.

EFFERCITRATE SACHETS

Use: Sachets of powder containing citric acid and potassium bicarbonate, for the treatment of cystitis.

Dose: One sachet should be dissolved in water three times a day and taken after meals.

EFFERCITRATE TABLETS

Use: An effervescent tablet that helps to reduce the acidity that causes cystitis, containing citric acid and potassium citrate

Dose: Two tablets should be dissolved in water and taken up to three times a day after meals.

EFFICO TONIC

Use: A liquid tonic for general fatigue, containing caffeine, Vitamin B1 and nicotinamide.

Dose: Adults should take 10 ml three times a day after food. Children should be given 2.5-5 ml, according to age, three times a day after food.

ELECTROLADE

Use: A powder solution for replacing the fluids and salts lost from the body during an attack of diarrhoea.

Dose: Adults should take 1-2 sachets dissolved in a measured amount of water (see instructions on the packet for correct measurements) after every loose bowel movement. Up to 16 sachets can be taken in 24 hours. Children should be given one sachet after every loose bowel movement, with up to 12 sachets in 24 hours. Consult a doctor before using this treatment on babies under two years. The product is available in a range of flavours.

ELLIMAN'S UNIVERSAL EMBROCATION

Use: An embrocation for easing muscular aches and pains, containing rubefacients.

Dose: The product should be applied to the affected area every three hours on the first day, then twice a day until the pain eases. This treatment is not recommended for children under 12 years.

ELUDRIL MOUTHWASH
Use: A mouthwash for the treatment of bad breath, sore gums and general infections of the mouth. It contains chlorhexidine, an anti-microbial.
Dose: The mouth should be rinsed with 10-15 ml of the mouthwash diluted with water, 2-3 times a day, taking care not to swallow the liquid. This treatment is not recommended for children. The product is also available as a spray.

EMULSIDERM EMOLLIENT
Use: An emollient bath additive for relieving the discomfort of eczema and dermatitis, containing various oils and an antiseptic.
Dose: The product can be added to bath water or applied directly onto the skin.

ENO
Use: A powder remedy for relieving indigestion, heartburn and gastritis, containing an antacid and sodium.
Dose: One sachet or one teaspoon should be dissolved in water every 2-3 hours or as required. Take a maximum of six doses in 24 hours. This treatment is not recommended for children under 12 years. The product is also available in lemon flavour.

ENTEROSAN TABLETS
Use: Tablets to help stop diarrhoea. They contain kaolin, morphine and belladonna.
Dose: Four tablets should be taken when diarrhoea starts, followed by two tablets every three to four hours. This treatment is not recommended for children under 12 years.

ENTROTABS
Use: Tablets for the treatment of diarrhoea, containing kaolin.
Dose: Adults should take four tablets at the start of diarrhoea, then two tablets every three to four hours. Children (6-12 years) should be given one

tablet every four hours. This treatment is not recommended for children under six years.

EQUILON

Use: Tablets for the treatment of irritable bowel syndrome that contain mebeverine, which helps calm intestinal spasms.

Dose: One tablet can be taken up to three times a day, preferably 20 minutes before meals. This treatment is not recommended for children under 10 years.

ESKAMEL CREAM

Use: A cream for the treatment of acne and spots, containing resorcinol and sulphur.

Dose: The cream should be applied once a day. This treatment is not recommended for children under 15 years.

ESKORNADE CAPSULES

Use: Capsules for relieving the symptoms of colds and flu. Each capsule contains phenylpropanolamine, a decongestant and diphenhydramine, an antihistamine.

Dose: One capsule should be taken every 12 hours. This treatment is not recommended for children under 12 years. The product is also available in a syrup form.

EURAX CREAM

Use: This is a cream containing crotamiton for relieving itching caused by stings, bites, hives, eczema, dermatitis and sunburn.

Dose: The product should be applied as required. The product is also available as a lotion.

EURAX HC CREAM

Use: This cream contains crotamiton and the steroid, hydrocortisone, for the treatment of eczema, dermatitis, stings, bites and hives.

Dose: The cream should be applied sparingly up to twice a day. This treatment is not recommended for children under 10 years.

EX-LAX SENNA
Use: Chocolate tablets for easing the discomfort of constipation, containing senna, a stimulant laxative.
Dose: Adults should take one tablet of chocolate when retiring. Children over six years should be given half to one tablet at bedtime. This treatment is not recommended for children under six years.

EXPULIN CHESTY COUGH LINCTUS
Use: A liquid remedy for relieving coughs, containing guaiphenesin, an expectorant.
Dose: Adults should take 10 ml every 2-3 hours. Children (3-12 years) should be given 5 ml every 2-3 hours. This treatment is not recommended for children under three years.

EXPULIN COUGH LINCTUS
Use: A liquid remedy for the treatment of coughs, containing pholcodine, a cough suppressant, chlorpheniramine, an antihistamine, and pseudoephedrine, a decongestant.
Dose: Adults should take 10 ml four times a day. Children (2-12 years) should be given 2.5-10 ml a day according to age. Read the label for the correct dosage. This treatment is not recommended for children under two years. A children's version is available.

EXPULIN CHESTY COUGH LINCTUS
Use: A liquid remedy for relieving coughs, containing guaiphenesin, an expectorant.
Dose: Adults should take 10 ml every 2-3 hours. Children (3-12 years) should be given 5 ml every 2-3 hours. This treatment is not recommended for children under three years.

EXPULIN DECONGESTANT FOR BABIES AND CHILDREN (LINCTUS)
Use: A sugar-free liquid remedy for relieving the symptoms of colds and flu in children. The liquid contains chlorpheniramine, an antihistamine, and ephedrine, a decongestant.

Dose: Children (3 months-12 years) should be given 2.5-15 ml, 2-3 times a day according to age. Read the label for the correct dosage. This treatment is not recommended for babies under three months.

EXPULIN DRY COUGH LINCTUS
Use: A liquid remedy for the treatment of coughs, containing pholcodine, a cough suppressant.
Dose: 5 ml should be taken three to four times a day. This treatment is not recommended for children under 12 years.

EX-LAX SENNA
Use: Chocolate tablets for easing the discomfort of constipation, containing senna, a stimulant laxative.
Dose: Adults should take one tablet of chocolate when retiring. Children over six years should be given half to one tablet at bedtime. This treatment is not recommended for children under six years.

EXTEROL EAR DROPS
Use: Ear drops for removing earwax, containing softening ingredients.
Dose: 5 drops should be applied into the affected ear once or twice a day, for 3-4 days.

FAMEL EXPECTORANT
Use: A liquid remedy for coughs, containing guaiphenesin, an expectorant.
Dose: Adults should take 20 ml every 2-4 hours if required. Children (1-12 years) should be given 5-10 ml, according to age. Read the label for the correct dosage. This treatment is not recommended for children under one year.

FAMEL ORIGINAL
Use: A liquid remedy for the treatment of coughs, containing codeine, a cough suppressant and creosote.
Dose: 10-15 ml should be taken three times a day. This treatment is not recommended for children under 12 years.

FEDRIL EXPECTORANT
Use: A liquid remedy for the treatment of coughs, containing

diphenhydramine, an antihistamine, ammonium chloride, an expectorant and menthol.

Dose: Adults should take 5-10 ml 3-4 times a day. Children (2-12 years) should be given 2.5-5 ml, according to age. Read the label for the correct dosage. This treatment is not recommended for children under two years.

FEDRIL TICKLY COUGH

Use: A liquid remedy for the treatment of coughs, containing cetylp yearidium, an antiseptic, ipecacuanha and ammonium chloride, which are both expectorants, lemon oil, purified honey, glycerin and citric acid.

Dose: Adults should take 15 ml every 2-3 hours. Children (2-12 years) should be given 5-10 ml, according to age. Read the label for the correct dosage. This treatment is not recommended for children under two years.

FELDENE P GEL

Use: This is a gel for the treatment of muscular aches and pains, containing piroxicam, a non-steroidal anti-inflammatory (NSAID).

Dose: The product should be applied to the affected area up to four times a day. This treatment is not recommended for children under 12 years.

FEMERON

Use: A cream for the treatment of thrush, containing 2 per cent miconazole nitrate.

Dose: The product should be applied to the external vaginal area morning and evening.

FEMERON SOFT PESSARY

Use: A pessary for the treatment of thrush, containing 1200 mg of miconazole nitrate.

Dose: One pessary should be inserted into the vagina at night. This is a single-dose treatment.

FEMINAX

Use: A tablet remedy for relieving period pain, containing paracetamol, codeine, caffeine and an antispasmodic.

Dose: 1-2 tablets should be taken every four hours when necessary. Take a maximum of six tablets in 24 hours.

FENBID GEL

Use: A gel containing ibuprofen, a non-steroidal anti-inflammatory (NSAID), for the treatment of muscular aches and pains.
Dose: The gel should be massaged into the affected area up to four times a day. This treatment is not recommended for children under 14 years. The product is also available as a cream.

FENNINGS CHILDREN'S COOLING POWDERS

Use: An analgesic powder which can be used for general pain relief, containing 50 mg of paracetamol in 1 ml.
Dose: Take a maximum of four doses in 24 hours. The powder should be dissolved in water. Babies (3 months-1 year) should be given one powder. Children (1-6 years) should be given two powders. Children (6-12 years) should be given four powders. This treatment is not recommended for babies under three months.

FENNINGS LITTLE HEALERS

Use: A tablet for the treatment of coughs, containing ipecacuanha, an expectorant.
Dose: Adults should take two tablets three times a day. Children (5-12 years) should take one tablet. This treatment is not recommended for children under five years.

FENOX NASAL DROPS

Use: Nasal drops for relieving nasal congestion caused by sinusitis or hayfever, containing phenylephrine, a decongestant.
Dose: Adults should take 4-5 drops into each nostril morning and night and every four hours if required. Children (5-12 years) should take two drops in each nostril night and morning, and every four hours if required. This treatment is not recommended for children under five years. Do not use longer than seven days. The product is also available as a spray.

FIERY JACK

Use: A cream rub for alleviating muscular aches and pains, containing rubefacients.

Dose: The product should be applied to the affected area twice a day. This treatment is not recommended for children under six years.

FRADOR

Use: A liquid treatment for mouth ulcers, containing antiseptic and astringent ingredients.

Dose: The liquid should be applied to the ulcer with the applicator provided, four times a day after meals and before retiring to bed. This treatment is not recommended for children.

FULL MARKS LIQUID

Use: A liquid treatment for head lice and other infestations, containing phenothrin.

Dose: The liquid should be rubbed into the scalp and the hair combed whilst wet, then allowed to dry naturally. The treatment should be left in for at least 12 hours, then washed out. This treatment is not recommended for babies under six months.

FULL MARKS LOTION

Use: A lotion for the treatment of head lice, containing phenothrin and alcohol.

Dose: The lotion should be rubbed into dry hair and left in for two hours or overnight. Wash and comb through hair while it is wet. This treatment is not recommended for babies under six months.

FYBOGEL

Use: These are granules for the treatment of constipation and irritable bowel syndrome, containing ispaghula husk, which is a bulking agent.

Dose: Adults should dissolve one sachet of the granules in water and drink after a meal, twice a day. Children (6-12 years) should be given 2.5-5 ml of granules twice a day. The product should be taken with plenty of liquid, and not before bedtime. This treatment is not recommended for children under six years. The product is available in various flavours.

FYNNON CALCIUM ASPIRIN

Use: A soluble analgesic which can be used for general pain relief, containing 500 mg of aspirin.

Dose: 1-2 tablets should be dissolved in water and taken every four hours if required. Take a maximum of eight tablets in 24 hours. This treatment is not recommended for children under 12 years.

FYNNON SALTS

Use: A powder remedy for relieving the symptoms of constipation. The powder contains sodium sulphate, an osmotic laxative.

Dose: 5 ml should be taken once or twice a day dissolved in water. This treatment is not recommended for children under 12 years.

GALENPHOL ADULT LINCTUS

Use: A liquid remedy for the treatment of coughs, containing pholcodine, a cough suppressant.

Dose: Adults should take 10-15 ml 3-4 times a day. Children (5-12 years) should be given one dose. This treatment is not recommended for children under five years.

GALENPHOL PAEDIATRIC

Use: A liquid remedy for the treatment of coughs, containing pholcodine, a cough suppressant.

Dose: Children (1-5 years) should be given 5-10 ml three times a day. Babies (3-12 months) should be given 2.5 ml. This treatment is not recommended for babies under three months.

GALLOWAY'S COUGH SYRUP

Use: A liquid remedy for coughs, containing ipecacuanha and squill, both expectorants.

Dose: Adults should take 10 ml three to four times a day. Children under 10 years should be given half the adult dose. Read the label for the correct dosage.

GALPSEUD

Use: Tablets for the treatment of sinusitis, containing pseudoephedrine, a decongestant.

Dose: Adults should take one tablet four times a day. This treatment is not recommended for children under 12 years. The product is also available as a liquid.

GASTROCOTE LIQUID

Use: A liquid remedy for the treatment of upset stomachs, indigestion and heartburn, containing sodium, an antacid, and an alginate.

Dose: 5-15 ml should be taken four times a day after meals and on retiring. This treatment is not recommended for children under six years. The product is also available in tablet form.

GAVISCON 250

Use: A tablet remedy for indigestion and heartburn, containing an antacid, sodium, and an alginate.

Dose: Two tablets should be chewed as needed. This treatment is not recommended for children under 12 years. The product is also available in extra strength form, Gaviscon 500, and in a liquid version, Gaviscon Advance.

GELCOTAR LIQUID

Use: A liquid for the treatment of dandruff, containing coal tar.

Dose: The liquid should be used as a shampoo twice a week.

GERMOLENE ANTISEPTIC WIPES

Use: Cleansing wipes for the treatment of minor wounds and skin irritations, impregnated with an antiseptic. The wipes contain benzalkonium chloride and chlorohexidine gluconate.

Dose: Use to clean wounds as required.

GERMOLENE CREAM

Use: An antiseptic cream for the treatment of minor wounds and irritations of the skin, containing phenol and chlorohexidine gluconate.

Dose: The cream should be applied to the affected area, and covered with a dressing if necessary.

GERMOLENE NEW SKIN
Use: A liquid that forms a water- and germ-proof barrier to protect minor wounds.
Dose: The liquid should be applied to the cut or graze and allowed to dry.

GERMOLENE OINTMENT
Use: An antiseptic ointment for the treatment of minor wounds and irritations of the skin. It contains zinc oxide, methyl salicylate, phenol lanolin and octaphonium chloride.
Dose: The product should be applied to the affected area or smeared onto a dressing.

GERMOLOIDS CREAM
Use: A cream treatment for piles, containing lidocaine, a mild local anaesthetic, and zinc oxide, an astringent.
Dose: The product should be applied to the affected area twice a day and after each bowel movement, with no more than four applications in one day. This treatment is not recommended for children under 12 years. The product is also available as suppositories and as an ointment.

GLUTAROL
Use: A liquid treatment for warts and verrucae, containing glutaraldehyde.
Dose: The product should be applied to the wart or verruca twice a day.

GODDARD'S EMBROCATION
Use: An embrocation for relieving muscular aches and pains, containing a rubefacient.
Dose: The product should be applied to the affected area once or twice a day or as required. This treatment is not recommended for children under six years.

GOLDEN EYE OINTMENT
Use: Eye ointment for treating infections of the eye including conjunctivitis and styes. It contains dibromopropamidine, an anti-microbial.

Dose: The product should be applied to the affected eye once or twice a day.

HALLS SOOTHERS
Use: Medicated sweets for easing sore throats, containing menthol and eucalyptus.
Dose: The sweets should be dissolved in the mouth as required.

HAY-CROM HAY FEVER EYE DROPS
Use: Eye drops for easing the symptoms of hayfever, containing sodium cromoglycate, an anti-inflammatory.
Dose: 1-2 drops should be applied into each affected eye up to four times a day. This treatment is not recommended for children under five years.

HAYMINE
Use: Tablets for relieving the symptoms of hayfever, containing chlorpheniramine, an antihistamine, and ephedrine, a decongestant.
Dose: One tablet should be taken in the morning, and another tablet can be taken at night if necessary. This treatment is not recommended for children under 12 years.

HC45 HYDROCORTISONE CREAM
Use: A hydrocortisone cream for the treatment of eczema, dermatitis, stings, bites and hives.
Dose: The product should be applied to the affected area sparingly once or twice a day. This treatment is not recommended for children under 10 years.

HEALTHY FEET
Use: A treatment for athlete's foot, containing undecylenic acid, an antifungal ingredient.
Dose: The product should be applied to the affected area as often as is necessary.

HEDEX
Use: Analgesic tablets that can be used for general pain relief, containing 500 mg of paracetamol.

Dose: Adults should take two tablets up to four times a day. Take a maximum of eight tablets in 24 hours. Children (6-12 years) should be given half of one tablet every four hours, with a maximum of four tablets in 24 hours. This treatment is not recommended for children under six years.

HEDEX EXTRA

Use: Analgesic tablets which can be used for general pain relief, containing 500 mg of paracetamol and caffeine.
Dose: Two tablets should be taken up to four times a day. Take a maximum of eight tablets in 24 hours. This treatment is not suitable for children under 12 years.

HEDEX IBUPROFEN

Use: Analgesic tablets for general pain relief, containing 200 mg of ibuprofen.
Dose: 1-2 tablets should be taken up to three times a day. Take a maximum of six tablets in 24 hours. This treatment is not recommended for children under 12 years.

HEMOCANE CREAM

Use: A cream treatment for the treatment of piles, containing lignocaine, a mild local anaesthetic and zinc oxide, an astringent.
Dose: The cream should be applied morning and night, and after each bowel movement. This treatment is not recommended for children under 12 years.

HERPETAD COLD SORE CREAM

Use: A cream for the treatment of cold sores, containing aciclovir, an antiviral.
Dose: The cream should be applied as soon as a cold sore tingling is felt, and applied to the sore every four hours, five times a day for five days.

HILL'S BALSAM CHESTY COUGH LIQUID

Use: A liquid remedy for the treatment of coughs, containing guaiphenesin, an expectorant.
Dose: 5-10 ml should be taken every two to four hours. Take a maximum

of 60 ml in 24 hours. This treatment is not recommended for children under 12 years.

HILL'S BALSAM CHESTY COUGH LIQUID FOR CHILDREN
Use: A liquid sugar-free remedy for relieving coughs, containing ipecacuanha, citric acid and capsicum, all expectorants, and benzoin, saccharin and orange oil.
Dose: 2.5-5 ml should be given three times a day and at bedtime, according to age. Read the label for the correct dosage.

HILL'S BALSAM DRY COUGH LIQUID
Use: A liquid remedy for the treatment of coughs, containing pholcodine, a cough suppressant.
Dose: 5 ml should be taken 3-4 times a day. This treatment is not recommended for children under 12 years.

HILL'S BALSAM EXTRA STRONG 2-IN-1 PASTILLES
Use: Herbal pastilles for soothing the symptoms of colds and flu, containing ipecacuanha, menthol and peppermint.
Dose: One pastille should be dissolved in the mouth as required, with a maximum of 10 pastilles in 24 hours. Children over 12 years should be given a maximum of seven pastilles in 24 hours. This treatment is not recommended for children under 12 years.

HIRUDOID CREAM
Use: A cream to aid the healing of minor bruises, containing heparinoid, an ingredient that helps resolve bruising.
Dose: The product should be applied to the bruise four times a day. This treatment is not recommended for children under four years. The product is also available as a gel.

HYDROMOL CREAM
Use: An emollient cream for relieving the discomfort of eczema and dermatitis, containing a mixture of oils including peanut oil.
Dose: The cream should be applied liberally and used as often as required.

HYDROMOL EMOLLIENT

Use: An emollient bath additive for relieving the discomfort of eczema and dermatitis, containing a mixture of oils.

Dose: 1-3 capfuls of the liquid should be added to a shallow bath.

IBULEVE GEL

Use: A gel for the treatment of muscular aches and pains, containing ibuprofen, a non-steroidal anti-inflammatory (NSAID).

Dose: The gel should be massaged into the affected area up to three times a day. This treatment is not recommended for children under 12 years. The product is also available in a spray and as a mousse.

IBULEVE SPORTS

Use: A gel for the treatment of muscular aches and pains, containing ibuprofen, a non-steroidal anti-inflammatory (NSAID).

Dose: The product should be massaged into the affected area up to three times a day. This treatment is not recommended for children under 12 years.

IBUSPRAY

Use: A spray for relieving muscular aches and pains, containing ibuprofen, a non-steroidal anti-inflammatory (NSAID).

Dose: The product should be sprayed onto the affected part and massaged in 3-4 times a day. This treatment is not recommended for children under 12 years.

IMODIUM CAPSULES

Use: Capsules to help stop diarrhoea, containing loperamide.

Dose: Two capsules should be taken at the start of an attack of diarrhoea, and then one capsule after every loose bowel movement. Take a maximum of eight capsules in 24 hours. This treatment is not recommended for children under 12 years. The product is also available in liquid form.

IMUDERM THERAPEUTIC OIL

Use: An emollient bath additive for the treatment of eczema and dermatitis, containing various oils.

Dose: 15-30 ml of the oil can be added to the bath water or applied directly to the skin.

INADINE
Use: A non-stick dressing to be applied to minor burns and scalds, containing povidone iodine - an anti-microbial.
Dose: The product should be applied as required.

INFACOL
Use: A liquid remedy for relieving wind and colic in babies, containing simethicone, an anti-wind ingredient. A measure is supplied.
Dose: One measured dose of 0.5 ml should be given before each feed. The liquid can be used from birth onwards.

INFADROPS
Use: An analgesic liquid for general pain relief, containing 100 mg of paracetamol. A measuring pipette is supplied.
Dose: A maximum of four doses can be given in 24 hours. Babies (3-12 months) should be given 0.8 ml. Babies (1-2 years) should be given 1.2 ml. Children (2-3 years) should be given 1.6 ml. This treatment is not recommended for babies under three months unless advised otherwise by a doctor.

INTRALGIN
Use: A gel for the treatment of muscular aches and pains, containing a rubefacient and a local anaesthetic.
Dose: The gel should be massaged gently into the affected area as required.

IONAX
Use: A facial scrub for treating spots and acne, containing abrasive and antibacterial ingredients.
Dose: The face should be moistened and the gel rubbed in for 1-2 minutes, then rinsed off. The treatment should be used once or twice a day. This treatment is not recommended for children under 12 years.

IONIL T

Use: A medicated shampoo for the treatment of dandruff, containing coal tar and an antiseptic.

Dose: Should be used as a shampoo once or twice a week.

ISOGEL

Use: A granule remedy for relieving the symptoms of constipation, diarrhoea and irritable bowel syndrome. The granules contain ispaghula husk, a bulking laxative.

Dose: Adults should take 10 ml dissolved in water once or twice a day. Children (6-12 years) should be given 5 ml once or twice a day. The granules should be taken with plenty of fluid and it is advisable not to take the treatment at bedtime. This treatment is not recommended for children under six years.

JACKSON'S ALL FOURS

Use: A liquid remedy for the treatment of coughs, containing guaiphesin, a cough suppressant.

Dose: 10-20 ml should be taken at bedtime or every four hours if necessary. This treatment is not recommended for children under 12 years.

JACKSON'S FEBRIFUGE

Use: This is a liquid remedy for relieving the symptoms of colds and flu, containing sodium salicylate, an ingredient related to aspirin.

Dose: Adults should take 5-10 ml in water every six hours or three times a day. The elderly should take half the adult dose. This treatment is not recommended for children under 12 years.

J COLLIS BROWNE'S MIXTURE

Use: This is a liquid remedy for the treatment of diarrhoea and digestive upsets, containing morphine.

Dose: Adults should take 10-15 ml every four hours. Children (6-12 years) should be given 5 ml every four hours. This treatment is not recommended for children under six years. The product is also available in tablet form.

JELONET

Use: A sterile gauze dressing for the treatment of burns and scalds. It is impregnated with soft paraffin which prevents fibres from sticking to the burn.
Dose: The product should be applied to the affected area as required.

JOY-RIDES

Use: Tablets for the prevention of travel sickness, containing hyoscine, an anti-spasmodic.
Dose: Adults should take two tablets 20 minutes before the start of a journey or at the onset of nausea. The dose may be repeated after six hours if necessary. Children over three years should be given half to two tablets depending on age, with a maximum of two doses in 24 hours. Check instructions on the label for the correct dosage. This treatment is not recommended for children under three years.

JUNGLE FORMULA BITE AND STING RELIEF CREAM

Use: This is a cream for the treatment of bites and stings. It contains a steroid.
Dose: The product should be applied sparingly to the affected area once or twice a day. Do not use for more than seven days. This treatment is not recommended for children under 10 years.

JUNIOR DISPROL PARACETAMOL TABLETS

Use: A lime flavoured, soluble analgesic tablet for general pain relief. Each tablet contains 120 mg of paracetemol.
Dose: A maximum of four doses may be taken in 24 hours. For children (1-6 years) dissolve 1-2 tablets in water every four hours if required. Children (6-12 years) should be given 2-4 tablets every four hours. This treatment is not recommended for babies under one year.

JUNIOR KAO-C

Use: A liquid remedy for stopping diarrhoea in children, containing kaolin.
Dose: Children should be given 5-20 ml according to age, three times a day. Check the label for the correct dosage. This treatment is not recommended for babies under one year.

JUNIOR MELTUS EXPECTORANT

Use: A liquid remedy for the treatment of coughs, containing guaiphesin, an expectorant, cetylp yearidium, an antiseptic, purified honey and sucrose.

Dose: Children over six years should be given 10 ml 3-4 times a day. Children (1-6 years) should be given 5 ml 3-4 times a day. This treatment is not suitable for children under one year. Sugar- and colour-free versions are also available.

JUNO JUNIPAH SALTS

Use: A powder remedy for relieving the discomfort of constipation. The powders contain sodium sulphate, an osmotic laxative.

Dose: 20 ml should be given once or twice a day. This treatment is not suitable for children under 12 years. The product is also available in tablet form.

KAMILLOSAN

Use: This is an ointment for the treatment of nappy rash, containing lanolin and camomile extract.

Dose: The cream should be applied to clean dry skin at each nappy change.

KARVOL DECONGESTANT TABLETS

Use: Capsules for relieving the symptoms of colds and flu, containing various decongestant oils.

Dose: For babies over three months, children, adults and the elderly, the capsules contents should be squeezed onto a pillow or onto sheets and should be inhaled while sleeping. Adults can also squeeze a capsule into a bowl of hot water and inhale. For young children a capsule can be squeezed onto a handkerchief or clothing.

KLN

Use: A liquid remedy for stopping diarrhoea in children, containing kaolin.

Dose: Children should be given 5-10 ml, according to age, after every loose bowel movement for up to 24 hours. Check the label for the correct dosage. This treatment is not recommended for babies under six months.

KOLANTICON

Use: A liquid gel solution for relieving gastritis, indigestion and heartburn, containing antacid and an antispasmodic.
Dose: 10-20 ml should be taken every four hours. This treatment is not recommended for children under 12 years.

KWELLS

Use: Tablets for preventing travel sickness, containing hyoscine, an antispasmodic.
Dose: Adults should take one tablet every six hours. Take a maximum of three tablets in 24 hours. Children over 10 years should be given half the adult dose. This treatment is not recommended for children under 10 years. The product is also available as a children's version.

KY JELLY

Use: A lubricating gel for alleviating vaginal dryness.
Dose: A little of the gel should be applied to the vagina as required. The product is also available as pessaries.

LABITON

Use: A liquid remedy for alleviating general fatigue, containing alcohol, caffeine, vitamin B1 and dried extract of kola nut.
Dose: 10-20 ml should be taken twice a day. This treatment is not recommended for children under 12 years.

LABOSEPT PASTILLES

Use: Pastilles for relieving sore throats, containing dequalinium, an antibacterial.
Dose: One pastille should be sucked every 3-4 hours. Take a maximum of eight pastilles in 24 hours. This treatment is not recommended for children under 10 years.

LACITOL

Use: A powder remedy for the treatment of constipation, containing lactitol, an osmotic laxative.
Dose: Adults should take 1-2 sachets twice a day, either mixed in a cold

drink or sprinkled over food. A maximum of four sachets should be taken in a day. Children (6-12 years) should be given half to one sachet a day. Children (1-6 years) should be given one quarter to half a sachet per day. This treatment is not recommended for babies under the age of one year.

LACTO-CALAMINE LOTION

Use: A lotion for soothing sunburn, containing calamine and zinc oxide.
Dose: The lotion should be applied as required

LANACANE CREME

Use: A cream for relieving bites, stings and sunburn, containing a local anaesthetic.
Dose: The product should be applied to the affected area three times a day.

LANACORT CREME

Use: A cream for the treatment of eczema and dermatitis, containing hydrocortisone, a steroid.
Dose: The cream should be applied sparingly once or twice a day. This treatment is not recommended for children under 10 years. The product is also available as an ointment.

LASONIL

Use: An ointment for the treatment of bruises containing heparinoid, an ingredient that helps to resolve bruising.
Dose: The product should be applied two to three times a day to the affected area.

LAXOBERAL

Use: This is a liquid remedy for constipation, containing sodium picosulphate, a stimulant laxative.
Dose: 2.5-15 ml should be given at night, depending on age. This treatment is not recommended for children under two years.

LEMSIP BREATHE EASY

Use: Sachets of powder for relieving the symptoms of colds and flu,

containing paracetamol, phenylephrine, a decongestant, and vitamin C.
Dose: One sachet should be dissolved in hot water every four hours or as required. Take a maximum of four sachets in 24 hours. This treatment is not recommended for children under 12 years.

LEMSIP CHESTY COUGH

Use: A liquid remedy for the treatment of coughs, containing guaiphenesin.
Dose: Adults should take 10-20 ml three to four times a day. Children (2-12 years) should be given 5-10 ml, according to age. Read the label for the correct dosage. This treatment is not recommended for children under two years.

LEMSIP COMBINED RELIEF CAPSULES

Use: Capsules for relieving the symptoms of colds and flu, containing paracetamol, phenylephrine, a decongestant, and caffeine.
Dose: Two capsules should be taken every 3-4 hours. Take a maximum of eight capsules in 24 hours. This treatment is not recommended for children under 12 years.

LEMSIP DRY COUGH

Use: A liquid remedy for relieving coughs, containing honey, lemon oil, glycerol and citric acid.
Dose: Adults should take 10 ml 3-4 times a day. Children under 12 years should be given 5 ml 3-4 times a day. Read the label for the correct dosage.

LEMSIP MAXIMUM STRENGTH

Use: A lemon flavoured powder in sachets, for relieving the symptoms of colds and flu. Each sachet contains paracetamol, phenylephrine, a decongestant, and vitamin C.
Dose: One sachet should be dissolved in hot water every 4-6 hours or as required. Take a maximum of four sachets in 24 hours. This treatment is not recommended for children under 12 years.

LEMSIP ORIGINAL

Use: A lemon flavoured powder for relieving the symptoms of colds and flu, containing paracetamol, phenylephrine, a decongestant and vitamin C.

Dose: One sachet should be dissolved in hot water every four hours or as required. Take a maximum of four sachets in 24 hours. This treatment is not recommended for children under 12 years.

LEMSIP PHARMACY POWDER + PARACETAMOL

Use: A lemon flavoured powder in sachets for relieving the symptoms of colds and flu. Each sachet contains paracetamol, pseudoephedrine, a decongestant, and vitamin C.

Dose: One sachet should be dissolved in hot water every four hours if required. Take a maximum of four sachets in 24 hours. This treatment is not recommended for children under 12 years.

LEMSIP PHARMACY POWER CAPS

Use: Capsules for relieving the symptoms of colds and flu, containing ibuprofen and pseudoephedrine, a decongestant.

Dose: Two capsules should be taken every four hours. Take a maximum of four capsules in 24 hours. This treatment is not recommended for children under 12 years.

LENIUM

Use: A medicated shampoo for the treatment of dandruff, containing selenium sulphide.

Dose: Should be used as a shampoo twice a week until the dandruff clears, then used as required. This treatment is not recommended for children under five years.

LIQUFRUTA GARLIC

Use: A liquid remedy for the treatment of coughs, containing guaiphenesin, an expectorant.

Dose: Adults should take 10-15 ml three times a day and at bedtime. Children (3-12 years) should be given 10 ml. Children (1-3 years) should be given 5 ml. This treatment is not recommended for children under one year.

LLOYDS CREAM

Use: A cream rub for the treatment of muscular aches and pains. It contains a rubefacient and a salicylate, an aspirin derivative.

Dose: The cream should be applied to the affected area up to three times a day. This treatment is not recommended for children under six years.

LYCLEAR CREME RINSE

Use: A lotion treatment containing permethrin for head lice and other similar infestations.

Dose: The lotion should be massaged into the hair and scalp after shampooing, then left for 10 minutes and washed out. The hair should be combed through while still wet. This treatment is not recommended for babies under six months.

LYPSYL COLD SORE GEL

Use: This is a gel for the treatment of cold sores. It contains lignocaine, a local anaesthetic, cetrimide, an antiseptic, and zinc sulphate, an astringent.

Dose: The cream should be applied to the cold sore 3-4 times a day.

MAALOX PLUS SUSPENSION

Use: A liquid remedy for relieving indigestion, heartburn and trapped wind. It contains an antacid and simethicone, an antiflatulent.

Dose: 5-10 ml should be taken four times a day after meals, and at bedtime. This treatment is not recommended for children under 12 years. The product is also available in tablet form.

MAALOX SUSPENSION

Use: A liquid for relieving indigestion and heartburn, containing antacids.

Dose: 10-20 ml should be taken four times a day 20-60 minutes after meals, and on retiring for the night. This treatment is not recommended for children under 12 years.

MACKENZIES SMELLING SALTS

Use: Liquid smelling salts for easing nasal congestion, containing ammonia with eucalyptus oil.

Dose: The vapour should be inhaled as required. This treatment is not recommended for babies under three months.

MACLEAN

Use: Antacid tablets for relieving indigestion and heartburn.

Dose: 1-2 tablets should be sucked or chewed as required. Take a maximum of 16 tablets in 24 hours. This treatment is not recommended for children under 12 years.

MAGNESIUM SULPHATE PASTE BP

Use: This is a non-brand name paste for 'drawing out' boils. It contains magnesium sulphate, phenol and glycerol.

Dose: The paste should be stirred and then applied to the boil. The area should then be covered with a clean, dry dressing.

MANEVAC

Use: A granular remedy for relieving constipation, containing fibre and senna, a stimulant laxative.

Dose: The granules should be placed on the tongue and swallowed with plenty of water, without chewing. Adults should take 5-10 ml once or twice a day. Children (5-12 years) should be given 5 ml once a day. Pregnant women should take 5-10 ml every morning and evening. This treatment is not recommended for children under five years.

MASNODERM

Use: A cream treatment for athlete's foot, containing the antifungal ingredient, clotrimazole.

Dose: The cream should be applied to the affected area twice a day for four weeks.

MAXIMUM STRENGTH ASPRO CLEAR

Use: An effervescent analgesic tablet for general pain relief, containing 500 mg of aspirin.

Dose: 1-2 tablets should be dissolved in water every four hours. Take a maximum of eight tablets in 24 hours. This treatment is not recommended for children under 12 years.

MEDIJEL

Use: A gel for the treatment of sore gums, bad breath and mouth ulcers, containing lidocaine, a local anaesthetic.

Dose: The gel should be applied every 20 minutes or as necessary.

MEDINOL OVER 6 PARACETAMOL ORAL SUSPENSION

Use: A strawberry flavoured analgesic liquid for general pain relief, which is sugar- and colour-free. It contains 250 mg of paracetamol in every 5 ml.

Dose: Take a maximum of four doses in 24 hours. Children (6-12 years) should be given 5-10 ml every four hours if required. For children under six years, use Medinol Under 6.

MEDINOL UNDER 6 PARACETAMOL ORAL SUSPENSION

Use: A strawberry flavoured analgesic liquid for general pain relief, which is sugar- and colour-free. It contains 120 mg of paracetamol in every 5 ml.

Dose: Take a maximum of four doses in 24 hours. Babies (3-12 months) should be given 2.5-5 ml every four hours if required. Children (1-5 years) should be given 10 ml every four hours. Children over five years should be given 15-20 ml. This treatment is not recommended for babies under three months unless advised otherwise by a doctor.

MEDISED

Use: A blackcurrant flavoured analgesic liquid for general pain relief, containing 120 mg of paracetamol in every 5 ml, and promethazine hydrochloride, an antihistamine.

Dose: Take a maximum of four doses in 24 hours. Children (1-6 years) should be given 10 ml every four hours if required. Children (6-12 years) should be given 20 ml every four hours. This treatment is not recommended for babies under one year. The product is also available in sugar- and colour-free versions.

MELTUS COUGH ELIXIR - See under Adult Meltus Cough Elixir

MENTHOLAIR

Use: An aromatic bath vapour for relieving sinusitis congestion, containing aromatic decongestants.

Dose: One measure should be added to bath water.

MENTHOLATUM

Use: An ointment for the treatment of muscular aches and pains, containing rubefacients and a salicylate, an aspirin derivative.

Dose: The product should be applied to the affected area 2-3 times a day. This treatment is not recommended for children under one year.

MEROCAINE LOZENGES

Use: Lozenges for relieving sore throats, containing cetylypridium, an antibacterial and benzocaine, an anaesthetic.

Dose: One lozenge should be dissolved in the mouth every two hours. Take a maximum of eight pastilles in 24 hours. This treatment is not recommended for children under 12 years.

MEROCETS LOZENGES

Use: Lozenges for relieving sore throats, containing cetylp yearidium, an antibacterial.

Dose: One lozenge should be dissolved in the mouth every three hours or as required. This treatment is not recommended for children under six years. The product is also available as a mouthwash.

MEROTHOL LOZENGES

Use: Lozenges for relieving sore throats, containing cetylp yearidium, an antibacterial with menthol and eucalyptus.

Dose: One lozenge should be dissolved in the mouth every three hours or as required. This treatment is not recommended for children under the age of six years.

METANIUM OINTMENT

Use: An ointment for relieving nappy rash, containing titanium salts, and an astringent.

Dose: The ointment should be applied to clean dry skin at each nappy change.

METATONE

Use: A liquid remedy for alleviating fatigue, containing calcium, potassium, sodium, manganese and vitamin B1.

Dose: Adults should take 5-10 ml 2-3 times a day. Children (6-12 years) should be given 5 ml two to three times a day. This treatment is not recommended for children under six years.

METED SHAMPOO
Use: A medicated shampoo for the treatment of dandruff, containing salicylic acid.
Dose: Should be used as a shampoo twice a week.

MIGRALEVE 1 (PINK)
Use: Pink tablets for relieving migraines that are accompanied by nausea and vomiting. The tablets contain 500 mg of paracetamol, 8 mg of codeine phosphate and 6.25 mg of buclizine hydrochloride, a sedative antihistamine.
Dose: Adults should take two tablets as soon as an attack is about to start. Take a maximum of two tablets in 24 hours. Children (10-14 years) should be given no more than one tablet in 24 hours. This treatment is not recommended for children under 10 years.

MIGRALEVE 2 (YELLOW)
Use: Yellow tablets that can be taken in the later stages of a migraine attack after Migraleve 1 has been taken. They contain 500 mg of paracetamol and 8 mg of codeine phosphate.
Dose: Adults should take two tablets every four hours. Take a maximum of six tablets in 24 hours. Children (10-14 years) should be given one tablet every four hours, with a maximum of three tablets in 24 hours. This treatment is not suitable for children under 10 years.

MIGRALEVE DUO
Use: Pink and yellow tablets for a complete migraine attack. The pink tablet contains 500 mg of paracetamol, 8 mg of codeine phosphate and 6.25mg of buclizine hydrochloride (a sedative antihistamine). The yellow tablet contains 500 mg of paracetamol and 8 mg of codeine phosphate.
Dose: Adults should take two pink tablets at the beginning of an attack. If required later, two yellow tablets should be taken every four hours. Take a maximum of two pink and six yellow tablets in 24 hours. Children (10-14 years) should be given one pink tablet at the beginning

of an attack. If required later, one yellow tablet can be given every four hours, with no more than one pink tablet and three yellow tablets in 24 hours. This treatment is not recommended for children under the age of 10 years.

MILK OF MAGNESIA

Use: A liquid remedy for relieving indigestion, heartburn, upset stomachs and constipation. It contains magnesium hydroxide, an osmotic laxative.
Dose: Adults should take 30-45 ml on retiring. Children over three years should be given 5-10 ml at bedtime. This treatment is not recommended for children under three years.

MIL-PAR

Use: A liquid remedy for easing constipation, containing magnesium sulphate, an osmotic laxative, and liquid paraffin, which helps to soften the stools.
Dose: Adults should take 15-30 ml a day. Children over three years should be given 5-15 ml a day, depending on age. Read the label for the correct dosage. This treatment is not recommended for children under three years of age.

MINADEX TONIC

Use: A liquid treatment for alleviating fatigue, containing the vitamins A and D3, calcium, copper, iron, magnesium and potassium.
Dose: Adults should take 10 ml, three times a day. Children (3-12 years) should be given 5 mls, three times a day. Children (6 months-3 years) should be given 5 ml twice a day. This treatment is not recommended for children under six years.

MINTEC

Use: These are capsules for the treatment of irritable bowel syndrome, containing peppermint oil, which can help to calm intestinal spasms.
Dose: One capsule should be taken three times a day just before a meal, swallowed whole to prevent the peppermint oil irritating the throat. This treatment is not recommended for children under 12 years.

MOLCER EAR DROPS

Use: Ear drops containing softening ingredients for the removal of earwax.

Dose: The ear should be filled with the drops and plugged with cotton wool. The treatment should be repeated for two nights, and then clear out the ear.

MONPHYTOL PAINT

Use: This is a liquid treatment for athlete's foot, containing a mixture of antifungals.

Dose: The liquid should be applied to the affected area twice a day. The treatment should be repeated until the infection has cleared.

MOORLAND

Use: Antacid tablets for relieving indigestion and heartburn.

Dose: Two tablets should be dissolved in the mouth as required, after meals and at bedtime. This treatment is not recommended for children under six years.

MORHULIN OINTMENT

Use: An emollient ointment relieving the discomfort of eczema, dermatitis and nappy rash, containing cod liver oil and zinc oxide, an astringent and an antiseptic.

Dose: The ointment should be applied to the affected area thinly. For nappy rash, apply after washing and drying baby's bottom.

MOTILIUM 10

Use: Tablets for easing digestive discomfort, containing domperidone, an ingredient to help speed up the digestive system.

Dose: One tablet should be taken three times a day and at night if required. This treatment is not recommended for children under 16 years.

MOVELAT RELIEF CREAM

Use: A cream for the treatment of muscular aches and pains, containing salicylic acid, an aspirin derivative, and an ingredient for reducing swelling.

Dose: The product should be applied to the affected area up to four times a day. This treatment is not recommended for children under 12 years. The product is also available as a gel.

MU-CRON

Use: A tablet for easing the congestion of colds and catarrh, containing paracetamol and phenylpropanolamine, a decongestant.

Dose: One tablet can be taken up to four times a day, allowing four hours between doses. Take a maximum of four tablets in 24 hours. This treatment is not recommended for children under 12 years.

MYCIL ATHLETE'S FOOT SPRAY

Use: This is a powder in a spray form for the treatment of athlete's foot. It contains tolnaftate, an antifungal ingredient.

Dose: The product should be applied morning and evening until the symptoms clear, and continued for a further seven days.

MYCIL GOLD CLOTRIMAZOLE

Use: A cream treatment for athlete's foot, containing the antifungal ingredient, clotrimazole.

Dose: The cream should be applied thinly to clean, dry feet, two to three times a day for up to one month.

MYCIL OINTMENT

Use: This is an ointment treatment for athlete's foot, containing the antifungal ingredient tolnaftate.

Dose: The product should be applied to the affected part morning and evening and continued for a further seven days once the infection has cleared.

MYCIL POWDER

Use: This is a powder treatment for athlete's foot, containing the antifungal ingredient tolnaftate.

Dose: The powder should be sprinkled over the affected area morning and evening. Treatment should be continued for a further seven days after the infection has cleared.

MYCOTA CREAM

Use: This is a cream treatment for athlete's foot, containing undecenoic acid, an antifungal ingredient.

Dose: Apply the cream to clean, dry skin. The treatment should be continued for a further seven days after the infection has cleared.

MYCOTA POWDER

Use: This is a powder for the treatment of athlete's foot. It contains undecenoic acid and zinc undecenoate, both antifungal ingredients.

Dose: Sprinkle the powder over the affected area morning and evening. The treatment should be continued for a further seven days after the infection has cleared up. This product is also available in spray form.

NASCIODINE

Use: A cream treatment for relieving muscular aches and pains, containing rubefacients and a salicylate, an aspirin derivative.

Dose: The cream should be massaged into the affected area 2-3 times a day. This treatment is not recommended for children under six years.

NASOBEC HAYFEVER

Use: A nasal spray for easing hayfever symptoms. The spray contains beclomethasone, a corticosteroid.

Dose: Two sprays should be directed into each nostril, with a maximum of eight sprays in 24 hours. This treatment is not recommended for children under 12 years.

NEO BABY CREAM

Use: A cream for the treatment of nappy rash, containing cetrimide and benzalkonium, both antiseptics.

Dose: The product should be applied to clean dry skin as required.

NEO BABY MIXTURE

Use: A liquid remedy for relieving infant wind and colic, containing sodium bicarbonate, an antacid, dill oil and ginger.

Dose: 2.5-15 ml, three times a day, according to age. Check the label for the correct dosage.

NERICUR

Use: A gel available in two strengths for the treatment of spots and acne, containing benzoyl peroxide.

Dose: The gel should be applied once a day to clean dry skin. Use the lower strength version first and progress to the stronger version if necessary. This treatment is not recommended for children under the age of 15.

NICORETTE

Use: A treatment for nicotine dependence (for those who smoke less than 20 cigarettes a day) in the form of chewing gum, containing 2 mg of nicotine per gum piece.

Dose: One piece of gum should be chewed for 30 minutes. Take a maximum of 15 pieces in 24 hours. After three months the dosage should be reduced. Nicorette Plus is also available, containing 4 mg of nicotine per piece of gum.

NICORETTE INHALER

Use: These are inhalable cartridges for nicotine dependence (for those who smoke more than 20 cigarettes a day). One cartridge contains 10 mg of nicotine.

Dose: The cartridge should be fixed into the inhaler and sucked when an urge to have a cigarette arises. Use a minimum of 12 cartridges in 24 hours. The amount should be reduced over three months.

NICORETTE PATCH

Use: This is a skin patch for treating nicotine dependence.

Dose: These patches are available in 5 mg, 10 mg and 15 mg strengths. One patch should be applied to the arm on waking and removed 16 hours later. The dose should be reduced gradually by using lower dosage patches.

NICOTINELL CHEWING GUM

Use: This is a chewing gum for treating nicotine dependence. Each piece of gum contains 2 mg of nicotine.

Dose: 8-12 pieces of gum should be chewed a day. Take a maximum of 25 pieces in 24 hours. The number of pieces of gum should be reduced gradually over a three- month period. The product is also available in 4 mg pieces.

NICOTINELL TTS (PATCH)
Use: This is a skin patch treatment for reducing nicotine dependence.
Dose: There are three strength doses available according to cigarette consumption. The dosage should be reduced gradually over a three-month period.

NIGHT NURSE
Use: A liquid remedy for easing cold and flu symptoms at night, containing paracetamol, promethazine, an antihistamine and dextromethorphan, a cough suppressant.
Dose: Adults should take 20 ml just before retiring. Children (6-12 years) should be given 10 ml just before retiring. This treatment is not recommended for children under six years.

NIZORAL DANDRUFF SHAMPOO
Use: A medicated shampoo for the treatment of dandruff, containing ketoconazole.
Dose: Should be used as a shampoo, left in for 2-3 minutes and then rinsed out. It should be used twice a week for 2-4 weeks, reducing use to once every 1-2 weeks as a preventive measure.

NOXACORN
Use: A liquid for the treatment of corns and calluses, containing salicylic acid.
Dose: The liquid should be applied every night to the affected area, for 3-6 nights. This treatment is not recommended for children under six years.

NULACIN TABLETS
Use: Antacid tablets for relieving indigestion, heartburn and general digestive discomfort.

Dose: One tablet should be sucked slowly as required. Take a maximum of eight tablets in 24 hours. This treatment is not recommended for children under 12 years.

NUPERCAINAL

Use: An ointment treatment for piles, containing cinchocaine, a mild local anaesthetic.

Dose: The ointment should be applied sparingly to the affected area up to three times a day. This treatment is not recommended for children under 12 years.

NUROFEN

Use: Analgesic tablets for pain relief, containing 200 mg of ibuprofen.

Dose: Two tablets should be taken initially, and a further 1-2 tablets every four hours if required. Take a maximum of six tablets in 24 hours. This treatment is not recommended for children under 12 years.

NUROFEN ADVANCE

Use: Analgesic tablets for general pain relief, containing 200 mg of ibuprofen.

Dose: Two tablets should be taken initially, and a further 1-2 tablets every 4-6 hours if required. Take a maximum of six tablets in 24 hrs. This treatment is not recommended for children under 12 years.

NUROFEN COLD AND FLU

Use: These are tablets for relieving the symptoms of cold and flu. Each tablet contains ibuprofen and pseudoephedrine, a decongestant.

Dose: Two tablets should be taken initially, followed by 1-2 tablets every four hours if required. Take a maximum of six tablets in 24 hours. This treatment is not recommended for children under 12 years.

NUROFEN FOR CHILDREN

Use: An orange flavoured analgesic liquid for general pain relief, which is sugar- and colour-free, containing 100 mg of ibuprofen in every 5 ml.

Dose: Take a maximum of four doses in 24 hours. Babies (6-12 months) should be given 2.5 ml up to three times in 24 hours. Babies (1-2 years) should be given 2.5 ml every four hours if required. Children (3-7 years) should be given 5 ml every four hours. Children (8-12 years) should be given 10 ml every four hours. This treatment is not recommended for babies under six months.

NUROFEN 400

Use: Analgesic tablets for general pain relief, containing 400 mg of ibuprofen.
Dose: One tablet should be taken initially, followed by one tablet every four hours if required. Take a maximum of three tablets in 24 hours. This treatment is not recommended for children under 12 years.

NUROFEN MICRO-GRANULES

Use: Effervescent analgesic granules for general pain relief. Each sachet contains 400 mg of ibuprofen.
Dose: One sachet should be dissolved in water and a further sachet can be taken every four hours if required. Take a maximum of three sachets in 24 hours. This treatment is not recommended for children under 12 years.

NUROFEN PLUS

Use: Analgesic tablets for general pain relief containing 200mg of ibuprofen and 12.5 mg of codeine phosphate.
Dose: Two tablets should be taken initially, and then 1-2 tablets every 4-6 hours if required. Take a maximum of six tablets in 24 hours. This treatment is not recommended for children under 12 years.

NURSE HARVEY'S GRIPE MIXTURE

Use: A liquid remedy for relieving infant colic and wind, containing sodium bicarbonate, an antacid, and dill oil and caraway oil.
Dose: 5-10 ml should be given according to age, after or during feeds. Give a maximum of six doses in 24 hours. This treatment is not recommended for babies under one month.

NURSE SYKES BRONCHIAL BALSAM

Use: A liquid remedy for relieving coughs, containing guaiphenesin, an expectorant.
Dose: 5-10 ml should be taken every four hours and at bedtime. This treatment is not recommended for children under 12 years.

NURSE SYKES POWDERS

Use: An analgesic powder for general pain relief, containing 165.3 mg of aspirin, 120 mg of paracetamol, and caffeine.

Dose: One powder should be dissolved in water and taken every four hours. Take a maximum of six powders in 24 hours. This treatment is not recommended for children under 12 years.

NYLAX

Use: A constipation remedy in the form of tablets. Each tablet contains senna, which is a stimulant laxative.

Dose: Adults should take two tablets on retiring. Children (5-12 years) should be given one tablet at bedtime. This treatment is not recommended for children under five years.

NYTOL

Use: A tablet remedy for insomnia, containing diphenhydramine, an antihistamine.

Dose: Two tablets should be taken 20 minutes before retiring. This treatment is not recommended for children under 16 years.

OCCLUSAL

Use: A liquid treatment for the removal of warts and verrucae, containing salicylic acid.

Dose: The product should be applied to the wart or verruca and allowed to dry. The treatment should be repeated daily. This treatment is not recommended for children under six years, unless advised otherwise by a doctor.

OILATUM EMOLLIENT

Use: An emollient liquid for the treatment of eczema and dermatitis, containing various oils.

Dose: The liquid can be added to the bath water, or applied to the skin directly and rinsed off afterwards. The product is also available as shower gel and hand gel.

OILATUM JUNIOR FLARE UP

Use: An emollient liquid for treating the discomfort of eczema and dermatitis in children, containing a mixture of oils and antiseptics.

Dose: The liquid should be added to bath water.

OILATUM PLUS

Use: An emollient liquid for relieving the discomfort of skin disorders such as eczema and dermatitis, containing a mixture of oils and antiseptics.

Dose: The liquid should be added to bath water.

OPAS

Use: Antacid tablets for easing indigestion and heartburn, containing sodium.

Dose: 1-2 tablets should be taken after each meal, or as required. This treatment is not recommended for children under 12 years.

OPAZIMES

Use: Tablets to help stop diarrhoea, containing kaolin, morphine and belladonna.

Dose: Adults should chew or suck two tablets every four hours, with a maximum of eight tablets in 24 hours. Children over six years should chew or suck one tablet every four hours, with a maximum of four tablets in 24 hours. This treatment is not recommended for children under six years.

OPTICROM ALLERGY EYE DROPS

Use: Eye drops for relieving itchy eyes caused by hayfever, containing sodium cromoglycate, an anti-inflammatory.

Dose: 1-2 drops should be applied to each eye four times a day. This treatment is not recommended for children under five years.

OPTREX HAYFEVER ALLERGY EYE DROPS

Use: Eye drops for relieving itchy eyes caused by hayfever, containing sodium cromoglycate, an anti-inflammatory.

Dose: 1-2 drops should be applied to each eye four times a day. This treatment is not recommended for children under five years.

ORALDENE

Use: This is a mouthwash for the treatment of mouth infections, sore gums and bad breath. It contains hexetidine, an anti-microbial.

Dose: 15 ml of the mouthwash should be rinsed or gargled 2-3 times a day. The product should not be diluted or swallowed. This treatment is not recommended for children under 5 years.

ORUVAIL

Use: This is a gel for the treatment of muscular aches and pains, containing ketoprofen, a non-steroidal anti-inflammatory (NSAID).

Dose: The gel should be massaged into the affected area three times a day. This treatment is not recommended for children under 12 years.

OTEX EAR DROPS

Use: Ear drops for the removal of earwax, containing softening ingredients.

Dose: 5 drops of the liquid should be put into the ear once or twice a day, for 3-4 days until the wax loosens.

OTRIVINE-ANTISTIN

Use: Eye drops for hayfever sufferers, containing xylometazeline, a decongestant and antazoline, a topical antihistamine.

Dose: Adults should take 1-2 drops into the affected eye/s, 2-3 times a day. Children over five years should be given one drop 2-3 times a day. This treatment is not recommended for children under five years.

OVEX TABLETS

Use: Tablets for the treatment of intestinal worms, containing mebendazole, an anti-worm ingredient.

Dose: For threadworms one dose of one tablet should be taken. This should be repeated after two weeks if the infestation is still present. Treatment is not recommended for children under two years.

OXY 5

Use: This is a lotion for the treatment of spots and acne, containing benzoyl peroxide.

Dose: The lotion should be applied once a day for one week. If no irritation occurs, it can be applied twice a day. The lower dose should be used first, progressing to the stronger version if required - Oxy 10. This treatment is not recommended for children under 15 years.

PACIFENE
Use: Analgesic tablets for general pain relief, containing 200 mg of ibuprofen.
Dose: 1-2 tablets should be taken three times a day. Take a maximum of six tablets in 24 hours. This treatment is not recommended for children under 12 years.

PACIFENE MAXIMUM STRENGTH
Use: Analgesic tablets for general pain relief, containing 400 mg of ibuprofen.
Dose: One tablet should be taken every four hours. Take a maximum of three tablets in 24 hours. This treatment is not recommended for children under 12 years.

PANADEINE
Use: Analgesic tablets for general pain relief, containing 500 mg of paracetamol and 8mg of codeine phosphate.
Dose: Adults should take two tablets up to four times a day. Take a maximum of eight tablets in 24 hours. Children (7-12 years) should be given half to one tablet every four hours. A maximum of four tablets should be taken in 24 hours. This treatment is not recommended for children under seven years.

PANADOL
Use: Analgesic tablets for general pain relief, containing 500mg of paracetamol.
Dose: Adults should take two tablets every four hours. Take a maximum of eight tablets in 24 hours. Children (6-12 years) should be given half to one tablet every four hours, with a maximum of four tablets in 24 hours. This treatment is not recommended for children under six years.

PANADOL CAPSULES

Use: Analgesic capsules for general pain relief, containing 500 mg of paracetamol.

Dose: Two capsules should be taken every four hours if required. Take a maximum of eight capsules in 24 hours. This treatment is not recommended for children under 12 years.

PANADOL EXTRA

Use: Analgesic tablets for general pain relief containing 500 mg of paracetamol, and caffeine.

Dose: Two tablets can be taken every four hours if required. Take a maximum of eight tablets in 24 hours. This treatment is not recommended for children under 12 years.

PANADOL EXTRA SOLUBLE

Use: Effervescent analgesic tablets for general pain relief, containing 500 mg of paracetamol, and caffeine.

Dose: Two tablets should be dissolved in water every four hours if required. Take a maximum of eight tablets in 24 hours. This treatment is not recommended for children under 12 years.

PANADOL NIGHT

Use: Analgesic capsules for general pain relief, containing 500 mg of paracetamol, and diphendydramine, an antihistamine.

Dose: Two tablets should be taken 20 minutes before retiring. This treatment is not recommended for children under 12 years.

PANADOL SOLUBLE

Use: An effervescent tablet for general pain relief, containing 500mg of paracetamol.

Dose: Adults should take two tablets dissolved in water every four hours if required. Take a maximum of eight tablets in 24 hours. Children (6-12 years) should be given half to one tablet dissolved in water every four hours if required, with a maximum of four tablets in 24 hours. This treatment is not recommended for children under six years.

PANADOL ULTRA

Use: Analgesic tablets for general pain relief, containing 500 mg of paracetamol and 12.8mg of codeine phosphate.

Dose: Two tablets should be taken up to four times a day if required. Take a maximum of four tablets in 24 hours. This treatment is not recommended for children under 12 years.

PANOXYL ACNEGEL

Use: This is a gel for the treatment of acne and spots available in two strengths, containing benzoyl peroxide.

Dose: The product should be applied to clean skin once a day, using the lower strength version first and then progressing to the higher strength version if necessary. This treatment is not recommended for children under 15 years.

PANOXYL AQUAGEL

Use: This is a gel available in three strengths for the treatment of acne and spots.

Dose: The product should be applied to clean skin once a day using the lower strength first, then progressing to the stronger version if required. This treatment is not recommended for children under 15 years.

PANOXYL 5 CREAM

Use: A cream for the treatment of acne and spots, containing benzoyl peroxide.

Dose: The product should be applied to clean skin once a day. This treatment is not recommended for children under 15 years.

PANOXYL LOTION

Use: This is a lotion for the treatment of acne and spots, available in two strengths. It contains benzoyl peroxide.

Dose: The product should be applied to clean skin once a day, using the lower dose first, then progressing to the higher strength version if required. This treatment is not recommended for children under 15 years.

PANOXYL WASH

Use: This is a wash for the treatment of acne and spots, containing benzoyl peroxide.

Dose: The wash should be applied to wet skin, rinsed with alternate warm and cold water and patted dry. Use once a day in the morning. This treatment is not recommended for children under 15 years.

PAPULEX

Use: This is a gel for the treatment of spots and acne, containing nicotinamide, an anti-inflammatory.

Dose: The gel should be applied twice a day after washing. This should be reduced to once every other day if there is an adverse skin reaction. This treatment is not recommended for children under 15 years.

PARACETS

Use: Analgesic tablets for general pain relief, containing 500 mg of paracetamol.

Dose: Adults should take two tablets up to four times a day if required. Take a maximum of eight tablets in 24 hours. Children (6-12 years) should be given half to one tablet up to four times a day, with a maximum of four tablets in 24 hours. This treatment is not recommended for children under six years.

PARACETS CAPSULES

Use: Analgesic capsules for general pain relief, containing 500 mg of paracetamol.

Dose: Adults should take 1-2 capsules every six hours. Take a maximum of eight capsules in 24 hours. Children (6-12 years) should be given one capsule every six hours. This treatment is not recommended for children under six years.

PARACLEAR

Use: Effervescent analgesic tablets for general pain relief, containing 500 mg of paracetamol.

Dose: Adults should take 1-2 tablets dissolved in water every four hours. Take a maximum of eight tablets in 24 hours. Children (6-12 years) should be given one tablet every four hours. Take a maximum of four tablets in 24 hours. This treatment is not recommended for children under six years.

PARACLEAR EXTRA STRENGTH

Use: Analgesic tablets for general pain relief, containing 500 mg of paracetamol, and caffeine.

Dose: 1-2 tablets should be taken every 4-6 hours. Take a maximum of eight tablets in 24 hours. This treatment is not recommended for children under 12 years.

PARACODOL

Use: Analgesic capsules for general pain relief, containing 500 mg of paracetamol and 8 mg of codeine phosphate.

Dose: 1-2 capsules should be taken every four to six hours. Take a maximum of eight capsules in 24 hours. This treatment is not recommended for children under 12 years. The product is also available in soluble tablet form.

PARAMOL

Use: Analgesic tablets for general pain relief, containing 500 mg of paracetamol and 7.46 mg dihydrocodeine tartrate.

Dose: 1-2 tablets should be taken during or after meals, every four to six hours as required. Take a maximum of eight tablets in 24 hours. This treatment is not recommended for children under 12 years.

PAVADOL D

Use: A sugar-free liquid remedy for relieving coughs, containing pholcodine, a cough suppressant.

Dose: Adults should take 5-10 ml four times a day if required. Children (1-12 years) should be given 2.5-5 ml three to five times a day according to age. Read the label for the correct dosage. This treatment is not suitable for children under one year.

PAXIDORM TABLETS

Use: Tablets for insomnia, containing diphenhydramine, an antihistamine.

Dose: 1-2 tablets should be taken just before retiring. This treatment is not recommended for children under 16 years.

PENTRAX

Use: A medicated shampoo for the treatment of dandruff, containing coal tar.
Dose: The treatment should be used as an ordinary shampoo twice a week.

PEPCID AC

Use: Tablets for relieving general stomach discomfort, indigestion and heartburn, containing famotidine, a histamine H2 antagonist that helps reduce stomach acid.
Dose: One tablet should be taken one hour before eating. Take a maximum of two tablets in 24 hours. This treatment is not recommended for children under 16 years, and should not be taken for more than two weeks.

PEPTO-BISMOL

Use: A liquid remedy for relieving indigestion, heartburn and general stomach discomfort. The liquid contains bismuth, an ingredient to coat the stomach lining.
Dose: Adults should take 30 ml every 30 minutes to one hour. Children (10-14 years) should be given 20 ml every 30 minutes to one hour. Children (6-10 years) should be given 10 ml every 30 minutes to one hour. Children (3-6 years), Up to eight doses in 24 hours. This treatment is not recommended for children under three years.

PERVARYL

Use: This is a cream for the treatment of athlete's foot, containing econazole, an antifungal ingredient.
Dose: The cream should be applied twice a day for as long as it is needed. This product is also available in lotion and powder forms.

PHENERGAN

Use: Tablets for preventing travel sickness, containing promethazine, an antihistamine. The tablets are available in two strengths, 10 mg and 25 mg.
Dose: Adults and children over 10 years should take 1-2 10 mg tablets,

or one 25 mg tablet, the night before the journey. The dose should be repeated after six to eight hours if necessary. Children (5-10 years) should be given one 10 mg tablet the night before the journey, and then again 6-8 hours later if necessary. The 25 mg tablets are not suitable for children under 10 years. A liquid version is available for younger children (2-5 years). This treatment is not recommended for children under two years.

PHENERGAN NIGHTIME
Use: A tablet remedy for insomnia, containing promethazine, an antihistamine.
Dose: Two tablets should be taken at night. This treatment is not recommended for children under 16 years.

PHENSEDYL PLUS LINCTUS
Use: A liquid remedy for the treatment of coughs, containing promethazine, an antihistamine, pholcodine, a cough suppressant and pseudoephedrine, a decongestant.
Dose: 5-10 ml should be taken 3-4 times a day. This treatment is not recommended for children under 12 years.

PHENSIC
Use: Analgesic tablets for general pain relief, containing 325 mg of aspirin and 22 mg of caffeine.
Dose: Two tablets should be taken every 3-4 hours as required. Take a maximum of 12 tablets in 24 hours. This treatment is not recommended for children under 12 years.

PICKLE'S OINTMENT
Use: An ointment for the treatment of corns and calluses, containing salicylic acid.
Dose: The product should be applied to the affected area at night for four nights. The skin should be allowed to fall off before reapplying the ointment.

PIRITON ALLERGY TABLETS
Use: A tablet for relieving hayfever symptoms, containing chlorpheniramine, an antihistamine.

Dose: Adults should take one tablet every 4-6 hours, with a maximum of six tablets in 24 hours. Children (6-12 years) should be given half a tablet every 4-6 hours, with a maximum of three tablets in 24 hours. This treatment is not recommended for children under six years.

PIRITON SYRUP

Use: A liquid remedy for relieving hayfever symptoms, containing chlorpheniramine, an antihistamine.
Dose: Adults should take 10 ml every 4-6 hours. Children (1-12 years) should be given 2.5-5 ml, according to age. Read the label for the correct dosage. This treatment is not recommended for babies under one year.

PLACIDEX SYRUP

Use: An analgesic liquid for general pain relief, containing 120 mg of paracetamol in every 5 ml.
Dose: A maximum of four doses can be given in 24 hours. Babies (3-12 months) should be given 2.5-5 ml every four hours if required. This treatment is not recommended for babies under three months unless advised otherwise by a doctor.

POLYTAR AF

Use: A liquid for the treatment of dandruff, containing peanut oil, zinc pyithione and coal tar.
Dose: The liquid should be massaged into the hair and scalp and left in for 2-3 minutes before rinsing out. Use 2-3 times a week.

POLYTAR EMOLLIENT

Use: A medicated treatment for dandruff, containing coal tar and peanut oil.
Dose: 2-4 capfuls should be added into a shallow bath.

POLYTAR LIQUID

Use: A liquid treatment for dandruff, containing coal tar and peanut oil.
Dose: The lotion should be applied to wet hair, massaged into the scalp and rinsed out. This should be carried out twice. The lotion should be used once or twice a week.

POLYTAR PLUS

Use: A liquid treatment for dandruff, containing coal tar, peanut oil and a hair conditioner.

Dose: The lotion should be applied to wet hair, massaged into the scalp and rinsed out. This should be carried out twice. The lotion should be used one to two times a week.

PREPARATION H OINTMENT

Use: An ointment for the treatment of piles, containing shark oil, a skin protectant.

Dose: The ointment should be applied morning and evening and after each bowel movement. This treatment is not recommended for children under 12 years. The product is also available in suppository form.

PR FREEZE SPRAY

Use: A spray for relieving muscular pain, containing cooling ingredients.

Dose: The spray should be applied to the affected area up to three times a day. This treatment is not recommended for children under six years.

PR HEAT SPRAY

Use: A spray for the treatment of muscular aches and pains, containing rubefacients and a salicylate, an aspirin derivative.

Dose: The product should be applied to the affected area twice a day. This treatment is not recommended for children under five years.

PRIODERM CREAM SHAMPOO

Use: A shampoo for the treatment of head lice, containing malathion.

Dose: The treatment should be shampooed into the hair and left for five minutes, then rinsed out. This should be carried out twice. Repeat this twice more at three-day intervals. The lotion can be also used for treating pubic lice. This treatment is not recommended for babies under six months.

PRIODERM LOTION

Use: A lotion for the treatment of lice and scabies, containing malathion and alcohol.

Dose: For head or pubic lice, the lotion should be applied to the affected area and left to dry for at least two hours, but preferably for 12 hours if possible. The treatment should then be washed off and the hair combed out while still wet. For scabies the lotion should be applied to the whole body and left on for 24 hours before washing off. This treatment is not recommended for babies under six months.

PRIPSEN MEBENDAZOLE TABLETS

Use: Tablets for removing intestinal worms, containing mebendazole, an anti-worm ingredient.

Dose: For threadworms one dose of one tablet should be taken. This can be repeated after two weeks if the infestation is still present. This treatment is not recommended for children under two years.

PRIPSEN PIPERAZINE CITRATE ELIXIR

Use: A liquid remedy for the removal of intestinal worms, containing piperazine citrate, an anti-worm ingredient.

Dose: For threadworms, adults should take 15 ml a day for seven days. This can be repeated after a seven-day interval if required. Children should be given 5-10 ml a day, depending on age, for seven days. The treatment should be repeated for a further seven days after a seven-day interval.

For roundworms, adults should take one single 30 ml dose, and then another 30 ml dose after 14 days. Children should be given 10-25 ml dose, according to age, and then another dose after 14 days. This treatment is not recommended for babies under one year unless advised otherwise by a doctor.

PRIPSEN PIPERAZINE PHOSPHATE POWDER

Use: A powder treatment for the removal of intestinal worms, containing piperazine phosphate, an anti-worm ingredient.

Dose: For threadworms and roundworms, adults and children over six years should take one sachet dissolved in a measured quantity of milk. Adults should take at bed-time, and children in the morning. Children (1-6 years) should be given 5 ml of the sachet contents in the morning. For threadworms, a repeat dose should be taken 14 days after the first dose. For roundworms, additional doses can be taken each month to avoid reinfestation. This treatment is not recommended for babies under one year unless advised otherwise by a doctor.

PROFLEX

Use: An analgesic for general pain relief containing 200 mg of ibuprofen.
Dose: 1-2 capsules to be taken three times a day. Take a maximum of six capsules in 24 hours. The treatment is not recommended for children under 12 years.

PROFLEX PAIN RELIEF

Use: A cream for the treatment of muscular pains, containing ibuprofen, a non-steroidal anti-inflammatory (NSAID).
Dose: The cream should be massaged into the affected area 3-4 times a day. This treatment is not recommended for children under 12 years.

PROFLEX SUSTAINED RELIEF CAPSULES

Use: Analgesic capsules for general pain relief, containing 300 mg of ibuprofen.
Dose: Two capsules should be taken twice a day. Take a maximum of four in 24 hours. This treatment is not recommended for children under 12 years.

PROPAIN

Use: Analgesic tablets for general pain relief, containing 400 mg of paracetamol, 10 mg of codeine phosphate, 5 mg of diphenhydramine, and caffeine.
Dose: 1-2 tablets should be taken every four hours. Take a maximum of 10 tablets in 24 hours. This treatment is not recommended for children under 12 years.

PSORIGEL

Use: A gel for the treatment of eczema and dermatitis, containing coal tar.
Dose: The gel should be rubbed into the affected area and allowed to dry, once or twice a day.

PULMO BAILLY

Use: A liquid remedy for relieving coughs, containing guaicol, an expectorant and codeine, a cough suppressant.

Dose: Adults should take up to 10 ml diluted in water, before food. Take a maximum of three doses in 24 hours. Children (5-15 years) should be given 5 ml. This treatment is not recommended for children under five years.

PYALVEX

Use: A liquid treatment for mouth ulcers, containing salicylic acid, an analgesic.
Dose: The liquid should be brushed onto the affected area 3-4 times a day. This treatment is not recommended for children under 12 years.

QUELLADA-M CREAM SHAMPOO

Use: A shampoo for the treatment for lice and scabies, containing malathion.
Dose: The shampoo should be applied to dry hair and scalp, and to the pubic area if necessary, left for four minutes, then lathered and rinsed off. This treatment is not recommended for babies under six months.

QUELLA-M LOTION

Use: A lotion for the treatment of lice and scabies, containing malathion and alcohol.
Dose: For head or pubic lice, the lotion should be applied to the affected area and left to dry for 2-12 hours. It should then be washed off and the hair combed out while wet. For scabies, the lotion should be applied to the whole body and left on for 24 hours before washing off. This treatment is not recommended for babies under six months.

QUINODERM CREAM

Use: This is a cream for the treatment of acne and spots available in two strengths, containing benzoyl peroxide.
Dose: The cream should be massaged into the affected area once to three times a day, starting with the lower dose version and progressing to the stronger dose version if required. This treatment is not recommended for children under 15 years. The product is available as a lotion, gel and face wash.

QUINOPED CREAM

Use: This is a cream for the treatment of athlete's foot, containing benzoyl peroxide.

Dose: The cream should be massaged into the affected part twice a day.

RALGEX IBUTOP GEL

Use: A gel for the treatment of muscular aches and pains, containing a non-steroidal anti-inflammatory (NSAID).

Dose: The gel should be applied to the affected area three to four times a day, allowing at least four hours between applications. It should not be used more than four times in 24 hours. This treatment is not recommended for children under 12 years.

RADIAN-B HEAT SPRAY

Use: A spray for relieving muscular aches and pains, containing rubefacients and a salicylate, an aspirin derivative.

Dose: The product should be sprayed onto the affected area, and a second dose applied 15 minutes later. This can be repeated up to three times a day if required. The number of applications should be reduced as symptoms subside. This treatment is not recommended for children under six years. The product is also available as a lotion.

RADIAN-B IBUPROFEN GEL

Use: A gel for the treatment of muscular aches and pains, containing ibuprofen, a non-steroidal anti-inflammatory (NSAID).

Dose: The product should be applied to the affected area, and used every four hours if necessary, with a maximum of four applications in 24 hours. This treatment is not recommended for children under 14 years.

RALGEX CREAM

Use: A cream for alleviating muscular aches and pains, containing rubefacients and a salicylate, an aspirin derivative.

Dose: The cream should be applied to the affected area up to four times a day. This treatment is not recommended for children under 12 years.

RALGEX FREEZE SPRAY

Use: A cooling spray for relieving muscle pain, containing a salicylate, an aspirin derivative.

Dose: The product should be applied to the affected area up to four times a day. This treatment is not recommended for children under five years.

RALGEX HEAT SPRAY

Use: A spray for relieving muscular pain, containing rubefacients and a salicylate, an aspirin derivative.

Dose: Two or three short bursts of spray should be applied to the affected area every two hours if required, no more than four times a day. This treatment is not recommended for children under five years.

RALGEX STICK

Use: An embrocation stick for relieving muscular aches and pains, containing rubefacients and a salicylate, an aspirin derivative.

Dose: The product should be applied to the affected area as required. It should not be massaged or rubbed in. This treatment is not recommended for children.

RAP-EZE

Use: Antacid tablets for relieving indigestion and heartburn.

Dose: Two tablets should be chewed or sucked as required. Take a maximum of 16 tablets in 24 hours. This treatment is not recommended for children under 12 years.

REGULAN

Use: A powder treatment for relieving constipation and irritable bowel syndrome. The powders consist of ispaghula husk, a bulk forming laxative.

Dose: Adults should take one sachet dissolved in water 1-3 times a day. Children (6-12 years) should be given half to one level teaspoonful dissolved in water 1-3 times a day. The powder should be taken with plenty of fluid and not before bedtime. This treatment is not recommended for children under six years. The product is also available in other flavours.

REGULOSE

Use: A liquid remedy for relieving constipation, containing lactulose, an osmotic laxative.

Dose: Adults and children over 12 years should take 15-30 ml daily for the first two or three days, reducing the dose to 10-15 ml daily thereafter. Children under 12 years should be given 10-25 ml for the first few days, reducing the dose to 5-15 ml thereafter.

REHIDRAT

Use: Powders to help replace the salts, minerals and water lost from the body during an attack of diarrhoea.

Dose: One sachet should be dissolved in a measured quantity of fluid (see pack for instructions) and taken after every loose bowel movement. Breast-fed babies should be given this fluid in place of their usual feed, but discuss with a doctor prior to use.

RELAXYL

Use: Capsules for relieving irritable bowel syndrome, containing alverine, an ingredient that helps control intestinal spasms.

Dose: 1-2 capsules should be taken up to three times a day. This treatment is not recommended for children under 12 years.

RELCOFEN

Use: Analgesic tablets for general pain relief, containing 200mg of ibuprofen.

Dose: 1-2 tablets should be taken three times a day. Take a maximum of six tablets in 24 hours. This treatment is not recommended for children under 12 years. A stronger version containing 400 mg of ibuprofen is also available.

REMEGEL ORIGINAL

Use: Square antacid tablets for easing indigestion and heartburn.

Dose: 1-2 squares should be chewed every hour. Take a maximum of 12 squares in 24 hours. This treatment is not recommended for children under 12 years. The product is available in several flavours.

RENNIE

Use: Antacid tablets for indigestion and heartburn.

Dose: Adults should suck or chew two tablets as required. Take a maximum of 16 tablets in 24 hours. Children (6-12 years) should be given one tablet as needed, with a maximum of eight tablets in 24 hours. This treatment is not recommended for children under six years. The product is available in several flavours.

REPLENS

Use: A gel to provide lubrication and ease itchiness and irritation of the vagina, for post-menopausal women.

Dose: One dose of the gel should be applied into the vagina three times a week.

RHINOLAST HAYFEVER SPRAY

Use: A nasal spray for relieving hayfever symptoms, containing azelastin, an antihistamine.

Dose: One spray should be applied into each nostril twice a day. This treatment is not recommended for children under 12 years.

RINSTEAD ADULT GEL

Use: A gel for the treatment of mouth ulcers, containing benzocaine, an anaesthetic, and chloroxylenol, an antiseptic.

Dose: The gel should be applied to the affected area up to six times a day. This treatment is not recommended for young children. The product is also available in pastille form.

RINSTEAD TEETHING GEL

Use: A gel for relieving teething pain in babies, containing lignocaine, an anaesthetic, and an antiseptic.

Dose: The gel should be applied every three hours as required. This treatment is not recommended for babies under three months.

ROBITUSSIN CHESTY COUGH MEDICINE

Use: A liquid remedy for the treatment of coughs, containing guaiphenesin, an expectorant.

Dose: Adults should take 10 ml four times a day. Children (1-12 years) should be 2.5-5 ml, according to age. Read the label for the correct dosage. This treatment is not recommended for children under one year.

ROBITUSSIN DRY COUGH

Use: A liquid remedy for the treatment of coughs, containing dextromethorphan, a cough suppressant.

Dose: Adults should take 10 ml four times a day. Children (6-12 years) should be given 5 ml four times a day. This treatment is not recommended for children under six years. A junior version is also available.

ROBITUSSIN FOR CHESTY COUGHS WITH CONGESTION

Use: A liquid remedy for the treatment of coughs, containing guaiphenesin, an expectorant and pseudoephedrine, a decongestant.

Dose: Adults should take 10 ml four times a day. Children (2-12 years) should be given 2.5-5 ml, according to age. Read the label for the correct dosage. This treatment is not recommended for children under two years.

ROBITUSSIN NIGHT TIME

Use: A liquid sugar-free remedy for relieving coughs, containing brompheniramine, an antihistamine, pseudoephedrine, a decongestant, and codeine, a cough suppressant.

Dose: Adults should take 5-10 ml four times a day. Children (4-12 years), should be given 5-7.5 ml three times a day, according to age. Read the label for the correct dosage. This treatment is not recommended for children under four years.

RYNACROM ALLERGY

Use: A nasal spray for relieving hayfever symptoms, containing sodium cromoglycate, an anti-inflammatory and xylometszoline, a decongestant.

Dose: One spray should be directed into each nostril four times a day. This treatment is not recommended for children under five years.

SALACTOL WART PAINT

Use: A paint for the treatment of corns and calluses, containing salicylic acid.

Dose: The product should be applied to the affected area daily and rubbed down with an emery board.

SALONAIR
Use: A spray for easing muscular aches and pains, containing rubefacients and a salicylate, an aspirin derivative.
Dose: The spray should be applied to the affected area once or twice a day. This treatment is not recommended for children under six years.

SALONPAS PLASTERS
Use: A plaster treatment for relieving muscular aches and pains. The plasters contain rubefacients and a salicylate, an aspirin derivative.
Dose: Plaster can be replaced up to three times a day for up to seven days. Not suitable for children under 12 years.

SAVLON ANTISEPTIC CREAM
Use: An antiseptic cream for the treatment of minor wounds and irritations of the skin, containing cetrimide and chlorohexidine gluconate.
Dose: The cream should be applied to the affected part as needed.

SAVLON ANTISEPTIC WOUND WASH
Use: A liquid spray antiseptic for the treatment of minor wounds and skin irritations, containing chlorohexidine gluconate.
Dose: The product should be sprayed onto the wound in order to help wash away any dirt.

SAVLON CONCENTRATED ANTISEPTIC
Use: A liquid antiseptic containing gluconate and cetrimide for the treatment of minor wounds and skin irritations.
Dose: The product should be diluted with water as appropriate for its use.

SAVLON DRY ANTISEPTIC
Use: An antiseptic aerosol powder in the form of a spray for the treatment of minor wounds and skin irritations. The spray contains povidone iodine.
Dose: A light dusting of the powder should be sprayed onto the affected part.

SCHOLL ANTISEPTIC FOOT BALM

Use: A foot balm for relieving sore feet, containing the antiseptic menthyl salicylate, and menthol.

Dose: The product should be applied to the affected area morning and evening, or as required.

SCHOLL ATHLETE'S FOOT CREAM

Use: This is a cream for the treatment of athlete's foot, containing tolnaftate, an antifungal ingredient.

Dose: The product should be applied twice a day to the affected area, and for a further two weeks after the infection has cleared.

SCHOLL CORN AND CALLUS REMOVAL LIQUID

Use: A liquid for the removal of corns and calluses.

Dose: The liquid should be applied to the affected area twice a day, for no longer than two weeks. This treatment is not recommended for children under 16 years.

SCHOLL CORN REMOVAL PADS

Use: Medicated pads for the removal of corns, containing salicylic acid.

Dose: A pad should be applied once a day to the affected area until the corn can be removed. This treatment is not recommended for children under 16 years. The product is also available as Scholl Soft Corn Removal Pads.

SCHOLL CORN REMOVAL PLASTERS

Use: Medicated plasters for the removal of corns, containing salicylic acid.

Dose: The medicated plasters should be applied to the affected area once a day until the corn can be removed. This treatment is not recommended for children under 16 years. Waterproof plasters also available.

SCHOLL POLYMER GEL CORN REMOVERS

Use: A gel for the treatment of corns and calluses, containing salicylic acid.

Dose: A new plaster should be applied each day to the affected area until the corn can be removed. This treatment is not recommended for children under 16 years.

SCHOLL SEAL AND HEAL VERRUCA REMOVAL GEL

Use: A liquid treatment for the removal of verrucae, containing salicylic acid.

Dose: 1-2 drops should be applied onto the affected area once a day and allowed to dry. The treatment should be applied daily until the verruca can be removed. This treatment is not recommended for children under 12 years.

SCHOLL VERRUCA REMOVAL SYSTEM

Use: Medicated plasters for the treatment of verrucae, containing salicylic acid.

Dose: An appropriately sized plaster should be applied to the verruca and left in position for 48 hours before repeating the treatment. The treatment may be continued for up to 12 weeks if necessary. This treatment is not recommended for children under six years unless advised otherwise by a doctor.

SCR

Use: An antiseptic cream treatment for cradle cap.

Dose: The cream should be applied sparingly onto the baby's head. Massage in gently, leave for 30 minutes and then rinse off. Leave for 2 minutes on babies under a year old. A second treatment can be applied seven days later if required. Do not apply to broken or inflamed skin.

SEA-LEGS

Use: Tablets for preventing travel sickness, containing meclozine, an antihistamine.

Dose: Adults should take two tablets one hour before a journey, or on the previous evening. Children over two years should be given half to one tablet, depending on age. Read the label for the correct dosage. This treatment is not recommended for children under two years.

SECADERM

Use: A salve for the treatment of boils and other minor skin infections. It contains an analgesic and an antiseptic.

Dose: The product should be applied to the boil or skin infection and covered with a clean, dry dressing, once or twice a day.

SECRON
Use: A liquid remedy for relieving colds and flu in children, containing ephedrine, a decongestant, and ipecacuanha, an expectorant.
Dose: Children over two years should be given 2.5-10 ml 2-3 times a day, according to age. Read the label for the correct dosage. This treatment is not recommended for children under two years.

SELSUN
Use: A liquid containing selenium sulphide for the treatment of dandruff.
Dose: The liquid should be applied twice a week for two weeks, then once a week for two weeks, until the dandruff has cleared. This treatment is not recommended for children under five years.

SENOKOT TABLETS
Use: Tablets for relieving constipation, containing senna, a stimulant laxative.
Dose: Two tablets should be taken on retiring. This treatment is not recommended for children under 12 years. The product is also available in granular and liquid forms.

SETLERS ANTACID TABLETS
Use: Antacid tablets for relieving indigestion.
Dose: 1-2 tablets should be sucked or chewed as required. Take a maximum of eight tablets in 24 hours. This treatment is not recommended for children under 12 years. The product is available in several different flavours.

SINUTAB TABLETS
Use: Tablets for relieving the symptoms of colds, flu and sinusitis. Each tablet contains paracetamol and phenylpropanolamine, a decongestant.
Dose: Adults should take two tablets three times a day. Take a maximum of six tablets in 24 hours. Children (6-12 years) should be given one tablet three times a day, with a maximum of three tablets in 24 hours. This treatment is not recommended for children under six years.

SIOPEL
Use: A cream for the treatment of nappy rash, containing dimethicone, a soothing barrier cream, and cetrimide, an antiseptic.

Dose: The cream should be applied 3-5 times a day to baby's bottom, after washing and drying. Repeat this for 3-4 days and then reduce the applications to 1-2 times a day.

SOLARCAINE CREAM

Use: A cream for the treatment of bites, stings, minor burns, scalds and sunburn, containing a mild anaesthetic.

Dose: The product should be applied to the affected area 3-4 times a day. This treatment is not recommended for children under three years. The product is also available in lotion and spray forms.

SOLPADEINE CAPSULES

Use: Analgesic capsules for general pain relief, containing 500 mg of paracetamol, 8 mg of codeine phosphate and 30 mg of caffeine.

Dose: Two capsules should be taken up to two times a day. Take a maximum of eight capsules in 24 hours. This treatment is not recommended for children under 12 years.

SOLPADEINE TABLETS

Use: Analgesic tablets for general pain relief, containing 500 mg of paracetamol, 8 mg of codeine phosphate, caffeine.

Dose: Two tablets should be taken up to four times a day if required. Take a maximum of eight tablets in 24 hours. This treatment is not recommended for children under 12 years. The product is also available in soluble form.

SOLPAFLEX

Use: Analgesic tablets for general pain relief, containing 200 mg of ibuprofen and 12.8 mg of codeine phosphate hemihydrate.

Dose: 1-2 tablets should be taken every 4-6 hours as required. Take a maximum of six tablets in 24 hours. This treatment is not recommended for children under 12 years.

SOLPAFLEX GEL

Use: This is a gel for the treatment of muscular aches and pains, containing ketoprofen, a non-steroidal anti-inflammatory (NSAID).

Dose: The gel should be massaged into the affected area 2-4 times a day. This treatment is not recommended for children under 15 years.

SOMINEX

Use: Tablets for insomnia, containing promethazine, an antihistamine.

Dose: One tablet should be taken at bedtime. This treatment is not recommended for children under 16 years.

SOOTHELIP

Use: A cream treatment for cold sores, containing aciclovir, an antiviral.

Dose: The cream should be applied as soon as the tingling of a cold sore is felt, and then every four hours, five times a day for five days. Repeat for a further five days if necessary.

STINGOSE

Use: A pump spray for relieving the discomfort of bites and stings, containing aluminium sulphate, a soothing ingredient.

Dose: The spray should be applied liberally to the affected area, as required. This treatment is not recommended for children under three years.

STREPSILS DIRECT ACTION SPRAY

Use: A spray for sore throats, containing lidocaine, an anaesthetic.

Dose: The spray should be directed into the back of the throat three times, every three hours as required. Take a maximum of six doses in 24 hours. This treatment is not recommended for children under 12 years.

STREPSILS DUAL ACTION LOZENGES

Use: Lozenges for sore throats, containing lidocaine, an anaesthetic, and amylmetacresol and dichlorobenzyl alcohol, both antibacterials.

Dose: One lozenge should be dissolved in the mouth every two hours. Take a maximum of eight tablets in 24 hours. This treatment is not recommended for children under 12 years.

STREPSILS ORIGINAL

Use: Lozenges for relieving sore throats, containing dichlorobenzyl alcohol and amylmetacresol, both antibacterials.

Dose: One lozenge should be dissolved in the mouth every 2-3 hours. Sugar-free and vitamin C versions are also available.

STURGERON TABLETS

Use: Tablets for the prevention of travel sickness, containing cinnarazine, an antihistamine.

Dose: Adults should take two tablets two hours before the journey, followed by one tablet every eight hours if required. Children (5-12 years) should be given half the adult dose. This product is not suitable for children under five years.

SUDAFED COLD AND FLU TABLETS

Use: Tablets for easing the symptoms of colds and flu, containing paracetamol and pseudoephedrine, a decongestant.

Dose: Adults should take one tablet every 4-6 hours. Take a maximum of four tablets in 24 hours. Children (6-12 years) should be given half a tablet every 4-6 hours, with a maximum of four doses in 24 hours. This treatment is not recommended for children under six years.

SUDAFED EXPECTORANT

Use: A liquid remedy for the treatment of coughs, containing guaiphenesin, an expectorant and pseudoephedrine, a decongestant.

Dose: Adults should take 10 ml four times a day. Children (6-12 years) should be given 5 ml. Children (2-5 years) should be given 2.5 ml. This treatment is not recommended for children under two years.

SUDAFED LINCTUS

Use: A liquid remedy for coughs, containing dextromethorphan, a cough suppressant, and pseudoephedrine, a decongestant.

Dose: Adults should take 10 ml four times a day. Children (6-12 years) should be given 5 ml. Children (2-5 years) should be given 2.5 ml. This treatment is not recommended for children under two years.

SUDAFED NASAL SPRAY

Use: A spray for easing nasal congestion caused by colds. The spray contains oxymetazoline, a decongestant.

Dose: 1-2 sprays should be directed into each nostril twice or three times a day. This treatment is not recommended for children under six years. Do not use for more than a week.

SUDAFED TABLETS
Use: Tablets for relieving cold and flu symptoms, containing pseudoephedrine, a decongestant.
Dose: One tablet should be taken every 4-6 hours. Take a maximum of four tablets in 24 hours. This treatment is not recommended for children under 12 years.

SUDOCREAM
Use: A cream for the treatment of nappy rash, containing zinc oxide, an antiseptic and astringent, and hypoallergenic lanolin.
Dose: The cream should be applied thinly to baby's bottom as required.

SULEO M LOTION
Use: A lotion for the treatment of lice and scabies, containing malathion and alcohol.
Dose: The lotion should be applied to dry hair and rubbed in well. The hair should be allowed to dry naturally, washed out after 12 hours and then combed through while still wet. This treatment is not recommended for babies under six months.

SWARM
Use: A cream for the treatment of bites and stings, containing witch hazel and an anti-microbial.
Dose: The product should be applied to the affected area as required.

SYNDOL
Use: Analgesic tablets for general pain relief, containing 450 mg of paracetamol, 10 mg of codeine phosphate, 30 mg of caffeine, and doxylamine succinate, an antihistamine.
Dose: 1-2 tablets should be taken every 4-6 hours as required. Take a maximum of eight in 24 hours. This treatment is not recommended for children under 12 years.

SYNTARIS HAYFEVER

Use: A nasal spray for relieving the symptoms of hayfever, containing flunisolide, a corticosteroid.

Dose: Adults should take two sprays into each nostril morning and evening, with a maximum of four sprays for each nostril in 24 hours. For children (12-16 years) direct one spray into each nostril up to three times a day, with a maximum of three sprays per nostril in 24 hours. This treatment is not recommended for children under 12 years.

TAGAMET 100

Use: Tablets for relieving indigestion, heartburn and general gastric discomfort. They contain cimetidine, a histamine H2 antagonist which reduces the production of stomach acid.

Dose: Two tablets should be taken when symptoms arise. For indigestion at night, one tablet should be taken one hour before retiring. Take a maximum of eight tablets in 24 hours. This treatment is not recommended for children under 16 years. Do not use for longer than two weeks. The product is also available in a liquid form.

TANCOLIN

Use: A liquid remedy for the treatment of coughs, containing dextromethorphan, a suppressant, and vitamin C.

Dose: Children (6 months -12 years) should be given 2.5-15 ml, three times a day according to age. Read the label for the correct dosage. This treatment is not recommended for babies under six months.

TCP ANTISEPTIC OINTMENT

Use: An antiseptic ointment for the treatment of minor wounds and skin irritations, containing iodine, methyl salicylate, salicylic acid, sulphur, tannic acid, camphor and TCP liquid antiseptic.

Dose: The product should be applied to the affected area as required.

TCP FIRST AID ANTISEPTIC CREAM

Use: An antiseptic cream for the treatment of minor wounds and irritations of the skin. It contains chloroxylenol, triclosan, sodium salicylate and TCP liquid antiseptic.

Dose: The product should be applied to the affected area as required.

TCP LIQUID

Use: A liquid antiseptic for the treatment of minor wounds and irritations of the skin, containing phenol and halogenated phenols.

Dose: The liquid should be diluted according to use, or applied undiluted to spots and mouth ulcers.

TCP SORE THROAT LOZENGES

Use: Lozenges for easing sore throats, containing antibacterial phenols.

Dose: One pastille should be sucked or chewed as required. This treatment is not recommended for children under six years.

T-GEL

Use: A medicated shampoo for the treatment of dandruff, containing coal tar.

Dose: The product should be massaged into wet hair and scalp and then rinsed. Repeat use once or twice a week.

TIGER BALM RED (REGULAR AND EXTRA STRENGTH)

Use: An ointment for easing muscle pain, containing various rubefacients.

Dose: The balm should be rubbed gently into the affected area 2-3 times a day. This treatment is not recommended for children under two years.

TINADERM CREAM

Use: An antifungal cream for the treatment of athlete's foot, containing tolnaftate.

Dose: The cream should be applied twice a day to the affected area.

TINADERM POWDER PLUS

Use: This is a powder treatment for athlete's foot, containing tolnaftate, an antifungal ingredient.

Dose: The powder should be sprinkled over the infected area and into socks and footwear, twice a day. The product is also available in spray form.

TIXYLIX CATARRH SYRUP

Use: This is a syrup for the treatment of catarrh, containing diphenhydramine, an antihistamine and menthol.

Dose: Children (6-10 years) should be given 10 ml four times a day. Children (1-5 years) should be given 5 ml four times a day.

TIXYLIX CHESTY COUGH

Use: A liquid remedy for relieving coughs, containing guaiphenesin, an expectorant.

Dose: Children should be given 2.5-10 ml according to age. Read the label for the correct dosage. This treatment is not recommended for babies under one year.

TIXYLIX DAYTIME

Use: A liquid remedy for the treatment of coughs, containing pholcodine, a cough suppressant.

Dose: Children should be given 2.5-10 ml every six hours, according to age. Read the label for the correct dosage. This treatment is not recommended for babies under one year. A night-time version is also available, containing promethazine, an antihistamine.

TIXYLIX INHALANT

Use: Capsules for relieving cold and flu symptoms in children. Each capsule contains menthol, eucalyptus oil, camphor and turpentine oil.

Dose: For babies (3-12 months), the capsule should be cut and its contents squeezed onto a handkerchief tied out of reach, so that the vapours can be inhaled. For children one year and over, the contents should be sprinkled over bed linen or night clothes. Alternatively the capsule can be emptied into a bowl of hot water and left out of reach but close enough for the vapours to be inhaled.

TOEPEDO

Use: This is a cream treatment for athlete's foot, containing keratolytics.

Dose: The cream should be applied sparingly to the affected area twice daily until the infection has cleared.

TOPAL

Use: Tablets for easing general digestive discomfort, containing an antacid and an alginate.

Dose: 1-3 tablets should be taken four times a day after meals and on retiring. This treatment is not recommended for children under 12 years.

TORBETOL

Use: A lotion for the treatment of acne and spots, containing cetrimide and chlorhexidine, both anti-microbials.

Dose: The lotion should be applied to the affected area up to three times a day. This treatment is not recommended for children under 15 years.

TRAMIL

Use: Analgesic capsules for general pain relief, containing 500mg of paracetamol.

Dose: Two capsules should be taken every four hours as required. Take a maximum of eight in 24 hours. This treatment is not recommended for children under 12 years.

TRANSVASIN HEAT RUB

Use: A cream for easing muscular aches and pains, containing rubefacients and a salicylate, an aspirin derivative.

Dose: The cream should be applied to the affected area up to three times a day. This treatment is not recommended for children under six years.

TRANSVASIN HEAT SPRAY

Use: A spray for the treatment of various muscular aches and pains, containing rubefacients and a salicylate, an aspirin derivative.

Dose: The product should be sprayed onto the affected area up to three times a day. This treatment is not recommended for children under five years.

TRAXAM PAIN RELIEF GEL

Use: A gel for relieving muscular aches and pains, containing felbinac, a non-steroidal anti-inflammatory (NSAID).

Dose: The gel should be rubbed into the affected area 2-4 times a day. This treatment is not recommended for children under 12 years.

TROSYL DERMAL CREAM

Use: A cream for the treatment of athlete's foot, containing tioconazole, an antifungal ingredient.

Dose: The product should be applied to the affected area once or twice a day.

TUMS

Use: Antacid tablets for relieving indigestion and heartburn.

Dose: 1-2 tablets should be taken as required. Take a maximum of 16 tablets in 24 hours. This treatment is not recommended for children under 12 years.

TYROZETS

Use: Lozenges for relieving sore throats, containing tyrothricin, an antibacterial and benzocaine, an anaesthetic.

Dose: One lozenge should be dissolved in the mouth every three hours. Take a maximum of eight in 24 hours. Children (3-11 years) should be given a maximum of six lozenges in 24 hours. This treatment is not recommended for children under three years.

ULTRABASE

Use: An emollient cream for the relief of eczema and dermatitis, containing a mixture of oils.

Dose: The product should be applied as required.

UNGUENTUM MERCK

Use: An emollient cream for relieving the discomfort of eczema, dermatitis and nappy rash, containing a mixture of various oils.

Dose: The cream should be applied as required.

UNIGEST

Use: Antacid tablets for relieving indigestion, heartburn and general digestive discomfort.

Dose: 1-2 tablets should be sucked or chewed after meals and at bedtime. This treatment is not recommended for children under 12 years.

VASOGEN CREAM

Use: A cream for the treatment of nappy rash, containing zinc oxide, an antiseptic and astringent, and calamine, a soothing ingredient.

Dose: The product should be applied to baby's bottom after washing and drying.

VEGANIN

Use: Analgesic tablets for general pain relief containing 250 mg of paracetamol, 250 mg of aspirin and 6.8 mg of codeine phosphate.

Dose: 1-2 tablets should be taken every three to four hours as required. Take a maximum of eight tablets in 24 hours. This treatment is not recommended for children under 12 years.

VENO'S DRY COUGH

Use: A liquid remedy for the treatment of coughs, containing glucose and treacle.

Dose: Adults should take 10 ml every two to three hours. Children (3-12 years) should be given 5 ml. This treatment is not recommended for children under three years.

VENO'S EXPECTORANT

Use: A liquid remedy for the treatment of coughs, containing guaiphenesin, an expectorant, glucose and treacle.

Dose: Adults should take 10 ml every two to three hours. Children (3-12 years) should be given 5 ml every 2-3 hours. This treatment is not recommended for children under three years.

VENO'S HONEY AND LEMON

Use: A liquid remedy for the treatment of coughs, containing lemon, glucose and treacle.

Dose: Adults should take 10 ml every 2-3 hours. Children (3-12 years) should be given 5 ml. This treatment is not recommended for children under three years.

VERACUR
Use: A gel for the treatment of verrucae and warts, containing formaldehyde.
Dose: Apply twice a day.

VERRUGON
Use: An ointment remedy for the treatment of verrucae, containing salicylic acid.
Dose: The felt ring should be placed on the verruca, and the ointment applied and covered with a plaster. This should be repeated daily. This treatment is not recommended for children under six years.

VICKS MEDINITE
Use: A liquid remedy for relieving coughs, containing dextromethorphan, a cough suppressant, ephedrine, a decongestant, doxylamine, an antihistamine and paracetamol.
Dose: Adults should take 30 ml on retiring. Children (10-12 years) should be given 15 ml. This treatment is not recommended for children under 10 years.

VICKS ORIGINAL COUGH SYRUP (CHESTY COUGH)
Use: A liquid remedy for the treatment of coughs, containing guaiphenesin and sodium citrate, both expectorants and cetylp yearidium, an antiseptic.
Dose: Adults should take 10 ml every three hours if required. Children (6-12 years) should be given 5 ml. This treatment is not recommended for children under six years.

VICKS SINEX DECONGESTANT NASAL SPRAY
Use: A nasal spray for clearing the congestion caused by colds, flu and sinusitis. It contains oxymetazoline, a decongestant.
Dose: 1-2 sprays should be directed into each nostril every six to eight

hours. This treatment is not recommended for children under six years. Do not use for longer than seven days.

VICKS ULTRA CHLORASEPTIC

Use: A throat spray for relieving sore throats, containing benzocaine, an anaesthetic.

Dose: Adults should take three sprays every 2-3 hours. Children (6-12 years) should be given one spray every 2-3 hours. Take a maximum of eight doses in 24 hours. This treatment is not recommended for children under six years, and should not be used for more than three consecutive days.

VICKS VAPORUB

Use: An inhalant rub for easing congestion caused by colds and flu, containing menthol, eucalyptus and camphor.

Dose: A small amount should be rubbed into the chest, throat and back at night. Alternatively, two teaspoons can be added to a bowl of hot water and the vapours inhaled. This treatment is not recommended for babies under six months.

VICKS VAPOSYRUP FOR CHESTY COUGHS

Use: A liquid remedy for relieving coughs, containing guaiphenesin, an expectorant.

Dose: Adults should take 15 ml up to six times a day. Children (6-11 years) should be given 10 ml. Children (2-5 years) should be given 5 ml. This treatment is not recommended for children under two years.

VICKS VAPOSYRUP FOR DRY COUGHS

Use: A liquid remedy for coughs, containing dextromethorphan, a cough suppressant.

Dose: Adults should take 15 ml up to four times a day. Children (6-11 years) should be given 5 ml. Children (2-5 years) should be given 2.5 ml. This treatment is not recommended for children under four years.

VICKS VAPOSYRUP FOR TICKLY COUGHS

Use: A liquid remedy for the treatment of coughs, containing menthol.

Dose: Adults should take 10 ml every 3-4 hours. Take a maximum of six doses in 24 hours. Children (6-12 years) should be given half the adult dose. This treatment is not recommended for children under six years.

VIRASORB

Use: A cream treatment for cold sores, containing aciclovir, an antiviral.
Dose: The cream should be applied as soon as a cold sore tingling is felt, and then every four hours, five times a day for five days. Repeat for a further five days if necessary.

VITATHONE

Use: An ointment for the treatment of chilblains. It contains menthyl nicotinate, which helps to relieve the itchiness by stimulating the circulation.
Dose: The ointment should be applied every 2-3 hours as required. This treatment is not recommended for children.

VOCALZONE

Use: Pastilles for easing sore throats.
Dose: One pastille should be dissolved in the mouth as needed, every two hours if necessary. This treatment is not recommended for children under 12 years.

WARTEX OINTMENT

Use: An ointment for the removal of warts, containing salicylic acid.
Dose: The product should be applied to the wart daily until the wart can be removed. This treatment is not recommended for children under six years.

WASP-EZE OINTMENT

Use: An ointment for the treatment of bites and stings, containing an antihistamine.
Dose: The product should be applied to the affected area immediately and then every hour if necessary, for up to 24 hours. This treatment is not recommended for children under one year. The product is also available as a spray.

WAXSOL EAR DROPS

Use: Ear drops for removing earwax, containing softening ingredients.
Dose: The ears should be filled with the liquid for two consecutive nights before syringe treatment.

WAX WANE EAR DROPS

Use: Ear drops for the removal of earwax, containing softening ingredients.
Dose: 4-5 drops should be directed into the ear and plugged with cotton wool. This should be repeated 2-3 times a day for several days or until the wax softens.

WITCH DOCTOR GEL

Use: An astringent gel for the treatment of bites, stings, minor burns, scalds, sunburn and bruises, containing witch hazel.
Dose: The product should be applied to the area as required. The product is also available as a stick.

WOODWARD'S BABY CHEST RUB

Use: An inhalant rub for easing congestion caused by colds and flu. It contains menthol, eucalyptus and turpentine.
Dose: A small amount should be rubbed onto the chest, throat and back so that the vapours can be inhaled during the night. This treatment is not recommended for babies under three months.

WOODWARD'S COLIC DROPS

Use: A liquid remedy for relieving infant colic and wind, containing dimethicone, an anti-wind ingredient. A measure is supplied.
Dose: For children under two years, one measured dose of 3 ml should be given before each feed.

WOODWARD'S GRIPE WATER

Use: A liquid remedy for relieving infant colic and wind, containing sodium bicarbonate, an antacid and dill oil.
Dose: 5-10 ml (according to age) should be given after or during feeds. Check the label for the correct dosage. Give a maximum of six doses in 24 hours. This treatment is not recommended for babies under one month.

WOODWARD'S NAPPY RASH OINTMENT

Use: An ointment for the treatment of nappy rash, containing zinc oxide, an antiseptic and an astringent, and cod liver oil, a moisturiser.

Dose: The product should be applied to baby's bottom three times a day after washing and drying.

WOODWARD'S TEETHING GEL

Use: A gel for relieving teething pain in babies, containing lignocaine, an anaesthetic, and an antiseptic.

Dose: The gel should be applied and then reapplied after 20 minutes. This can be repeated every three hours if necessary.

WRIGHT'S VAPOURIZING FLUID

Use: An inhalant to be used in conjunction with Wright's Vaporizer, containing chlorocesol. Its vapours help to ease congestion caused by colds and flu.

Dose: 10 ml should be added to the vaporizer block every eight hours. This treatment is not recommended for children under two years.

YEAST-VITE

Use: A tablet remedy for alleviating fatigue, containing caffeine, vitamin B1 and nicontamide.

Dose: Two tablets should be taken every 3-4 hours as required. Take a maximum of 12 tablets in 24 hours. This treatment is not recommended for children.

YESTAMIN PLUS TABLETS

Use: A tablet remedy for relieving fatigue, containing caffeine, yeast and glucose.

Dose: Two tablets should be taken three times a day. This treatment is not recommended for children.

ZANTAC 75 TABLETS

Use: Tablets for easing digestive discomfort, containing rantidine, a histamine H2 antagonist which helps to reduce the production of stomach acid.

Dose: One tablet should be taken initially, followed by one more if necessary. Take a maximum of four tablets in 24 hours. This treatment is not recommended for children under 16 years. Do not use for more than two weeks.

ZIRTEK

Use: A tablet for relieving the symptoms of hayfever, containing cetirizine, an antihistamine.

Dose: One tablet should be taken each day. This treatment is not recommended for children under 12 years.

ZOVIRAX COLD SORE CREAM

Use: A cream treatment for cold sores containing aciclovir, an antiviral.

Dose: The cream should be applied as soon as the tingling of a developing cold sore is felt. Continue to apply every four hours, five times a day for up to ten days.

ALTERNATIVE REMEDIES

Alternative or complementary medicine is a designation for any medical system which is based on a theory other than that taught in traditional Western medical schools. The popularity of alternative medicine has grown dramatically over the last decade and it is estimated that 80 per cent of people in the UK have either taken a complementary remedy or consulted a complementary practitioner at some time or another.

The most widely used types of remedies are homeopathic and herbal, and for this reason we have focused on them in this section.

HOMEOPATHY

Homeopathy is a system of medicine which is based on the principle that that the substance which causes a medical problem can also be used to cure it. This is known as the 'like cures like' theory. The patient is treated with minute amounts of substances that are themselves capable of producing the symptoms of the problem in question. For example, the homeopathic remedy recommended to treat diarrhoea may be a very dilute laxative.

Homeopathic remedies derive from vegetable, animal and mineral substances which are diluted in water or alcohol. Critics say the substances are diluted to the point where they cannot be of any medical value. However, homeopaths argue that another principle of homeopathy is 'less is more', so the more dilute a preparation, the more powerful its action. Following the dilution process, the substance is shaken rapidly until the desired strength is achieved.

The dosage for homeopathic remedies relates to the amount of times the original substance has been diluted and shaken.

Three dosages are commonly available:

• 6x, which has been diluted in a 1 to 9 ratio with 6 repeats of the shaking process

• 6c, which has been diluted in a 1 to 99 ratio with 6 repeats of the shaking process

• 30c, which has been diluted in a 1 to 99 ratio with 30 repeats of the shaking process

Many homeopathic remedies can be bought over the counter from chemists and health food shops, but the very strong preparations can only be prescribed by a registered homeopath who will take a holistic approach to treatment, bearing in mind the patient's personality as well as symptoms.

As with any type of medication, you should always read the label carefully before taking or administering any homeopathic remedy - the number of tablets you should take depends on a range of factors. The remedies should be dissolved on the tongue and taken when your mouth is as clean as possible. It is not advisable to ingest any other substance - especially tea, coffee or toothpaste - within 30 minutes of taking homeopathic remedies, as this may affect their action. Avoid touching the tablets with your hands. Women who are pregnant or breastfeeding should consult a doctor or pharmacist before embarking on treatment.

HERBAL MEDICINE

Herbal medicine is a system of treatment in which different plants are used in order to treat symptoms of illness and to promote health. Herbal medicine has been the most common form of medical treatment in many cultures for centuries.

Although some traditional herbalists claim that it is crucial for extracts of the whole plant to be used in order for the maximum benefit of herbs to be realised, modern herbal remedies are made from the leaves, bark, roots, flowers or oils of plants. They can be taken as tablets, drops that are added to water, or teas. Some are also available as creams or ointments.

Herbal remedies can now be bought from most pharmacies and healthfood shops. As with all kinds of medicine it is vital to read the instructions carefully before taking or administering any herbal remedy. They can be harmful if not taken appropriately and they can have unwanted side effects. Breastfeeding or pregnant women should not take any kind of remedy without prior consultation with a doctor or pharmacist. Many herbal remedies are not suitable for children.

SELF-TREATMENT WITH COMPLEMENTARY REMEDIES

There is a widely held belief that complementary medicines are always harmless. This is not the case. Some of the most potent and dangerous medicines used in orthodox medicine are derived from natural substances, for instance the heart drug digoxin is derived from the common foxglove.

It is important therefore to approach complementary medicine with the same caution as you would orthodox medication, and observe the following guidelines:

• Only attempt to treat minor ailments yourself - if in doubt, speak to a GP or pharmacist

• Ask for advice if you are not sure which is the most suitable preparation for your need

• Read the packet very carefully and take note of how much to take, when and how - if in doubt, ask an expert

• Be extra vigilant when treating children - particularly with the dosage

• Check the use-by date

• Seek advice first if you are pregnant or breastfeeding

• Do not take without seeking advice if you have been prescribed prescription medicines

• Keep away from children

• If symptoms do not improve, seek further advice.

HOW TO USE THIS SECTION

Included in this part of the book is a selection of many of the basic herbal and homeopathic remedies that are most widely available. The list is not exhaustive and you will find other brands of many of the substances. The organization in this section differs from the alphabetical arangement adopted in the sections for prescription and over-the-counter medicines. The entries are arranged firstly by the disorder for which treatment is being sought, then alphabetically by name. The name may be the title of a specific preparation (for example, bryonia) or the name of the product's originator or manufacturer (for example, Potter's or Weleda).

The disorders for which treatments are given are for those affecting -
• *Throat and lungs*
• *Head and neck*
• *Stomach and digestive system*
• *Ears, eyes and mouth*
• *Blood and circulatory system*
• *Mental health*
• *Female reproductive system*
• *The skin*
• *Bones and muscles*
• *Children*

REMEDIES FOR THROAT AND LUNG DISORDERS
ACONITE
What it is: A homeopathic remedy which should be taken during the early stages of a cold. Also suitable for sore throats, fevers or dry, persistent coughs.
Dose: Ainsworth's 30c, Nelsons 6c, Weleda 6c and 30c.

ALLIUM CEPA
What it is: A homeopathic remedy for the treatment of colds and catarrh. It can also be used for hayfever and laryngitis.
Dose: Ainsworth's 30c, Weleda 6c.

APIS MELLIFICA
What it is: A homeopathic remedy for relieving a sore and burning throat.
Dose: Weleda 6c and 30c, Nelsons 6c.

ARGENTUM NITRICUM

What it is: A homeopathic remedy for treating hoarseness and a sore throat.

Dose: Weleda 6c and 30c, Nelsons 6c, Ainsworth's 30c.

BELLADONNA

What it is: A homeopathic remedy for the treatment of sudden fevers.

Dose: Nelsons 6c, Weleda 6c and 30c.

BIO-STRATH CHAMOMILE FORMULA

What it is: A herbal liquid remedy which can be used to ease the symptoms of sore throats. It contains camomile, sage and yeast.

Dose: 20 drops should be diluted in water three times a day before meals. This treatment is not suitable for children.

BIO-STRATH THYME FORMULA

What it is: A liquid herbal cough remedy containing thyme, primula and yeast.

Dose: 20 drops should be taken in water three times a day before meals.

BRYONIA

What it is: A homeopathic remedy for the treatment of dry, irritating coughs.

Dose: Ainsworth's 30c, Nelsons 6c, Weleda 6c and 30c.

BUTTERCUP POL 'N' COUNT

What it is: A herbal remedy for relieving the symptoms of hayfever. It contains garlic and echinacea.

Dose: Two tablets should be taken three times a day. This treatment is not suitable for children.

CALCAREA FLUORICA

What it is: A homeopathic remedy for the treatment of coughs which are accompanied by yellow mucus.

Dose: Nelsons 6c, New Era 6x, Weleda 6c and 30c.

CALCAREA PHOSPHORICA

What it is: A homeopathic remedy for the treatment bronchial asthma and catarrh.

Dose: Nelsons 6c, New Era 6x, Weleda 6c and 30c.

CALCAREA SULPHURICA

What it is: This is a homeopathic remedy for the treatment of catarrh.

Dose: New Era 6x.

CARBO VEGETABILIS

What it is: A homeopathic remedy for relieving violent coughing.

Dose: Nelsons 6c, Weleda 6c and 30c.

CATARRH CREAM

What it is: An aromatic herbal decongestant which can be used to ease the congestion and inflamed nasal passages caused by catarrh. It contains camphor, eucalyptus, echinacea, thyme, barberry, blackthorn, bryonia, aesculin and mercurius sulphuratus.

Dose: A small amount of cream should be inserted into each nostril as required. It is not advisable to combine this treatment with homeopathic remedies. This treatment is not suitable for use on children under three years.

CATARRH-EEZE

What it is: This is a traditional herbal remedy which can be used to relieve the congestion caused by catarrh. It contains inula, horehound and yarrow.

Dose: Adults should take two tablets three times a day. Children (8-12 years) should take one tablet three times a day.

COLD-EEZE

What it is: A tablet herbal remedy for relieving colds, containing garlic and echinacea.

Dose: Two tablets should be swallowed whole, three times a day. This treatment is not suitable for children.

COUGH EEZE

What it is: An expectorant herbal cough remedy available in the form of tablets. It contains ipecacuanha, inula and horehound.

Dose: Adults should take two tablets, three times a day. Children (8-12 years) should take one tablet a day.

DROSERA

What it is: A homeopathic remedy for the treatment of tickly, irritating coughs and violent coughing attacks. It is also useful for laryngitis and sore throats where swallowing is painful.

Dose: Ainsworth's 30c, Nelsons 6c, Weleda 6c and 30c.

ECHINACEA AND GARLIC

What it is: A herbal tablet remedy for the relief and treatment of colds and flu.

Dose: 1- 2 tablets should be taken three times a day. This treatment is not suitable for children.

ERNEST JACKSON'S CATARRH PASTILLES

What it is: These are herbal pastilles for the treatment of catarrh. They contain menthol, creosote, abietis pine oil and sylvestris pine oil.

Dose: Dissolve one pastille in the mouth when required.

ERNEST JACKSON'S CHILDREN'S COUGH PASTILLES

What it is: These are expectorant herbal pastilles containing ipecacuanha, citric acid, honey, and squill.

Dose: One pastille should be dissolved in the mouth. Read the label for the maximum amount that can be taken in 24 hours.

EUPHRASIA

What it is: A homeopathic remedy for the treatment of daytime coughs which produce mucus.

Dose: Ainsworth's 30c, Nelsons 6c, Weleda 6c and 30c.

FERRUM PHOSPHORICUM

What it is: A homeopathic remedy to be used during the early stages of a cold or fever, after using aconite.

Dose: Ainsworth's 30c, Nelsons 6c, New Era 6x, Weleda 6c and 30c.

GARLODEX

What it is: A herbal tablet remedy for the treatment and relief of colds and catarrh, containing garlic, parsley and marshmallow.

Dose: One tablet should be taken three times a day. Children (5-12 years) should take one tablet at bedtime. This treatment is not suitable for children under five years.

GELSEMIUM

What it is: A homeopathic remedy for sore throats where swallowing is painful or difficult.

Dose: Weleda 6c and 30c, Nelsons 6c, Ainsworth's 30c.

GENCYDO

What it is: This is an ointment containing quince, lemon juice and boric acid and is used for relieving the symptoms of hayfever.

Dose: The ointment should be applied to the inside of the nostrils several times a day and before retiring. It is also available as a nasal paint that can be diluted with water and used as a nasal spray.

HEATH & HEATHER BALM OF GILEAD COUGH PASTILLES

What it is: These are herbal expectorant cough pastilles for treating general coughs. They contain balm of Gilead, lobelia and squill.

Dose: One pastille should be dissolved in the mouth as required. Take a maximum of 12 pastilles over 24 hours.

HEATH & HEATHER CATARRH TABLETS

What it is: Herbal tablets which can be used to relieve the symptoms of catarrh. The tablets contain white horehound and squill.

Dose: One tablet should be taken three times a day. This treatment is not suitable for children.

HEPAR SULPHURIS

What it is: A homeopathic remedy for the treatment of coughs that are brought on by cold air.

Dose: Ainsworth's 30c, Nelsons 6c, Weleda 6c and 30c.

HERBELIX

What it is: A liquid herbal expectorant which can relieve the symptoms of catarrh. It contains lobelia, tolu solution and sodium bicarbonate.

Dose: 5 ml should be taken at bedtime. Children (7-14 years) should be given half the adult dose. This treatment is not suitable for children under seven years.

HOFELS GARLIC AND PARSLEY ONE-A DAY TABLETS

What it is: A herbal remedy for the relief of colds, catarrh and hayfever. The tablets contain garlic oil. This remedy is also available as Hofels Garlic One-A-Day Garlic Pearles, and Original Garlic Pearles.

Dose: One tablet should be taken with food. This treatment is not suitable for children under seven years.

IGNATIA

What it is: A homeopathic remedy for the treatment of dry, irritating coughs and sore throats.

Dose: Nelsons 6c, Weleda 6c and 30c.

KALIUM BICHROMICUM

What it is: A homeopathic remedy for the treatment of stringy, persistent catarrh and sore throats.

Dose: Ainsworth's 30c, Nelsons 6c, Weleda 6c and 30c.

KALIUM MURIATICUM

What it is: A homeopathic remedy for the treatment of white, sticky catarrh and tonsillitis.

Dose: New Era 6x.

KALIUM PHOSPHORICUM

What it is: A homeopathic remedy for the treatment of asthma in cases where breathing is particularly difficult, or for nervous asthma accompanied by hoarseness.

Dose: Nelsons 6c, New Era 6x, Weleda 6c and 30c.

KALIUM SULPHURICUM

What it is: A homeopathic remedy for the treatment of asthma accompanied by bronchitis, and yellow catarrh.

Dose: New Era 6x.

LACHESIS

What it is: A homeopathic remedy for sore throats that extend to the ear and tonsillitis.

Dose: Weleda 6c.

LANES HONEY AND MOLASSES COUGH MIXTURE

What it is: A liquid herbal expectorant remedy containing ipecacuanha, horehound and squill.

Dose: Adults should take 5 ml three times a day. Children (2-14 years) should be given 2.5 ml. Read the label for the maximum dose.

LOBELIA COMPOUND

What it is: A herbal remedy available in the form of tablets that act as an anti-spasmodic, expectorant and respiratory stimulant. They contain lobelia, gum ammoniacum and squill.

Dose: One tablet should be taken three times a day.

LUSTY'S GARLIC PERLES

What it is: Herbal capsules for the treatment of colds, runny nose, catarrh and coughs. The capsules contain garlic.

Dose: One capsule should be taken three times a day with meals. Children (5-12 years) should be given one capsule a day. This treatment is not suitable for children under five years.

MERCURIUS SOLUBILIS

What it is: A homeopathic remedy for relieving feverish head colds which are accompanied by catarrh.

Dose: Nelsons 6c, Weleda 6c and 30c.

NATRUM MURIATICUM

What it is: A homeopathic remedy for relieving the symptoms of hayfever.

Dose: Ainsworth's 30c, Nelsons 6c, New Era 6x, Weleda 6c and 30c.

NEW ERA COMBINATION H

What it is: A homeopathic remedy for relieving the symptoms of hayfever and allergic rhinitis. It contains mag phos, nat mur and silica.

Dose: One dose contains 6x each of the above ingredients.

NEW ERA COMBINATION Q

What it is: A homeopathic remedy for the treatment of catarrh and sinus disorders. It contains calc fluor, calc phos, kali phos and mag phos.

Dose: Each dose contains 6x each of the above ingredients.

NUX VOMICA

What it is: A homeopathic remedy which can be used to treat violent coughing fits and raw sore throats.

Dose: Ainsworth's 30c, Nelsons 6c, Weleda 6c and 30c.

OLBAS INHALER

What it is: An inhalant for relieving nasal congestion caused by colds and flu. It can also help to relieve congestion caused by catarrh, hayfever and blocked sinuses. It contains menthol, eucalyptus, peppermint and cajuput.

Dose: Place the inhaler in each nostril and inhale. Repeat up to four times in one hour. This treatment is not recommended for children under seven years.

OLBAS OIL

What it is: This is a liquid inhalation which can help to relieve nasal congestion caused by colds, flu, catarrh, hayfever, sinusitis and any infections of the upper respiratory tract. It contains menthol, eucalyptus, wintergreen, juniper berry, clove, mint and cajuput.

Dose: Put 2-3 drops on a handkerchief and inhale as required. The liquid can be added to hot water and used as a steam inhalant. For children aged three months to two years, use one drop on a tissue and tie out of reach on clothing or bedhead at night. This treatment is not suitable for babies under three months.

OLBAS PASTILLES

What it is: Pastilles for the relief of cold and flu symptoms, containing menthol, eucalyptus, wintergreen, juniper berry, peppermint and cloves.

Dose: One pastille should be dissolved in the mouth as required. Take a maximum of eight pastilles over 24 hours. This treatment is not suitable for children under seven years.

OLEUM RHINALE

What it is: A herbal oil remedy which can help to relieve the symptoms of sinus congestion, dry rhinitis and catarrh. It contains eucalyptus, peppermint, marigold and mercurius sulphuratus.

Dose: 2-4 drops should be applied into each nostril twice a day. This treatment should not be combined with any other herbal or homeopathic remedies.

PHOSPHORUS

What it is: A homeopathic remedy for the treatment of a cough which causes breathing difficulties, laryngitis and hoarseness.

Dose: Ainsworth's 30c, Nelsons 6c, Weleda 6c and 30c.

PHYTOLACCA

What it is: A homeopathic remedy for the treatment of dry sore throats.

Dose: Weleda 6c.

POLLENNA

What it is: A homeopathic remedy for the treatment of hayfever, containing 6c each of Allium cepa, Euphrasia officinallis and Sabadilla officinarum.

Dose: Adults should take two tablets every two hours for six doses, then two tablets three times a day. Children should be given half the adult dose. Stop the treatment when symptoms cease.

POTTER'S ANTIBRON

What it is: A herbal tablet remedy that can be used as an anti-spasm, expectorant, soothing and sedative cough treatment. It contains lobelia, euphorbia, coltsfoot, pleurisy root, senega and wild lettuce.

Dose: Adults should take two tablets three times a day. Children over seven years should take one tablet as directed.

POTTER'S ANTISMOKING TABLETS
What it is: A herbal remedy for reducing nicotine dependence. The tablets contain lobelia.
Dose: One tablet should be taken every hour. Take a maximum of 10 tablets over 24 hours.

POTTER'S BALM OF GILEAD
What it is: A liquid herbal expectorant for the treatment of general coughs. It contains balm of Gilead, lobelia, lungwort and squill.
Dose: Adults should take 10 ml diluted in water 3-4 times a day. Children over five years should take 5 ml.

POTTER'S CATARRH MIXTURE
What it is: A liquid herbal remedy used to relieve nasal and throat catarrh. It contains capsicum, burdock, boneset, hyssop and blue flag.
Dose: Adults should take 5 ml three times a day. Children over seven years should be given 5 ml twice a day. This treatment is not suitable for children under seven years.

POTTER'S CHEST MIXTURE
What it is: An expectorant liquid herbal cough and catarrh remedy, containing lobelia, horehound, pleurisy root, senega and squill.
Dose: Adults should take 5 ml every three hours. This treatment is not suitable for children.

POTTER'S ELDERMINT LIFE DROPS
What it is: A homeopathic liquid remedy for the treatment of colds, flu, fevers and sore throats. It contains capsicum, elderflower and peppermint.
Dose: Adults should take 11 drops diluted in warm water every hour. Children over seven years should be given 11 drops every two hours. This treatment is not suitable for children under seven years. Do not combine this treatment with other homeopathic remedies.

POTTER'S GARLIC TABLETS

What it is: A herbal tablet remedy for the treatment of colds and flu, containing garlic.

Dose: Adults should take two tablets three times a day. Children over eight years should be given one tablet 3-4 times a day.

POTTER'S LIGHTNING COUGH REMEDY

What it is: A liquid herbal cough remedy containing liquorice and anise.

Dose: Adults should take 10 ml 3-4 times a day. Children over five years should be given 5 ml every 5-6 hours.

POTTER'S VEGETABLE COUGH REMOVER

What it is: A herbal liquid remedy that is an expectorant and an anti-spasmodic for relieving cough symptoms. It contains ipecacuanha, lobelia, hyssop, horehound, elecampane, black cohosh, pleurisy root and skullcap.

Dose: Adults, 10ml 3-4 times a day. Children over eight years, 5 ml three times a day. Children (5-7 years) 5 ml twice a day.

PULSATILLA

What it is: A homeopathic remedy for the treatment of thick, yellow catarrh.

Dose: Ainsworth's 30c, Nelsons 6c, Weleda 6c and 30c.

RESOLUTION

What it is: Lozenges for reducing nicotine dependence. They contain the vitamins A, C, E and nicotine.

Dose: One lozenge should be dissolved in the mouth when the urge to smoke a cigarette arises.

SILICA

What it is: A homeopathic remedy for relieving the symptoms of persistent colds and hayfever.

Dose: Ainsworth's 30c, Nelsons 6c, New Era 6x, Weleda 6c and 30c.

SINOTAR

What it is: A herbal tablet remedy that is an antiseptic and decongestant for relieving the symptoms of catarrh and sinusitis. It contains echinacea, marshmallow and elderflower.

Dose: Two tablets should be taken three times a day before meals. Children (5-12 years) should be given half the adult dose. This treatment is not suitable for children under five years.

STOPPERS
What it is: Lozenges containing nicotine for reducing nicotine dependence.
Dose: One lozenge should be dissolved in the mouth when the urge to smoke a cigarette arises.

THUJA
What it is: A homeopathic remedy for relieving catarrh.
Dose: Nelsons 6c, Weleda 6c and 30c.

WELEDA COUGH DROPS
What it is: A liquid herbal remedy containing aqua cherry laurel, angelica, cinnamon, coriander, clove, nutmeg, lemon balm and lemon oil.
Dose: 10-20 drops should be dissolved in warm water and swallowed every two hours.

WELEDA HERB AND HONEY COUGH ELIXIR
What it is: A liquid herbal cough remedy containing thyme, horehound, elderflower, Iceland moss, marshmallow and aniseed.
Dose: Adults should take 10 ml diluted in water every 3-4 hours. Take a maximum of four doses over 24 hours. Children over six years should be given half the adult dose.

WELEDA MIXED POLLEN
What it is: A homeopathic remedy for relieving the symptoms of hayfever. It contains a wide range of pollens.
Dose: 30c.

REMEDIES FOR HEAD AND NECK DISORDERS
ACTAEA RACEMOSA
What it is: A homeopathic remedy used for the treatment of headaches that

begin with severe pain at the back of the head and tend to spread upwards.
Dose: Nelsons 6c, Weleda 6c.

BELLADONNA

What it is: A homeopathic remedy for relieving severe throbbing headaches.
Dose: Ainsworth's 30c, Nelsons 6c, Weleda 6c.

BRYONIA

What it is: A homeopathic remedy for relieving splitting headaches that occur over the eyes.
Dose: 30c, one tablet every four hours for a maximum of six doses.

CALCAREA PHOSPHORICA

What it is: A homeopathic remedy for relieving headaches caused by long periods of study.
Dose: Nelsons 6c, New Era 6x, Weleda 6c.

COFFEA

What it is: A homeopathic remedy for relieving nervous headaches occurring on one side of the head.
Dose: Weleda 6c.

FEVERFEW

What it is: A homeopathic remedy which can be used to reduce the severity and frequency of migraine headaches.
Dose: Weleda 6x.

GELSEMIUM

What it is: A homeopathic remedy for the treatment of general headaches, it is especially effective for those brought on by colds and flu.
Dose: Ainsworth's 30c, Nelsons 6c, Weleda 6c.

GLONOINE

What it is: A homeopathic remedy that can be used to treat thumping headaches.

Dose: One tablet every 30 minutes until an improvement occurs, for a maximum of six doses.

IGNATIA
What it is: A homeopathic remedy for relieving sharp, painful headaches.
Dose: Nelsons 6c, Weleda 6c or 30c.

KALIUM BICHROMICUM
What it is: A homeopathic remedy for relieving migraines which are preceded by blurred vision.
Dose: Nelsons 6c, Weleda 6c and 30c.

KALIUM PHOSPHORICUM
What it is: A homeopathic remedy for the treatment of stress-related headaches.
Dose: Nelsons 6c, New Era 6x, Weleda 6c.

LACHESIS
What it is: A homeopathic remedy for relieving throbbing headaches.
Dose: Weleda 6c.

NATRUM MURIATICUM
What it is: A homeopathic remedy for relieving severe headaches.
Dose: Ainsworth's 30c, Nelsons 6c, New Era 6x, Weleda 6c and 30c.

NEW ERA COMBINATION F
What it is: A combination of kali phos, mag phos, nat mur and silica for the treatment of migraine headaches.
Dose: One tablet containing 6x of each of the above ingredients.

NUX VOMICA
What it is: A homeopathic remedy for headaches which are accompanied by dizziness, nausea and sickness.
Dose: Nelsons 6c, Weleda 6c and 30c.

SILICA
What it is: A homeopathic remedy for the relief and treatment of migraine.

Dose: Ainsworth's 30c, Nelsons 6c, New Era 6x, Weleda 6c and 30c.

THUJA
What it is: A homeopathic remedy for severe headaches or migraine.
Dose: Nelsons 6c, Weleda 6c.

REMEDIES FOR DISORDERS AFFECTING THE STOMACH AND DIGESTIVE SYSTEM
ARGENTIUM NITRICUM
What it is: A homeopathic remedy for the treatment of nervous diarrhoea and heartburn.
Dose: Weleda 6c and 30c, Nelsons 6c, Ainsworth's 30c.

ARSENICUM ALBUM
What it is: A homeopathic remedy for the treatment of sudden diarrhoea with vomiting.
Dose: Weleda 6c and 30c, Nelsons 6c, Ainsworth's 30c.

BIOBALM POWDER
What it is: A herbal powder remedy for relieving indigestion, containing slippery elm, camomile, Irish moss and marshmallow.
Dose: 1-2 level teaspoons should be mixed with water and taken up to four times a day. Children (5-12 years) should be given half the adult dose. This treatment is not suitable for children under five years.

BIO-STRATH ARTICHOKE FORMULA
What it is: A herbal liquid remedy for relieving indigestion particularly after eating fatty foods.
Dose: Take two drops diluted in water three times a day before meals This treatment is not suitable for children and should not be combined with other homeopathic remedies.

BIO-STRATH LIQUORICE FORMULA
What it is: A herbal liquid remedy for aiding digestion. It contains liquorice, camomile, gentian and yeast.

Dose: Take 2 ml diluted in water three times a day. This treatment is not suitable for children.

CALCAREA CARBONICA

What it is: A homeopathic remedy for relieving constipation, containing senna and aloes.

Dose: Nelsons 6c, Weleda 6c and 30c. This treatment is not suitable for children under seven years.

CARBO VEGETABILIS

What it is: A homeopathic remedy for treating indigestion with flatulence.

Dose: Weleda 6c and 30c, Nelsons 6c, Ainsworth's 30c.

CATASSIUM HERBAL TRAVEL SICKNESS TABLETS

What it is: A herbal tablet remedy for relieving travel sickness, containing ginger.

Dose: Adults should take three tablets 30 minutes before starting a journey. Children (6-12 years) should be given 1-2 tablets. This treatment is not suitable for children under six years.

CAUSTICUM

What it is: A homeopathic remedy to help relieve constipation where there is ineffectual urging.

Dose: Weleda 6c.

CLAIRO TEA

What it is: A herbal tea for relieving constipation. It contains senna (a stimulant laxative), aniseed, peppermint and clove.

Dose: Adults should take 2.5 ml dissolved in boiling water at night. Children over six years should be given half the adult dose in the morning. This treatment is not suitable for children under six years.

COCCULUS

What it is: A homeopathic remedy for relieving travel sickness and jetlag.

Dose: Weleda 6c, Ainsworth's 30c.

COLOCYNTHIS
What it is: A homeopathic remedy for relieving diarrhoea that is accompanied by abdominal cramps and spasms.
Dose: Weleda 6c.

CRANESBILL
What it is: A herbal tablet that provides astringent relief for non-persistent diarrhoea. It contains cranesbill.
Dose: 1-2 tablets should be taken as required, up to three times a day. Children over 12 years should take one tablet twice a day. This treatment is not suitable for children under 12 years.

DIGEST
What it is: A herbal tablet remedy for relieving indigestion and wind. It contains centaury, parsley and marshmallow.
Dose: Two tablets should be taken three times a day before meals. This treatment is not suitable for children under 12 years.

DUAL-LAX
What it is: A herbal tablet remedy for relieving constipation. The tablets contain senna and aloes, both of which are stimulant laxatives.
Dose: Adults should take 1-2 tablets at night. Children (7-14 years) should be given one tablet at night. This treatment is not suitable for children under seven years. An extra strength version is also available.

GINGER TABLETS
What it is: A herbal tablet remedy for calming nauseous sensations.
Dose: Take one tablet three times a day. This treatment is not suitable for children.

GLADLAX
What it is: A herbal tablet remedy for relieving constipation. It contains senna and aloes, both of which are stimulant laxatives.
Dose: Adults should take 1-2 tablets at night. Children (7-14 years) should be given one tablet at night. This treatment is not suitable for children under seven years.

GOLDEN SEAL COMPOUND

What it is: A herbal tablet remedy which can help to soothe and relieve nausea, containing golden seal, cranesbill, marshmallow root and dandelion.

Dose: Two tablets should be taken three times a day between meals. This treatment is not suitable for children under 12 years.

GRAPHITES

What it is: A homeopathic remedy for relieving constipation.

Dose: Weleda 6c and 30c, Nelsons 6c.

HERBULAX

What it is: A herbal tablet remedy for relieving constipation, containing dandelion and frangula.

Dose: Adults should take 1-2 tablets at bedtime. Children (5-12 years) should be given half to one tablet at bedtime. This treatment is not suitable for children under five years.

IGNATIA

What it is: A homeopathic remedy for relieving constipation.

Dose: Weleda 6c and 30c, Nelsons 6c.

INDIAN BRANDEE

What it is: A liquid mixture for relieving digestive discomfort, containing ginger, rhubarb and capsicum.

Dose: 5 ml should be taken in or with water, once or twice daily as required. This treatment is not suitable for children.

IPECACUANHA

What it is: A homeopathic remedy for relieving nausea and travel sickness.

Dose: Weleda 6c and 30c, Nelsons 6c.

KALIUM MURIATICUM

What it is: A homeopathic remedy for relieving indigestion caused by fatty foods.

Dose: New Era 6x.

LUSTY'S HERBALENE

What it is: A herbal mixture for relieving constipation, containing senna, fennel, frangula and elder.

Dose: 2.5 ml should be taken twice a day. The dose should be placed on the tongue and swallowed with water. This treatment is not suitable for children under seven years.

MELISSA COMPOUND

What it is: A herbal liquid remedy for relieving occasional diarrhoea, containing alcohol, archangelica, cinnamon, cloves, coriander, lemon, lemon balm and nutmeg.

Dose: 10-20 drops should be diluted in a little water, as required, up to eight times a day. Children over eight years should take 5-10 drops up to eight times a day. This treatment is not suitable for children under eight years. Do not combine with other homeopathic remedies without seeking advice first.

MERCURIUS SOLUBILIS

What it is: A homeopathic remedy for relieving diarrhoea with straining.

Dose: Weleda 6c and 30c, Nelsons 6c, Ainsworth's 30c.

NATRALEZE

What it is: A herbal tablet remedy for heartburn, indigestion and wind. It contains slippery elm, liquorice and meadowsweet.

Dose: 2.5-15ml should be taken three times a day, according to age. This treatment is not suitable for children under seven years.

NATRUM MURIATICUM

What it is: A homeopathic remedy to relieve constipation.

Dose: Weleda 6c and 30c, Nelsons 6c, New Era 6x, Ainsworth's 30c.

NATRUM PHOSPHORICUM

What it is: A homeopathic remedy for relieving indigestion.

Dose: New Era 6x.

NATRUM SULPHURICUM

What it is: A homeopathic remedy for relieving yellow diarrhoea.

Dose: New Era 6x.

NELSONS TRAVELLA

What it is: A homeopathic remedy for relieving travel sickness.

Dose: Adults should take two tablets every hour for two hours before starting on a journey, followed by two tablets every hour during the journey. Children should take half the adult dose.

NEW ERA COMBINATION C

What it is: A homeopathic remedy for relieving indigestion and heartburn. Contains mag phos, nat phos, nat sulp and silica.

Dose: One dose contains 6x of each of the above ingredients.

NEW ERA COMBINATION E

What it is: A homeopathic remedy for relieving indigestion, containing a combination of calc phos, mag phos, nat phos and nat sulph.

Dose: One dose contains 6x of each of the above ingredients.

NUX VOMICA

What it is: A homeopathic remedy for relieving constipation where there is ineffectual urging.

Dose: Weleda 6c and 30c, Nelsons 6c, New Era 6x, Ainsworth's 30c.

PAPAYA PLUS

What it is: A herbal tablet remedy for relieving heartburn, indigestion and wind. It contains papain, slippery elm, golden seal and charcoal.

Dose: One tablet should be taken before meals three times a day. This treatment is not suitable for children.

PILEWORT COMPOUND

What it is: A herbal tablet remedy for relieving constipation and piles, containing senna, cascara, cranesbill and pilewort.

Dose: 1-2 tablets should be taken at night. This treatment is not suitable for children under 12 years.

POTTER'S CLEANSING HERB

What it is: A herbal tablet remedy for relieving occasional constipation, containing fennel, valerian, aloes and holly thistle.

Dose: 1-2 tablets should be taken at bedtime. This product should not be taken during the day, as valerian has a sedative effect. This treatment is not suitable for children under 12 years.

POTTER'S CLEANSING HERB TABLETS

What it is: A herbal tablet remedy for relieving constipation, containing senna, cascara, aloes, fennel and dandelion.

Dose: 1-2 tablets should be taken at bedtime. This treatment is not suitable for children.

POTTER'S INDIGESTION MIXTURE

What it is: A herbal liquid remedy for relieving indigestion, heartburn and wind, containing meadowsweet, gentian and wahoo.

Dose: 5 ml should be taken 3-4 times a day after meals. This treatment is not suitable for children.

POTTER'S LION CLEANSING HERBAL TABLETS

What it is: A herbal tablet remedy for relieving constipation, containing cascara, aloes, fennel and dandelion.

Dose: 1-2 tablets should be taken at bedtime. This treatment is not suitable for children.

POTTER'S OUT OF SORTS TABLETS

What it is: A herbal tablet remedy for relieving constipation, containing senna, cascara, aloes fennel and dandelion.

Dose: 1-2 tablets should be taken at bedtime. This treatment is not suitable for children.

POTTER'S SLIPPERY ELM TABLETS

What it is: A herbal tablet remedy for relieving indigestion, heartburn and wind, containing slippery elm, peppermint, cinnamon and cloves.

Dose: 5 ml should be taken 3-4 times a day after meals. This treatment is not suitable for children.

POTTER'S SPANISH TUMMY MIXTURE

What it is: A herbal astringent mixture which can be used to relieve non-persistent diarrhoea, containing blackberry root and catechu.

Dose: 5 ml should be taken every hour, as required. This treatment is not suitable for children.

RHUAKA HERBAL SYRUP

What it is: A herbal syrup for relieving constipation, containing rhubarb, senna and cascara.

Dose: Adults should take 20 ml at bedtime. Children over seven years should be given 5 ml at bedtime. This treatment is not suitable for children under seven years.

SILICA

What it is: A homeopathic remedy for relieving constipation.

Dose: Weleda 6c and 30c, Nelsons 6c, New Era 6x, Ainsworth's 30c.

SULPHUR

What it is: A homeopathic remedy for relieving early morning diarrhoea.

Dose: Nelsons 6c, New Era 6c and 30c, Ainsworth's 30c.

REMEDIES FOR DISORDERS AFFECTING EARS, EYES AND MOUTH
ACONITE

What it is: A homeopathic remedy for relieving earaches which occur after exposure to cold, dry wind.

Dose: Weleda 6c and 30c, Nelsons 6c, Ainsworth's 30c.

ARGENTUM NITRICUM

What it is: A homeopathic remedy for earaches which cause buzzing in the ears.

Dose: Weleda 6c and 30c, Nelsons 6c, Ainsworth's 30c.

BELLADONNA

What it is: A homeopathic remedy for relieving throbbing earaches.

Dose: Weleda 6c and 30c, Nelsons 6c, Ainsworth's 30c.

CALCAREA SULPHURICA
What it is: A homeopathic remedy for treating abscesses which have begun to emit a discharge.
Dose: New Era 6x.

CHAMOMILLA
What it is: A homeopathic remedy which can be used for children's earaches. It can also be used for toothaches that worsen after taking a warm drink.
Dose: Weleda 3x and 30c, Ainsworth's 30c.

COFFEA
What it is: A homeopathic remedy for treating toothaches with shooting pains.
Dose: Weleda 6c.

EUPHRASIA
What it is: A homeopathic remedy for conjunctivitis with tears.
Dose: Nelsons 6c, Weleda 6c and 30c.

GRAPHITES
What it is: A homeopathic remedy for the treatment of a sty.
Dose: Weleda 6c and 30c, Nelsons 6c.

HEPAR SULPHURIS
What it is: A homeopathic remedy for relieving earaches.
Dose: Weleda 6c, Nelsons 6c, Ainsworth's 30c.

LALIUM MURIATICUM
What it is: A homeopathic remedy for relieving earaches caused by blocked Eustachian tubes.
Dose: New Era 6c.

MERCURIUS SOLUBILIS

What it is: A homeopathic remedy for the treatment of earaches, abscesses and bad breath.
Dose: Weleda 6c and 30c, Nelsons 6c, Ainsworth's 30c.

NATRUM MURIATICUM

What it is: A homeopathic remedy which can be used to treat viral skin conditions.
Dose: Weleda 6c, New Era 6x, Nelsons 6c, Ainsworth's 30c.

NELSONS CANDIDA

What it is: A treatment which can be used for Candida albicans (thrush) infections, including those affecting the mouth.
Dose: Adults should take two 6c tablets every hour for six doses, followed by two tablets three times a day. Children should be given half the adult dose.

PICKLE'S SOOTHAKE GEL

What it is: A gel for relieving toothache, containing clove oil and an antiseptic.
Dose: Apply to the tooth as required. Seek dental treatment if symptoms persist. This treatment is not suitable for children.

PICKLE'S SOOTHAKE TOOTHACHE TINCTURE

What it is: A tincture for relieving toothache, containing a mild anaesthetic.
Dose: Apply to the tooth to ease the pain as required.

RHUS TOXICODENDRON

What it is: A homeopathic remedy which can be used to treat viral skin conditions.
Dose: Weleda 6c and 30c, Nelsons 6c, Ainsworth's 30c.

SILICA

What it is: A homeopathic remedy for the treatment of abscesses.

Dose: Weleda 6c and 30c, Nelsons 6c, New Weleda 6c and 30c, Nelsons 6c, New Era 6x, Ainsworth's 30c.

THUJA

What it is: A homeopathic remedy for tooth decay which occurs at the roots.

Dose: Weleda 6c and 30c, Nelsons 6c.

REMEDIES FOR DISORDERS AFFECTING THE BLOOD AND CIRCULATORY SYSTEM

CALCAREA FLUORICA

What it is: A homeopathic remedy for the treatment of piles and varicose veins that promotes tissue elasticity.

Dose: Weleda 6c and 30c, Nelsons 6c, New Era 6x. This treatment is not suitable for children.

FERRUM PHOSPHORICUM

What it is: A homeopathic remedy for anaemia.

Dose: Weleda 6c and 30c, New Era 6x, Nelsons 6c. If anaemia persists, consult your doctor.

HAMAMELIS

What it is: A homeopathic remedy for the treatment of chilblains, piles and varicose veins.

Dose: Weleda 6c and 30c, Nelsons 6c. This treatment is not suitable for children.

LANES HEEMEX

What it is: An astringent ointment for relieving the discomfort of piles, containing witch hazel.

Dose: Apply the ointment morning and evening and after each bowel movement. Can cause allergy in some people. This treatment is not suitable for children.

NELSONS HAEMORRHOID CREAM

What it is: A herbal cream which can be used to soothe and treat the symptoms of piles, containing calendula, horse chestnut, witch hazel and paeonia officinalis.

Dose: Apply as needed. This treatment is not suitable for children.

NELSONS OINTMENT FOR CHILBLAINS

What it is: A homeopathic ointment for the treatment of unbroken chilblains, containing tamus communis 6x.

Dose: Weleda 6c and 30c, Nelsons 6c. This treatment is not suitable for children.

NEW ERA COMBINATION L

What it is: A homeopathic remedy for the treatment of varicose veins, containing calc fluor, ferr phos and nat mur.

Dose: The prepared remedy contains 6x of each of the above ingredients.

NUX VOMICA

What it is: A homeopathic remedy for itchy piles.

Dose: Weleda 6c and 30c, Nelsons 6c, Ainsworth's 30c. This treatment is not suitable for children.

PICKLE'S CHILBLAIN CREAM

What it is: A herbal cream for the treatment of chilblains, containing a rubefacient.

Dose: The cream should be applied sparingly morning and night and more frequently if required. This treatment is not suitable for pregnant or breastfeeding women.

PICKLE'S SNOWFIRE

What it is: A herbal ointment for the treatment of chilblains, containing benzoin, citronella and oils of thyme, clove and cade.

Dose: Apply to the affected area as required.

POTTER'S PILE TABS

What it is: A herbal tablet for relieving the symptoms of piles. The tablets have an astringent and laxative effect, and contain pilewort, cascara, agrimony and stone root.

Dose: Two tablets should be taken three times a day. The elderly should take two tablets twice a day. This treatment is not suitable for children or pregnant women.

POTTER'S PILEWORT OINTMENT

What it is: A herbal ointment for relieving the symptoms of piles, containing pilewort and lanolin.

Dose: The ointment should be applied twice a day. This treatment is not suitable for children and should not be used by anyone sensitive to lanolin.

POTTER'S VARICOSE OINTMENT

What it is: A herbal ointment for the treatment of varicose veins, containing cade oil, witch hazel and zinc oxide.

Dose: The ointment should be applied to the affected area twice a day. It should not be used on broken skin.

PULSATILLA

What it is: A homeopathic remedy for the treatment of varicose veins associated with poor circulation.

Dose: Weleda 6c and 30c, Nelsons 6c, Ainsworth's 30c.

WELEDA FROST CREAM

What it is: A homeopathic cream for relieving the symptoms of chilblains, containing balsam of Peru, rosemary oil and stibium metallicum.

Dose: The cream should be applied to the affected area several times a day. Can cause allergy, so a skin test should be carried out first.

REMEDIES FOR DISORDERS AFFECTING MENTAL HEALTH
ACTAEA RACEMOSA

What it is: A homeopathic remedy for the treatment of depression.

Dose: Weleda 6c, Nelsons 6c.

ARGENTUM NITRICUM

What it is: A homeopathic remedy for treating anxiety caused by nervousness or anticipatory fear.

Dose: Nelsons 6c, Weleda 6c and 30c.

ARSENICUM ALBUM

What it is: A homeopathic remedy for treating insomnia caused by an overactive mind and for anxiety with fear.

Dose: Weleda 6c and 30c, Nelsons 6c, Ainsworth's 30c.

AVENA SATIVA COMP

What it is: A liquid herbal remedy that has a sedative and analgesic effect. It can be used to treat irritability, tension, tension-induced aches and pains and sleep problems. Contains coffea, oats, passionflower and valerian.

Dose: Adults should take 10-20 drops in water 30 minutes before retiring. Children (2-12 years) should be given 5-10 drops. This treatment is not suitable for children under two years.

BIOPHYLLIN

What it is: A herbal tablet remedy which helps promote sleep and can be used to treat tension, restlessness and irritability. The tablets contain valerian, black cohosh, Jamaican dogwood and skullcap.

Dose: Two tablets should be taken after meals three times a day. This treatment is not suitable for children.

BIO-STRATH ELIXIR

What it is: A herbal elixir for alleviating fatigue and tiredness, containing yeast.

Dose: 5 ml should be taken three times a day before meals. This treatment is not suitable for children under 12 years.

BIO-STRATH VALERIAN FORMULA

What it is: A herbal liquid remedy which promotes natural sleep and can be used for relieving tension, irritability, stress and emotional strain. Contains passionflower, valerian, peppermint and yeast.

Dose: 20 drops should be diluted in water and taken three times a day before meals. This treatment is not suitable for children, and should not be combined with other homeopathic remedies.

CALCAREA CARBONICA

What it is: A homeopathic remedy for the treatment of insomnia.
Dose: Nelsons 6c, Weleda 6c and 30c.

CALCAREA PHOSPHORICA

What it is: A homeopathic remedy for alleviating fatigue in adolescents.
Dose: Weleda 6c, Nelsons 6c, New Era 6x.

CHAMOMILLA

What it is: A homeopathic remedy for treating insomnia which occurs as a result of pain or anger. This remedy is also available in drops.
Dose: Ainsworth's 30c, Weleda 3x and 30c.

COFFEA

What it is: A homeopathic remedy for treating insomnia caused by an overactive mind.
Dose: Weleda 6c.

CURZON

What it is: A herbal stimulant in tablet form for relieving nervous strain. Contains damiana.
Dose: Two tablets should be taken at night and two in the morning. This treatment is not suitable for children under 12 years. This stimulant can cause side effects - always read the label.

FRAGADOR

What it is: A tablet remedy for relieving temporary irritability and emotional unrest, containing aniseed, conchae, lovage, sage, scurvy grass, stinging nettle, wheatgerm, wild strawberry, glycogen 10x, ferrum phosphoricum 4x, natrum carbonicum 1x and radix mel 1x.
Dose: Two tablets should be taken three times a day. This treatment is not suitable for children, and should not be combined with other homeopathic remedies.

GELSEMIUM

What it is: A homeopathic remedy for alleviating fatigue.

Dose: Weleda 6c, Nelsons 6c, Ainsworth's 30c.

HEATH & HEATHER BECALM

What it is: A tablet remedy with a sedative effect for relieving stress. The tablets contain hops, passionflower and valerian.

Dose: One tablet should be taken three times a day. This treatment is not suitable for children.

HEATH & HEATHER QUIET NIGHT TABLETS

What it is: A tablet remedy to aid sleep, containing hops, passionflower and valerian.

Dose: Two tablets one hour before bedtime. This treatment is not suitable for children.

HYPERICUM

What it is: A herbal remedy for treating mild depression made from the St John's wort plant.

Dose: Weleda 6c and 30c, Nelsons 6c, Ainsworth's 30c.

KALIUM PHOSPHORICUM

What it is: A homeopathic remedy for treating mild depression and nervous exhaustion.

Dose: Weleda 6c and 30c, Nelsons 6c, New Era 6x.

KALMS

What it is: A herbal tablet remedy which promotes natural sleep. Can be used to relieve the symptoms of anxiety, irritability and stress. Contains gentian, hops and valerian.

Dose: Two tablets should be taken three times a day after meals. This treatment is not suitable for children.

MOTHERWORT COMPOUND

What it is: A tablet remedy with a sedative effect for treating the symptoms of emotional stress and strain. Contains motherwort, limeflower and passionflower.

Dose: Two tablets should be taken three times a day after meals. This treatment is not suitable for children.

NATRACALM

What it is: A tablet remedy for relieving stress, strain and nervous tension, containing passionflower.

Dose: One tablet should be taken three times a day. This treatment is not suitable for children.

NATRASLEEP

What it is: A herbal tablet which promotes natural sleep, containing hops and valerian.

Dose: 1-3 tablets should be taken 30 minutes before bedtime. This treatment is not suitable for children.

NATRUM MURIATICUM

What it is: A homeopathic remedy for the treatment of mild depression.

Dose: Weleda 6c and 30c, New Era 6x, Nelsons 6c, Ainsworth's 30c.

NATUREST

What it is: A herbal tablet remedy for the treatment of temporary insomnia which occurs as a result of stress. Contains passiflora.

Dose: Two tablets should be taken three times a day and 1-3 tablets at bedtime. This treatment is not suitable for children.

NEW ERA COMBINATION B

What it is: A homeopathic remedy for alleviating general debility, containing calc phos, kali phos and ferr phos.

Dose: One tablet contains 6x of each of the above ingredients.

NOCTURA

What it is: A tablet remedy for treating insomnia, containing kali brom, coffea, passiflora, avena sativa, alfalfa and valeriana.

Dose: Two tablets should be taken four hours before bedtime followed by two tablets immediately before bedtime. A further two tablets should be taken during the night, if required. One tablet contains 6c of each of the ingredients above. This treatment is not suitable for children.

NYTOL HERBAL
What it is: A tablet remedy for relieving temporary insomnia. Contains hops, passiflora, Jamaican dogwood, pulsatilla and wild lettuce.
Dose: Two tablets should be taken before bedtime. This treatment is not suitable for children.

POTTER'S ANA-SED
What it is: A sedative herbal remedy with an analgesic action that can be used to treat irritability, emotional stress and tension. Contains valerian, vervain, skullcap and hops.
Dose: Two tablets should be taken three times a day. This treatment is not suitable for children.

POTTER'S CHLOROPHYLL
What it is: A herbal stimulant in tablet form for relieving temporary tiredness. Contains chlorophyll and kola nut.
Dose: 1-2 tablets should be taken three times a day.

POTTER'S ELIXIR OF DAMIANA AND SAW PALMETTO
What it is: A restorative elixir containing saw palmetto, damiana and cornsilk.
Dose: 10 ml should be taken three times a day for seven days, reducing dose by half for the following seven days. This treatment is not suitable for children. This treatment can cause side effects - always read the label.

POTTER'S NODOFF PASSIFLORA TABLETS
What it is: A herbal tablet remedy which promotes sleep. The tablets contain passiflora.
Dose: Two tablets should be taken in early evening and two tablets before bedtime. This treatment is not suitable for children.

POTTER'S STRENGTH TABLETS

What it is: A herbal tablet stimulant for treating fatigue after illness. Contains damiana, kola and saw palmetto.

Dose: Two tablets should be taken three times a day. This treatment is not suitable for children. These tablets can cause side effects - always read the label.

QUIET LIFE

What it is: A tablet remedy with a mild sedative action for the treatment of irritability, nervousness, tension and sleeplessness. The tablets contain hops, motherwort, passionflower, valerian, wild lettuce and vitamins B1, B2 and B3.

Dose: Two tablets should be taken twice a day, and 2-3 tablets before bedtime. This treatment is not suitable for children.

SEPIA

What it is: A homeopathic remedy for treating mild depression and tiredness.

Dose: Weleda 6c and 30c, Nelsons 6c, Ainsworth's 30c.

SERENITY

What it is: A tablet remedy for relieving emotional stress, strain and irritability. The tablets contain hops, passionflower and valerian.

Dose: Two tablets should be taken three times a day after food. This treatment is not suitable for children.

SOMNUS

What it is: A herbal tablet remedy which promotes natural sleep, containing hops, valerian and wild lettuce.

Dose: Two tablets should be taken one hour before bedtime. This treatment is not suitable for children.

SULPHUR

What it is: A homeopathic remedy which promotes deep natural sleep.
Dose: Ainsworth's 30c, Nelsons 6c, New Era 6c and 30c.

SUNERVEN

What it is: A tablet remedy for relieving anxiety, irritability, emotional stress, fatigue and insomnia. The tablets contain motherwort, passionflower, valerian and vervain.

Dose: Two tablets should be taken three times a day after meals and two tablets before bedtime. This treatment is not suitable for children.

VALERIAN COMPOUND

What it is: A herbal tablet remedy which promotes natural sleep, containing valerian, hops, Jamaican dogwood, passionflower and wild lettuce.

Dose: Two tablets should be taken in early evening followed by two just before retiring. This treatment is not suitable for children.

VALERINA DAY TABLETS

What it is: Tablets which relieve tension and irritability, containing valerian and lemon balm.

Dose: Two tablets should be taken three times a day. This treatment is not suitable for children. Also available as Valerian Night Tablets.

REMEDIES FOR DISORDERS AFFECTING THE FEMALE REPRODUCTIVE SYSTEM

ATHERA

What it is: A traditional herbal remedy for the relief of minor conditions associated with the menopause, such as water retention and constipation. It has a mild tonic effect and contains vervain, senna leaf, clivers and parsley root.

Dose: 2-3 tablets should be taken three times a day after meals. This treatment should not be used by pregnant or breastfeeding women.

CASCADE

What it is: A herbal tablet remedy for relieving pre-menstrual water retention. It has a diuretic action and contains clivers, burdock root and uva ursi.

Dose: Two tablets should be taken three times a day before meals.

HEATH & HEATHER WATER RELIEF
What it is: A herbal tablet remedy for relieving pre-menstrual water retention. It has a diuretic action and contains bladderwrack, burdock root, clivers and ground ivy.
Dose: 1-2 tablets up to three times a day for up to seven days, before a period is expected.

POTTER'S ANTITIS
What it is: A herbal tablet remedy for relieving the symptoms of cystitis.
Dose: Two tablets should be taken three times a day for a maximum of 10 days. The fluid intake should be increased while taking this remedy.

POTTER'S PREMENTAID
What it is: A diuretic and antispasmodic herbal tablet remedy with a mild, sedative effect for relieving pre-menstrual bloating and abdominal discomfort. It contains valerian, vervain, motherwort, uva ursi and wild anemone.
Dose: Two tablets should be taken three times a day when symptoms start prior to a period. Should not be used while taking sedative medications or alcohol.

POTTER'S RASPBERRY LEAF
What it is: A herbal tablet remedy for relieving painful menstrual cramps, with a toning and relaxing effect. Contains raspberry leaf.
Dose: Two tablets should be taken three times a day after meals.

POTTER'S WELLWOMAN
What it is: A herbal tablet remedy which promotes wellbeing in middle-aged women in pre-menopause and menopause. It contains valerian, lime flowers, motherwort, skullcap and yarrow.
Dose: Two tablets should be taken three times a day. This treatment should not be used while taking other sedative medications, and should not be used by pregnant women.

REMEDIES FOR DISORDERS AFFECTING THE SKIN
APIS MELLIFICA
What it is: A homeopathic remedy for relieving burning and stinging pains, and bites and stings that are red and swollen. It is made from honeybee venom.
Dose: Weleda 6c and 30c, Nelsons 6c, Ainsworth's 30c.

ARNICA
What it is: A homeopathic remedy for treating bruising.
Dose: Weleda 6c and 30c, Nelsons 6c, Ainsworth's 30c.

BELLADONNA
What it is: A homeopathic remedy for treating acne.
Dose: Weleda 6c and 30c, Nelsons 6c, Ainsworth's 30c.

BLUE FLAG ROOT COMPOUND
What it is: An antiseptic, anti-inflammatory herbal tablet remedy that is used to treat eczema and other skin conditions, containing blue flag root, burdock and sarsaparilla.
Dose: One tablet should be taken three times a day after meals. This treatment is not suitable for children under 12 years. Pregnant women should consult their doctor before using this product.

CALCAREA CARBONICA
What it is: A homeopathic remedy for the treatment of itchy and cracked skin.
Dose: Weleda 6c and 30c, Nelsons 6c.

CALCAREA FLUORICA
What it is: A homeopathic remedy which is used to promote tissue elasticity, scar and adhesion healing.
Dose: Weleda 6c and 30c, Nelsons 6c, New Era 6x.

CALCAREA PHOSPHORICA
What it is: A homeopathic remedy for the treatment of acne.
Dose: Weleda 6c and 30c, Nelsons 6c, Ainsworth's 30c.

CALCAREA SULPHURICA

What it is: A homeopathic remedy for treating acne, abscesses which have begun to emit discharge and any wounds that are healing slowly.

Dose: New Era 6x.

CANTHARIS

What it is: A homeopathic remedy for the treatment of minor burns.

Dose: Weleda 6c and 30c, Nelsons 6c, Ainsworth's 30c.

CAUSTICUM

What it is: A homeopathic remedy for the treatment of minor burns.

Dose: Weleda 6c.

DERMATODORON OINTMENT

What it is: A herbal ointment for relieving the symptoms of eczema, containing loosestrife and woody nightshade.

Dose: The ointment should be applied to the affected area two or three times a day.

GRAPHITES

What it is: A homeopathic remedy for the treatment of eczema where there is weeping and cracked skin.

Dose: Weleda 6c and 30c, Nelsons 6c.

HAMAMELIS

What it is: A homeopathic remedy for relieving sore, bruised skin.

Dose: Weleda 6c and 30c, Nelsons 6c.

HEATH & HEATHER SKIN TABLETS

What it is: A herbal tablet remedy for relieving the symptoms of skin blemishes and dry eczema, containing burdock root and wild pansy.

Dose: Two tablets should be taken three times a day. This treatment is not suitable for children. Pregnant women should consult their doctor before use.

HEPAR SULPHURIS

What it is: A homeopathic remedy which acts as a healing aid for eczema and for wounds that ooze.

Dose: Weleda 6c and 30c, Nelsons 6c, Ainsworth's 30c.

HERBHEAL OINTMENT

What it is: A soothing herbal ointment for relieving itchy skin complaints, containing chickweed, colophony, lanolin, marshmallow, sulphur and zinc oxide.

Dose: The ointment should be applied to the affected area twice a day. This treatment is not suitable for children under five years.

HYPERICUM

What it is: A homeopathic remedy which promotes the healing of wounds which affect nerve endings.

Dose: Weleda 6c and 30c, Nelsons 6c.

KLEER TABLETS

What it is: A herbal tablet for the treatment of minor skin conditions and eczema. It contains burdock root, echinacea and stinging nettle.

Dose: Adults should take two tablets three times a day before meals. Children (5-12 years) should be given one tablet three times a day before meals. This treatment is not suitable for children under five years or for pregnant or breastfeeding women.

LEDUM

What it is: A homeopathic remedy for relieving the symptoms of insect bites, bee stings and puncture wounds.

Dose: Weleda 6c, Ainsworth's 30c.

MERCURIUS SOLUBILIS

What it is: A homeopathic remedy for the treatment of abscesses and boils.

Dose: Weleda 6c and 30c, Nelsons 6c, New Era 6x, Ainsworth's 30c.

NATRUM MURIATICUM

What it is: A homeopathic remedy for the treatment of eczema.

Dose: Weleda 6c and 30c, Nelsons 6c, New Era 6x, Ainsworth's 30c.

NELSONS ARNICA CREAM

What it is: A herbal cream remedy for relieving bruises, containing arnica.

Dose: The cream should be applied to the affected area as required.

NELSONS BURNS OINTMENT

What it is: A herbal ointment remedy for the treatment of minor burns. It contains calendula, echinacea, hypericum and urtica urens.

Dose: The ointment should be applied as required to the affected area which should then be covered with a dry dressing.

NELSONS CANDIDA

What it is: A homeopathic tablet remedy for the treatment of athlete's foot, containing Candida albicans 6c.

Dose: Adults should take two tablets every hour for six doses, then reduce the dose to two tablets three times a day. Children should be given half the adult dose.

NELSONS GRAPHITES CREAM

What it is: A homeopathic remedy for the treatment of dermatitis, containing Graphites 6x.

Dose: The cream should be applied to the affected area as required.

NELSONS HYPERCAL

What it is: A herbal cream and tincture remedy for soothing and promoting the healing of sore skin and cuts. The cream contains calendula and hypericum.

Dose: The cream should be applied to the affected area. Can be diluted 1 part cream to 10 parts water and then applied to larger wounds.

NELSONS PYRETHRUM

What it is: A herbal liquid remedy for soothing hives, insect bites and stings, containing pyrethrum, arnica, calendula, echinacea, hypericum, ledum palustre and rumex crispus.

Dose: The liquid should be applied to the affected area as soon as possible after a bite or sting has occurred. This treatment is also available in spray form.

NEW ERA ELASTO
What it is: A homeopathic remedy to promote the formation of elastic, responsible for the repair and health of tissues in the body. Contains 6x of each of the following - calc fluor, calc phos, ferr phos and mag phos.
Dose: One tablet provides 6x of each of the above ingredients.

PHOSPHORUS
What it is: A homeopathic remedy which can be used to prevent bruising, particularly in those who are prone to it.
Dose: Weleda 6c and 30c, Nelsons 6c, Ainsworth's 30c.

POTTER'S ADIANTINE
What it is: A herbal remedy for the treatment of dandruff and for improving hair condition. It contains bay oil, rosemary, southernwood and witch hazel.
Dose: The liquid should be massaged into the scalp morning and evening. This treatment is not suitable for children.

POTTER'S COMFREY OINTMENT
What it is: A herbal ointment remedy for the relief and treatment of sprains and bruises. It contains comfrey.
Dose: The ointment should be applied to the affected area twice a day after bathing. This treatment should not be used for more than 10 days.

POTTER'S ECZEMA OINTMENT
What it is: A herbal ointment for relieving the symptoms of eczema, containing benzoic acid, salicylic acid, zinc oxide, lanolin and chickweed.
Dose: The ointment should be applied to the affected area twice a day. This treatment is not suitable for children under five years.

POTTER'S ERUPTIONS MIXTURE
What it is: A herbal mixture for treating the symptoms of mild eczema,

containing blue flag, buchu, burdock root, cascara, sarsaparilla and yellow dock.

Dose: Adults should take 5 ml three times a day. Children over eight years should be given 5 ml every 12 hours. This treatment is not suitable for children under eight years. Pregnant or breastfeeding women should consult their doctor before using this product.

POTTER'S EXTRACT OF ROSEMARY

What it is: A herbal liquid for improving general hair condition which can also be used to treat mild dandruff. Contains bay oil, rosemary, rose geranium and methyl salicylate.

Dose: The liquid should be massaged into the scalp twice a day until symptoms clear. This treatment is not suitable for children.

POTTER'S SKIN CLEAR OINTMENT

What it is: An astringent and mild antiseptic ointment for relieving the symptoms of mild acne and eczema. It contains sulphur, tea tree oil and zinc oxide.

Dose: The ointment should be applied twice a day to the affected areas. This treatment is not suitable for children under five years.

POTTER'S SKIN CLEAR TABLETS

What it is: A herbal tablet remedy for the relief and prevention of minor skin blemishes and acne. It contains echinacea.

Dose: Two tablets should be taken three times a day. This treatment is not suitable for children, or for pregnant or breastfeeding women.

RHUS TOXICODENDRON

What it is: A homeopathic remedy for the treatment of eczema.

Dose: Weleda 6c and 30c, Nelsons 6c, Ainsworth's 30c.

SILICA

What it is: A homeopathic remedy for the treatment of abscesses, boils and athlete's foot.

Dose: Weleda 6c and 30c, Nelsons 6c, New Era 6x, Ainsworth's 30c.

SULPHUR

What it is: A homeopathic remedy for the treatment of eczema, acne and slow healing burns.

Dose: Weleda 6c and 30c, Nelsons 6c, Ainsworth's 30c.

THUJA

What it is: A homeopathic remedy for the treatment of warts.

Dose: Weleda 6c and 30c, Nelsons 6c.

URTICA URENS

What it is: A homeopathic remedy for the treatment of minor burns where blistering has not occurred.

Dose: Weleda 6c.

WELEDA ARNICA OINTMENT

What it is: A herbal ointment which can be used to relieve muscular pains, stiffness, strains and bruises. It contains arnica.

Dose: The ointment should be massaged into the affected area three to four times a day. This treatment is also available in lotion form.

WELEDA BALSAMICUM OINTMENT

What it is: A herbal ointment which promotes the healing of boils and minor wounds. It contains balsam of Peru, marigold, dog's mercury, metallicum preparatum and stibium.

Dose: The ointment should be applied directly to the affected area or placed on a dressing which will be applied to the boil or wound. Repeat as necessary. The treatment should be discontinued immediately if there is any adverse reaction of the skin.

WELEDA CALENDOLON OINTMENT

What it is: An antiseptic herbal remedy for the treatment of cuts and minor wounds, containing marigold.

Dose: The ointment should be applied to the affected area 2-3 times a day. It should not be applied to infected wounds. Pregnant women should consult their doctor prior to use.

WELEDA CALENDULA LOTION

What it is: A herbal lotion for the treatment of minor skin wounds, containing marigold.

Dose: 5 ml of the liquid should be added to boiled water and allowed to cool. The lotion can be used to clean wounds or applied to dressings over the affected area. It should not be used on wounds which are infected. Pregnant women should consult a pharmacist or doctor before using this product.

WELEDA COMBUDORON LOTION

What it is: A herbal lotion for the treatment and relief of minor burns, containing arnica and small nettle.

Dose: 5 ml of the lotion should be added to a cup of cooled boiled water, then used to moisten a pad which should be applied to the burn as a compress and kept moist. This treatment is also available in ointment form.

WELEDA WCS DUSTING POWDER

What it is: A herbal powder remedy for the treatment of minor burns. It contains arnica, echinacea, marigold, silica, stibium and metallicum praep.

Dose: The powder should be applied to the affected area and covered with a dry dressing. The dressing should be changed twice a day.

REMEDIES FOR DISORDERS AFFECTING BONES AND MUSCLES
ACTAEA RACEMOSA

What it is: A homeopathic remedy for relieving stiff neck, rheumatic pains in the back and neck and muscle ache brought on by exercise.

Dose: Weleda 6c and 30c, Nelsons 6c.

APIS MELLIFICA

What it is: A homeopathic remedy for the treatment of arthritis with red and swollen joints and hot, red swellings in the body.

Dose: Weleda 6c and 30c, Nelsons 6c, Ainsworth's 30c.

ARNICA

What it is: A homeopathic remedy for relieving sprains and aching muscles.

Dose: Weleda 6x, 6c and 30c, Nelsons 6c, Ainsworth's 30c.

BELLADONNA PLASTER

What it is: An adhesive plaster impregnated with a rubefacient for relieving muscular and rheumatic pains, strains, stiffness and lumbago. Contains belladonna alkaloids.

Dose: The plaster should be applied to the affected area and left on for two to three days. This treatment is not suitable for children under 10 years.

BIO-STRATH WILLOW FORMULA

What it is: A herbal liquid remedy for relieving muscular pain, backache, lumbago, sciatica and fibrosis. It contains willow bark, primula and yeast.

Dose: 1.5 ml should be diluted in water three times a day before meals. This treatment is not suitable for children.

BRYONIA

What it is: A homeopathic remedy for relieving arthritis and sharp pains.

Dose: Weleda 6c and 30c, Nelsons 6c, Ainsworth's 30c.

CALCAREA FLUORICA

What it is: A homeopathic remedy for relieving arthritis that responds to warmth and movement.

Dose: Weleda 6c and 30c, Nelsons 6c, New Era 6x.

COLOCYNTHIS

What it is: A homeopathic remedy for alleviating cramps and spasms, particularly those occurring in the calves.

Dose: Weleda 6c.

DRAGON BALM OINTMENT

What it is: A herbal ointment for relieving rheumatism and other joint problems. It contains balsam of Peru, camphor, cassia, eucalyptus, guaiacum, nutmeg, turpentine and thymol.

Dose: The ointment should be applied to the affected area as required. This treatment is not suitable for children under six years.

FERRUM PHOSPHORICUM

What it is: A homeopathic remedy for relieving rheumatism.

Dose: Weleda 6c and 30c, Nelsons 6c, New Era 6x, Ainsworth's 30c.

GERARD HOUSE CELERY TABLETS

What it is: A herbal tablet for relieving the symptoms of rheumatic pain, containing celery.

Dose: Should be used according to the instructions on the label, according to symptoms. This treatment is not suitable for children.

GERARD HOUSE LIGVITES

What it is: A herbal tablet for relieving the symptoms of rheumatic pain, stiffness, backache and lumbago. Each tablet contains black cohosh, guaiacum, poplar bark, sarsaparilla and white willow bark.

Dose: Two tablets should be taken twice a day with food. This treatment is not suitable for children under 12 years.

GONNE BALM

What it is: A herbal remedy for relieving muscular aches and pains such as general stiffness, backache, sciatica and lumbago. The balm contains camphor, eucalyptus oil, levo-menthol, methyl salicylate (an aspirin derivative) and turpentine.

Dose: The balm should be massaged into the affected area two to three times a day, and once during the night if necessary. This treatment is not suitable for children under 12 years.

HEATH & HEATHER RHEUMATIC PAIN TABLETS

What it is: A herbal tablet remedy for relieving the symptoms of backache, lumbago, fibrositis and rheumatic pain. Each tablet contains bogbean, guaiacum and celery.

Dose: One tablet should be taken three times a day. This treatment is not suitable for children.

KALIUM MURIATICUM

What it is: A homeopathic remedy for the treatment of rheumatic swelling.

Dose: New Era 6x.

KALIUM SULPHURICUM

What it is: A homeopathic remedy for the treatment of rheumatism that moves from joint to joint.
Dose: New Era 6x.

LEDUM

What it is: A homeopathic remedy for the treatment of rheumatism that moves from joint to joint.
Dose: New Era 6x.

MAGNESIA PHOSPHORICA

What it is: A homeopathic remedy for relieving sciatica, cramp and muscular spasms.
Dose: New Era 6x.

NATRUM PHOSPHORICUM

What it is: A homeopathic remedy which assists the removal of excess lactic acid in the body in order to ease rheumatic conditions.
Dose: New Era 6x.

NELSONS OINTMENT FOR STRAINS

What it is: A herbal ointment for relieving strains and sprains, containing ruta graveolens.
Dose: The ointment should be applied to the affected area as required.

NELSONS RHEUMATICA

What it is: A homeopathic remedy for relieving rheumatic pains, containing rhus toxicodendron 6c.
Dose: Adults should take two tablets every hour for six doses, followed by two tablets three times a day. Children should be given half the adult dose.

NELSONS RHUS TOX CREAM

What it is: A herbal cream for relieving rheumatic pains and strains, containing rhus toxicodendron.
Dose: The cream should be massaged into the affected area as required.

NEW ERA COMBINATION A

What it is: A homeopathic remedy for relieving sciatica, containing ferr phos, kali phos and mag phos.

Dose: Contains 6x of each of the above ingredients.

NEW ERA COMBINATION G

What it is: A homeopathic remedy for the treatment of backache and lumbar pain, containing calc fluor, calc phos, kali phos and nat mur.

Dose: Contains 6x of each of the above ingredients.

NEW ERA COMBINATION 1

What it is: A homeopathic remedy for the treatment of muscular pain and fibrositis, containing ferr phos, kali sulph and mag phos.

Dose: Contains 6x of each of the above ingredients.

NEW ERA COMBINATION P

What it is: A homeopathic remedy for relieving aching legs and feet, containing calc fluor, calc phos, kali phos and mag phos.

Dose: Contains 6x of each of the above ingredients.

OLBAS OIL

What it is: An oil for the treatment of muscular pain and stiffness. It contains oils of cajuput, clove, eucalyptus, juniper berry, menthol, mint and wintergreen and acts as an analgesic and rubefacient.

Dose: The oil should be massaged into the affected area three times a day. This treatment is not suitable for children.

PHYTOLACCA

What it is: A homeopathic remedy for relieving rheumatism and shooting pains in the body.

Dose: Weleda 6c.

POTTER'S BACKACHE TABLETS

What it is: A herbal tablet remedy for relieving back pain. Each tablet contains buchu, gravel root, hydrangea and uva ursi.